AF669492

# Cervical Myelopathy

*Editor*
**Peter G Passias** MD
New York Spine Institute
Hospital for Joint Diseases
New York University Langone Medical Center
New York, New York, USA

JAYPEE *The Health Sciences Publisher*
Philadelphia | New Delhi | London | Panama

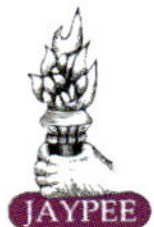

**Jaypee Brothers Medical Publishers (P) Ltd**

**Headquarters**
Jaypee Brothers Medical Publishers (P) Ltd.
4838/24, Ansari Road, Daryaganj
New Delhi 110 002, India
Phone: +91-11-43574357
Fax: +91-11-43574314
E-mail: jaypee@jaypeebrothers.com

**Overseas Offices**
J.P. Medical Ltd.
83, Victoria Street, London
SW1H 0HW (UK)
Phone: +44-20 3170 8910
Fax: +44(0)20 3008 6180
E-mail: info@jpmedpub.com

Jaypee-Highlights Medical Publishers Inc.
City of Knowledge, Bld. 237, Clayton
Panama City, Panama
Phone: +1 507-301-0496
Fax: +1 507-301-0499
E-mail: cservice@jphmedical.com

Jaypee Medical Inc.
325 Chestnut Street
Suite 412
Philadelphia, PA 19106, USA
Phone: +1 267-519-9789
E-mail: support@jpmedus.com

Jaypee Brothers Medical Publishers (P) Ltd.
17/1-B, Babar Road, Block-B, Shaymali
Mohammadpur, Dhaka-1207
Bangladesh
Mobile: +08801912003485
E-mail: jaypeedhaka@gmail.com

Jaypee Brothers Medical Publishers (P) Ltd.
Bhotahity, Kathmandu, Nepal
Phone: +977-9741283608
E-mail: kathmandu@jaypeebrothers.com

Website: www.jaypeebrothers.com
Website: www.jaypeedigital.com



**Inquiries for bulk sales may be solicited at:** jaypee@jaypeebrothers.com

***Cervical Myelopathy***

*First Edition:* **2016**

ISBN: 978-93-5152-492-2

*Printed at* Replika Press Pvt. Ltd.

## *Dedication*

*I would like to dedicate the completion of this work to the memory of my grandparents, Konstantinos and Eleni Passias, whose memory lives with us constantly.*

# Contributors


**John A Bendo** MD
Associate Professor of Clinical Orthopedic Surgery
Department of Orthopedic Surgery
New York University
New York, New York, USA

**Carolina G Benjamin** MD
Department of Neurosurgery
New York University Langone Medical Center
New York, New York, USA

**Aleksandar Beric** MD DSc
Professor of Neurology, Neurosurgery, Orthopedic Surgery, and Rehabilitation
Department of Neurology
New York University School of Medicine
New York, New York, USA

**Akwasi Ofori Boah** MD
Chief Resident
Department of Neurosurgery
New York University Langone Medical Center
New York, New York, USA

**John A Buza III** MD
Resident Physician
Department of Orthopedic Surgery
Hospital for Joint Diseases
New York University Langone Medical Center
New York, New York, USA

**Mohamad Bydon** MD
Assistant Professor
Department of Neurosurgery
Mayo Clinic
Rochester, Minnesota, USA

**Jerry Cheriyan** MD
Resident Physician
Department of Surgery
Marshfield Clinic
Chippewa Falls, Wisconsin, USA

**Thomas Cheriyan** MD
Research Scientist
Division of Spine Surgery
Hospital for Joint Diseases
New York University Langone Medical Center
New York, New York, USA

**Michael G Fehlings** MD PhD FRCS
Professor of Neurosurgery
Vice Chair Research, Halbert Chair in Neural Repair and Regeneration
Co-Chairman of Spinal Program
Department of Neurosurgery
University of Toronto
Head of Spinal Program
Senior Scientist, McEwen Centre for Regenerative Medicine
Toronto Western Hospital
University Health Network
Toronto, Ontario, Canada

**Anthony K Frempong-Boadu** MD
Associate Professor
Department of Neurosurgery
New York University Langone Medical Center
New York, New York, USA

**Rafael De la Garza-Ramos** MD
Postdoctoral Fellow
Department of Neurosurgery
Johns Hopkins University School of Medicine
Baltimore, Maryland, USA

**Michael Gerling** MD
Clinical Assistant Professor
Department of Orthopedic Surgery
New York University School of Medicine
New York, New York, USA

**Ziya L Gokaslan** MD FAANS FACS
Gus Stoll, MD Professor and Chair
Department of Neurosurgery
The Warren Alpert Medical School of Brown University
Providence, Rhode Island, USA

**Andrew J Grossbach** MD
Chief Resident
Department of Neurosurgery
University of Iowa Hospitals and Clinics
Iowa City, Iowa, USA

**Cyrus M Jalai** BA
Research Associate
Department of Orthopedic Surgery
Spine Research Center
Hospital for Joint Diseases
New York University Langone Medical Center
New York, New York, USA

**Han Jo Kim** MD
Assistant Professor
Department of Orthopedic Surgery
Hospital for Special Surgery
New York, New York, USA

**Yong Kim** MD
Assistant Clinical Professor
Department of Orthopedic Surgery
New York University Langone Medical Center
New York, New York, USA

**Virginie Lafage** PhD
Scientist
Orthopedic/Spine Division
New York University
New York, New York, USA

**Athena Lolis** MD
Assistant Professor
Department of Neurology
Division of Clinical Neurophysiology
New York University School of Medicine
New York, New York, USA

**Arnold H Menezes** MD
Professor and Vice Chairman
Department of Neurosurgery
University of Iowa Hospitals and Clinics
Iowa City, Iowa, USA

**Emmanuel N Menga** MD
Assistant Professor of Spine Surgery
Department of Orthopedic Surgery
University of Texas Health Science Center
San Antonio, Texas, USA

**Venu M Nemani** MD PhD
Fellow, Adult and Pediatric Spine Surgery
Department of Orthopedic Surgery
Washington University in St. Louis
St. Louis, Missouri, USA

**Lana Nirenstein** MD
Resident, PGY4
Department of Orthopedics
Maimonides Medical Center
New York, New York, USA

**Donato Pacione** MD
Assistant Professor
Department of Neurosurgery
New York University School of Medicine
New York, New York, USA

**Peter G Passias** MD
New York Spine Institute
Hospital for Joint Diseases
New York University Langone
Medical Center
New York, New York, USA

**Themistocles S Protopsaltis** MD
Assistant Professor
Department of Orthopedic Surgery
New York University Langone
Medical Center
New York, New York, USA

**Kristen Radcliff** MD
Associate Professor
Department of Orthopedic Surgery
Thomas Jefferson University
Philadelphia, Pennsylvania, USA

**Afshin E Razi** MD
Clinical Assistant Professor
Department of Orthopedic Surgery
Hospital for Joint Diseases
New York University Langone
Medical Center
New York, New York, USA

**Nikhil A Sahasrabudhe** MD
Resident
Department of Neurosurgery
New York University Langone
Medical Center
New York, New York, USA

**Ahmed Saleh** MD
Resident
Department of Orthopedics
Maimonides Medical Center
New York, New York, USA

**Frank Schwab** MD
Clinical Professor
Department of Orthopedics/Spine
Weill Cornell Medical College
New York, New York, USA

**Daniel M Sciubba** MD
Associate Professor
Department of Neurosurgery
Johns Hopkins University
Baltimore, Maryland, USA

**Anna Shor** MD
Assistant Professor
Department of Neurology
New York University School of Medicine
New York, New York, USA

**Michael L Smith** MD
Assistant Professor
Department of Neurosurgery
New York University School of Medicine
New York, New York, USA

**Matthew A Spiegel** BA
Medical Student
Spine Research Fellow, Spine Division
Hospital for Joint Diseases
New York University Langone
Medical Center
New York, New York, USA

**Russell G Strom** MD
Chief Resident
Department of Neurosurgery
New York University Langone
Medical Center
New York, New York, USA

**Hideki Sudo** MD
Associate Professor
Department of Advanced Medicine for
Spine and Spinal Cord Disorders
Hokkaido University Graduate
School of Medicine
Kita-Ku, Sapporo, Japan

**Elizabeth Tanzi** ARNP
Research Associate
Department of Orthopedic Surgery
Spine Research Center
Hospital for Joint Diseases
New York University Langone
Medical Center
New York, New York, USA

**Shaleen Vira** MD
Resident Physician
Department of Orthopedic Surgery
Hospital for Joint Diseases
New York University Langone
Medical Center
New York, New York, USA

**Brett M Walker** DO
Department of Orthopedic Surgery
Michigan State University
Pontiac, Michigan, USA

**Chao Wang** MD
Orthopedic Department
Peking University Third Hospital
Haidian, Beijing, China

**Shaobai Wang** PhD
Professor
Department of Orthopedic Surgery
Massachusetts General Hospital/
Harvard Medical School
Boston, Massachusetts, USA

**Shenglin Wang** MD
Orthopedic Department
Peking University
Third Hospital
Haidian, Beijing, China

**Christopher D Witiw** MD
Neurosurgery Resident
Division of Neurosurgery
University of Toronto
Toronto, Ontario, Canada

**Nancy Worley** MS
Research Associate
Department of Orthopedic Surgery
Spine Research Center
Hospital for Joint Diseases
New York University
Langone Medical Center
New York, New York, USA

**Hiroyuki Yoshihara** MD PhD
Assistant Professor
Department of
Orthopedic Surgery
SUNY Downstate Medical Center
Brooklyn, New York, USA

**Hisashi Yoshimoto** MD PhD
Vice Director
Department of
Orthopedic Surgery
Shin Sapporo Orthopedic Hospital
Sapporo, Japan

# Preface

In a rapidly advancing field, such as spine surgery, editing a textbook that retains relevance and contains up-to-date references is a major challenge. With this reality in mind, we attempted to illustrate underlying principles that can be applied to approaching patients with cervical myelopathy. These principles can be applied regardless of any specific treatment plan, which are rapidly evolving based on ever-expanding technologies and devices.

Cervical myelopathy remains a challenging clinical entity, both in terms of diagnosis and management. A recurrent theme throughout this book is the importance of understanding and restoring sagittal alignment. The importance of sagittal alignment in terms of achieving successful patient outcomes in patients with cervical myelopathy has enjoyed growing appreciation in the literature. This textbook seeks to reflect this trend and provide instructions as to how to incorporate diagnostic factors, such as alignment in designing treatment for this complex pathology.

*Cervical Myelopathy* is appropriate for surgeons in training seeking to understand how to diagnose and treat cervical myelopathy, as well as for experienced clinicians who seek a thorough review of the pertinent etiologic, diagnostic, and therapeutic aspects of cervical myelopathy.

To achieve this goal of providing a comprehensive overview of this complex pathology, we have assembled a multidisciplinary team of neurosurgeons, orthopedic surgeons, and research scientists. They have generously provided both insights and practical experiences in order to make this work both scientifically rigorous and relevant to clinical practice. I hope to incorporate your suggestions and comments in future editions of *Cervical Myelopathy*.

**Peter G Passias** MD

# Acknowledgments

The process of writing and publishing this first book dedicated to cervical myelopathy could not have been accomplished without contributions from many individuals. I would like to thank my loving family, who have always supported me and have enabled me to pursue my goals. I would also like to give thanks to my many mentors in my previous and continued path of learning, as well as the numerous researchers at the beginning stages of their careers, who often are unappreciated, yet holding the future of medicine in their hands.

I would also like to thank the Senior Management team and production staff of Jaypee Brothers Medical Publishers (P) in Philadelphia, USA and in New Delhi, India.

# Contents

## Section 1: Introduction


1. **Anatomy and Embryology of the Skull Base and Cervical Spine** 3
   *Carolina G Benjamin, Donato Pacione*
2. **Cervical Biomechanics and Clinical Instability** 15
   *Shaobai Wang*
3. **Cervical Alignment** 25
   *Shaleen Vira, Matthew A Spiegel, Virginie Lafage, Frank Schwab*
4. **Clinical Diagnosis of Cervical Myelopathy** 33
   *Brett M Walker, Kristen Radcliff*
5. **Electrodiagnostics** 43
   *Athena Lolis, Anna Shor, Aleksandar Beric*


## Section 2: Outcomes


6. **Natural History of Cervical Spondylotic Myelopathy** 57
   *Christopher D Witiw, Michael G Fehlings*
7. **Influence of Conservative Management on Outcomes** 67
   *Jerry Cheriyan, Elizabeth Tanzi, Peter G Passias, Thomas Cheriyan*
8. **Influence of Surgical Intervention on Outcomes** 73
   *Hisashi Yoshimoto*


## Section 3: Distinct Diagnostic Etiologies


9. **Cervical Amyotrophy** 87
   *Venu M Nemani, Han Jo Kim*
10. **Rheumatologic Disorders of the Cervical Spine** 93
    *Afshin E Razi, Lana Nirenstein, Yong Kim*
11. **Ossification of the Posterior Longitudinal Ligament** 103
    *Nikhil A Sahasrabudhe, Russell G Strom, Michael L Smith*
12. **Os Odontoideum** 109
    *Peter G Passias, Cyrus M Jalai*
13. **Atlantoaxial Dislocations** 117
    *Shenglin Wang, Chao Wang*
14. **Basilar Invagination** 133
    *Andrew J Grossbach, Arnold H Menezes*
15. **Congenital Anomalies of the Cervical Spine** 143
    *Peter G Passias, Cyrus M Jalai, Nancy Worley*

## Section 4: Surgical Management


**16. Surgical Management of Cervical Spondylotic Myelopathy: Anterior Techniques** **149**
*Michael Gerling, Nancy Worley*

**17. Cervical Laminectomy with or without Fusion** **157**
*Hiroyuki Yoshihara*

**18. Cervical Laminoplasty: Techniques and Outcomes** **167**
*John A Buza III, Themistocles S Protopsaltis*

**19. Instrumentation Techniques of the Occiput, Upper Cervical Spine, and Subaxial Spine** **177**
*Afshin E Razi, Yong Kim, Ahmed Saleh*

**20. Neurological and Vascular Complications after Surgery for Cervical Myelopathy** **189**
*Hideki Sudo*


## Section 5: Cervical Myelopathy in the Setting of Cervical Deformities


**21. Cervical Myelopathy in the Setting of Cervical Deformities** **201**
*Shaleen Vira, Matthew A Spiegel, Virginie Lafage, Frank Schwab*


## Section 6: Cervical Myelopathy in the Setting of Spine Tumors


**22. Cervical Myelopathy in the Setting of Metastatic Tumors in the Spine** **213**
*Mohamad Bydon, Rafael De la Garza-Ramos Daniel M Sciubba, Ziya L Gokaslan*

**23. Cervical Myelopathy in the Setting of Intramedullary Spinal Cord Tumors** **221**
*Akwasi Ofori Boah, Donato Pacione, Anthony K Frempong-Boadu*

**24. Role of Total Disk Replacement for the Treatment of Cervical Myelopathy** **237**
*Emmanuel N Menga, Shaleen Vira, John A Bendo*

*Index* *243*

# Section 1

# Introduction

Chapter 1

# Anatomy and Embryology of the Skull Base and Cervical Spine

*Carolina Benjamin, Donato Pacione*

## EMBRYOLOGY

The normal development of the spine is an intricate process that involves the influence of multiple genes and proteins. One of the guiding principles in the embryology of the spine is segmentation, also known as metamerism. This is a phenomenon by which part of an organism is created by multiple consecutive anatomically similar sections.[1] Two important genes implicated in the embryonic development of the spine are the Hox and Pax genes. In particular, the Hox genes control rostrocaudal specification and the Pax genes control resegmentation. These genes code for proteins that directly guide normal developmental processes (such as shh, FGF8, BMP) or activate transcription factor pathways that alter the genetic code directly.[2-6]

An understanding of the embryology of the developing spine allows for an appreciation of normal anatomy as well as pathologic conditions that occur when these processes go awry. This section will focus on the development of the skull base, the atlas, and the axis, which together constitute the craniovertebral junction. Given its function as the transitional zone between the cranium and the remainder of the axial skeleton, the craniovertebral junction plays an important role in the stability and functionality of the spine.

### Mesenchymal Stage

The three separate stages involved in the formation of the cervicocranium include the mesenchymal or membranous stage, the chondrification or cartilaginous stage, and the ossification stage. The mesenchymal stage takes place during the first 6 weeks of embryonic development. Under the influence of factors secreted by Hensen's node, the notochord develops and induces the formation of the neural plate. As the neural plate involutes to form the neural tube, mesodermal cells migrate laterally and develop into 42–44 paired somites in the rostral-caudal direction. Each somite further differentiates to an outer dermatome, an inner myotome, and a medial sclerotome, which are precursors for skin, paraspinal musculature, and vertebrae, respectively. As the somitic cells proliferate, they surround the notochord and neural tube to form a continuous layer of paraxial mesoderm that can be referred to as the membranous vertebral column. The proliferation of the cells that make up each sclerotome occurs unevenly such that there is a larger concentration of cells cranially and a smaller concentration of cells caudally. When developing into the vertebral column, the more dense caudal mass of one sclerotome joins with the less dense rostral mass of the following sclerotome to form a single vertebral body. This process is termed resegmentation. The dense caudal zone and loose rostral zone are separated by a fissure of von Ebner. The loose rostral zone will line up with the fissure of von Ebner to form the intervertebral boundary zone, which contributes to the intervertebral disks (Fig. 1.1).[1,3,7] The embryologic process of somite differentiation accounts for the fact that there are eight cervical somites and nerve roots but only seven resegmented sclerotomes and thus only seven cervical vertebrae. This explains why the C1 nerve root exits above the C1 neural arch and the C8 nerve root exits above the C7 neural arch, which is in fact derived from the eighth somite.[1,2]

The somites that serve as the embryologic precursors of the cranial base, the atlas, and the axis include the occipital somites and the first two cervical somites. The first three occipital somites do not undergo the aforementioned process of resegmentation. Instead, the first two occipital somites fuse to form the basiocciput and the third occipital somite forms the exoccipital bone, which gives rise to the jugular tubercles (Table 1.1).[1,6]

The fourth occipital sclerotome is unique and is termed the pro atlas. It is further subdivided into a hypocentrum, a centrum, and a neural arch, which has both a

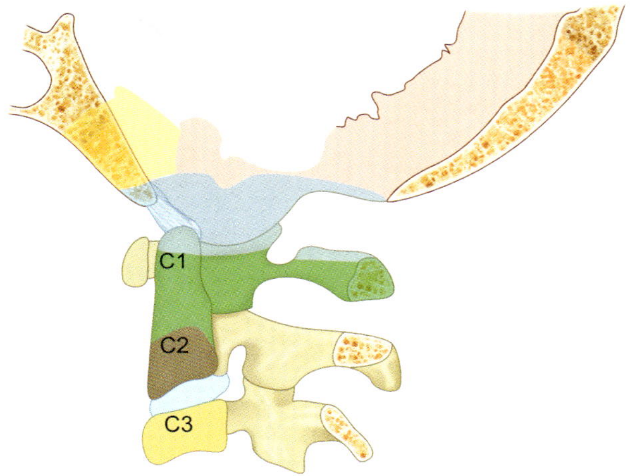


**Fig. 1.1:** Bones of craniovertebral junction separated by colors based on which somite and sclerotome it differentiates from (*see* Table 1.1).

**Table 1.1:** List of first four occipital and two cervical sclerotomes and their contributions to bones of craniovertebral junction.

| *Sclerotome* | *Structure* |
|---|---|
| Occipital 1 | Basiocciput |
| Occipital 2 | Basiocciput |
| Occipital 3 | Exoccipital centers (jugular tubercles) |
| Occipital 4 (Proatlas) | Anterior tubercle clivus<br>Apical ligament<br>Apex of dens<br>Occipital condyles<br>Alar and cruciate ligaments<br>Posterior arch of atlas<br>Lateral masses of atlas |
| Cervical 1 | Anterior arch atlas<br>Dens<br>Posterior inferior arch atlas |
| Cervical 2 | Body of axis<br>Facets, posterior arch axis |

dorsal and a ventral component. The hypocentrum gives rise to the anterior tubercle of the clivus, and the centrum forms the apical cap of the dens and the apical ligament. The ventral neural arch forms the anterior margin of the foramen magnum, the occipital condyle, and the midline third occipital condyle. It also gives rise to the alar and cruciate ligaments. The caudal neural arch forms the lateral masses of the atlas as well as the posterior arch of the atlas (Table 1.1).[1,6]

The first cervical sclerotome is also further subdivided into a hypocentrum, a centrum, and a neural arch. In most scenarios, the hypocentrum disappears. In rare cases, it can persist and give rise to an abnormal joint between the clivus and anterior arch of the atlas. The centrum contributes to the axis body, which is joined by the apical tip that originates from the hypocentrum of the fourth occipital sclerotome to form the ondontoid process. The fusion between the tip and the body of the dens does not occur until around 8 years of life. Until that point, they are joined by a cartilaginous band called the neural central synchrondrosis. The neural arch forms the posterior and inferior portion of the arch of the atlas (Table 1.1).[1,6]

Similarly, the second cervical sclerotome is subdivided into a hypocentrum, centrum, and a neural arch. The hypocentrum involutes. The centrum becomes the body of the axis. The neural arch gives rise to the facets and the posterior arch of the axis (Table 1.1).[1,6]

This same process of somite differentiation into segmented sclerotomes that then contribute to different components of each vertebra guides the development of the rest of the spine from C3 to C7. There are eight cervical somites but only seven resegmented sclerotomes, which explains the fact that there are only seven cervical vertebrae.[1]

## Chondrification and Ossification Stages

The chondrification stage occurs starting the 6th embryonic week. This is followed by the ossification stage, which occurs in chronologic waves.

The atlas usually has three primary ossification centers at birth, although sometimes it can have two (Fig. 1.2A). Ossification of the atlas initiates in utero with the lateral masses and fuses around the 7–10th year of life (Fig. 1.2B).[1,6-9]

The axis has six primary ossification centers at birth (Fig. 1.3A). The ossification of the axis begins in utero, occurs in three different waves, and is usually complete by the 7th year of life. The first wave of ossification takes place at 4 months of gestation and begins with the ossification of bilateral centers within the neural arches and a center within the body of the axis. The second wave of ossification takes place at 6 months of gestation as two centers on each side of the basal dens. These two centers typically fuse by birth (Fig. 1.3B).[1,6-9] Rarely, these two centers fail to fuse, causing a bifid dens or dens bicornis.[1,10,11] The third wave of ossification takes place postnatally at 3–5 years of life at the ossification center at the apical tip of the dens. Failure of this apical dental synchondrosis to ossify causes ossiculum terminale pesistens.[1,7,10]

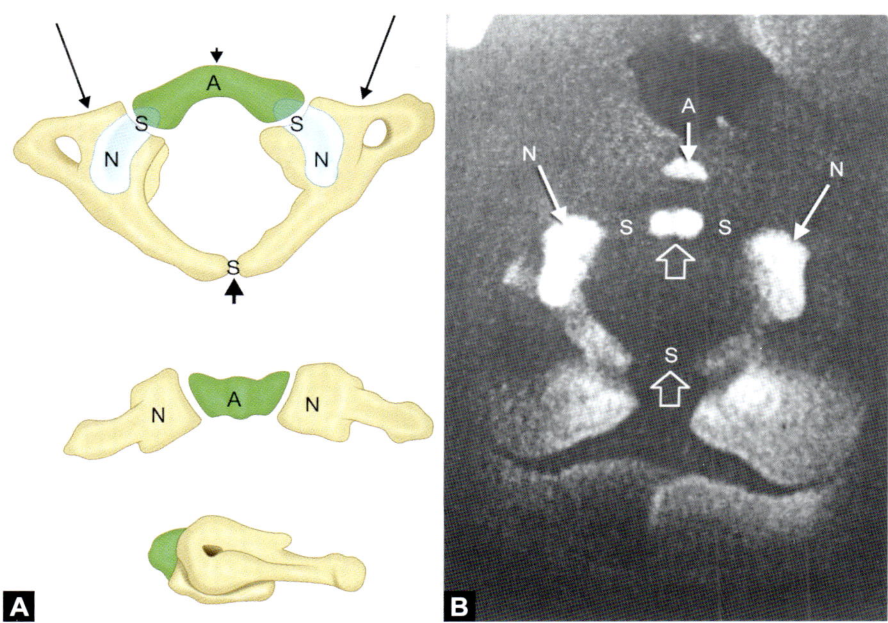


**Figs. 1.2A and B:** (A) Schematic representation of the three ossification centers of C1 at birth, one in the anterior arch (A) and two neurocentral ossification centers (N). In between the ossification centers, the synchondroses (S) can be visualized. (B) Axial computed tomography scan of C1 ossification centers, one in the anterior arch (A) and two neurocentral ossification centers (N). The syndrondroses are visualized as gaps. The small arrowhead points to the tip of the dens. The large arrowhead points to the space in between unfused laminae of C1.

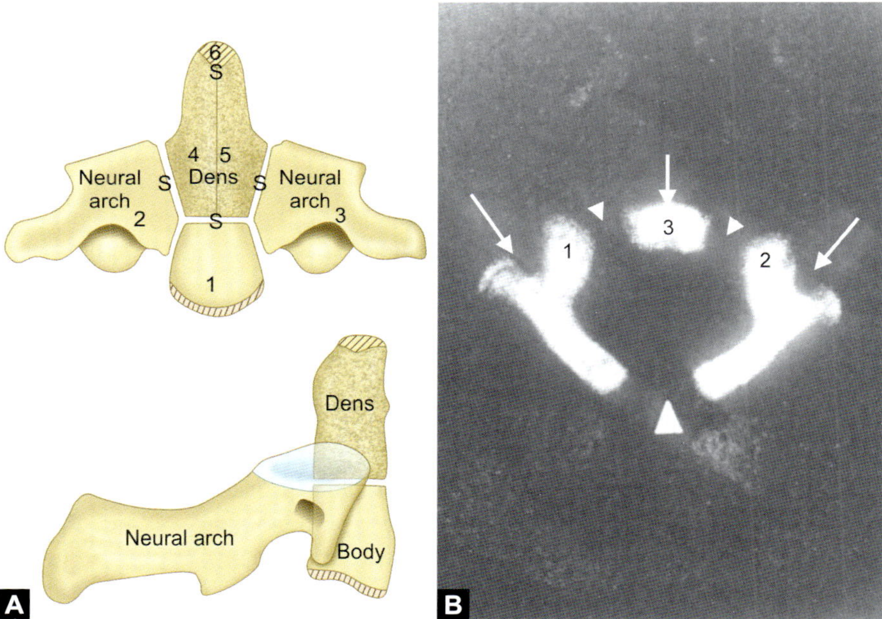


**Figs. 1.3A and B:** (A) Schematic representation of the six ossification centers of C2, including one in the body of the axis, one in the bilateral neural arches, two in the body of the dens, and one in the tip of the dens. (B) Axial computed tomography scan of C2 ossification centers. Three of the six ossification centers can be visualized here, including the two in the neural arches and the one in the tip of the dens. The two ossification centers in the base of the dens and the ossification center in the body of the axis are not visualized here. The syndrondroses are visualized as gaps (arrowheads).

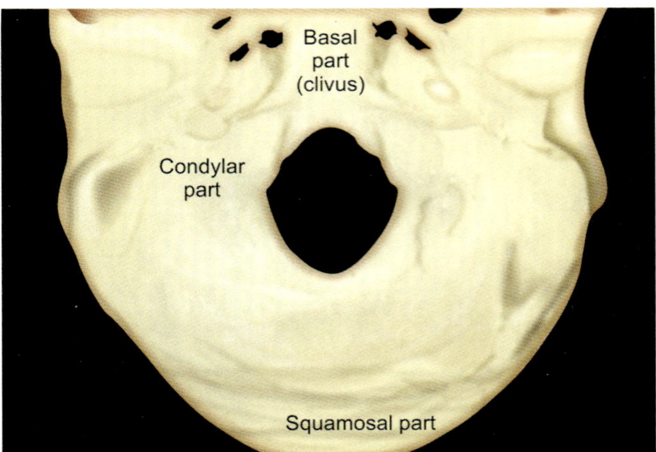


**Fig. 1.4:** The three parts of the occipital bone that make up the foramen magnum: the clival part anteriorly, the squamosal part posteriorly, and the condylar parts laterally.

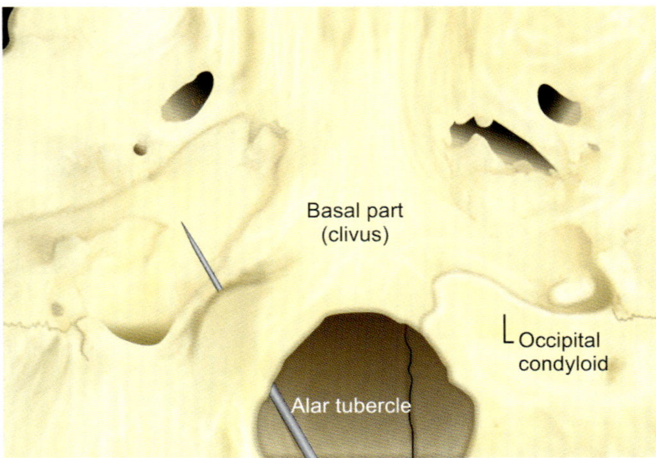


**Fig. 1.5:** The relationship between the occipital condyles and the hypoglossal canal.

# ANATOMY

## Foramen Magnum and Hypoglossal Canal

The foramen magnum is a structure whose margins are made up from the three different parts of the occipital bone. The basal or clival portion of the occipital bone is anterior to the foramen magnum, the squamosal portion is posterior to the foramen magnum, and the condylar portions are lateral on either side (Fig. 1.4). On average, the foramen magnum is 35 mm in the sagittal diameter and 28 mm in the transverse diameter.[8,12] The occipital condyles are oval structures that face anteromedially and articulate with the superior facet of the atlas. The average condylar length is 21 mm, though longer variants can be >26 mm and shorter variants can be <20 mm (Fig. 1.5).[8,13-16] On the medial aspect of each condyle, there is an alar tubercle that is attached to the alar ligament of the odontoid process. Superior to each condyle at the middle third is the hypoglossal canal, which transmits the hypoglossal nerve. The hypoglossal canal has an intracranial end and an extracranial end. The intracranial end can be found 5 mm above the junction of the posterior and middle third of the occipital condyle, and the extracranial end can be found 5 mm above the junction of the anterior and middle third of the occipital condyle. Given this orientation, the hypoglossal nerve travels anterolaterally from intracranial to extracranial (Fig. 1.5). From a surgical standpoint, the distance between the posterior margin of the occipital condyle and the intracranial end of the hypoglossal canal is important to avoid violation of the canal and injury to the hypoglossal nerve when drilling. This distance is approximately 10 mm and should be measured with computed tomography (CT) scans preoperatively for confirmation.[16-18] The oval shape of the occipital condyle that faces inferolaterally allows for articulation with the convex superior articulating process of the atlas.

## Atlas

The atlas is the first cervical vertebrae and is unique in its shape and anatomy. Unlike other cervical vertebrae, the atlas lacks a vertebral body and a spinous process. Instead, it is composed of a shorter anterior arch and a longer posterior arch, which come together to form a ring. Two oval-shaped lateral masses are located at the anteromedial border of the ring on either side (Figs. 1.6A and B). In the midway point of the anterior arch, there is an anterior tubercle. Similarly, in the midway point of the posterior arch there is a posterior tubercle. There are also two tubercles medial to the lateral masses where the transverse ligament of the atlas will attach (Fig. 1.7). The transverse process of the atlas extends from the lateral masses. In comparison to adjacent cervical vertebrae, the transverse process of the atlas extends further out. In between the lateral masses and the transverse process is the foramen transversarium through which the vertebral arteries (VAs) course. The VA will be discussed separately below.

Closely related to the VA at the level of the atlas is the C1 nerve root, also known as the suboccipital nerve.

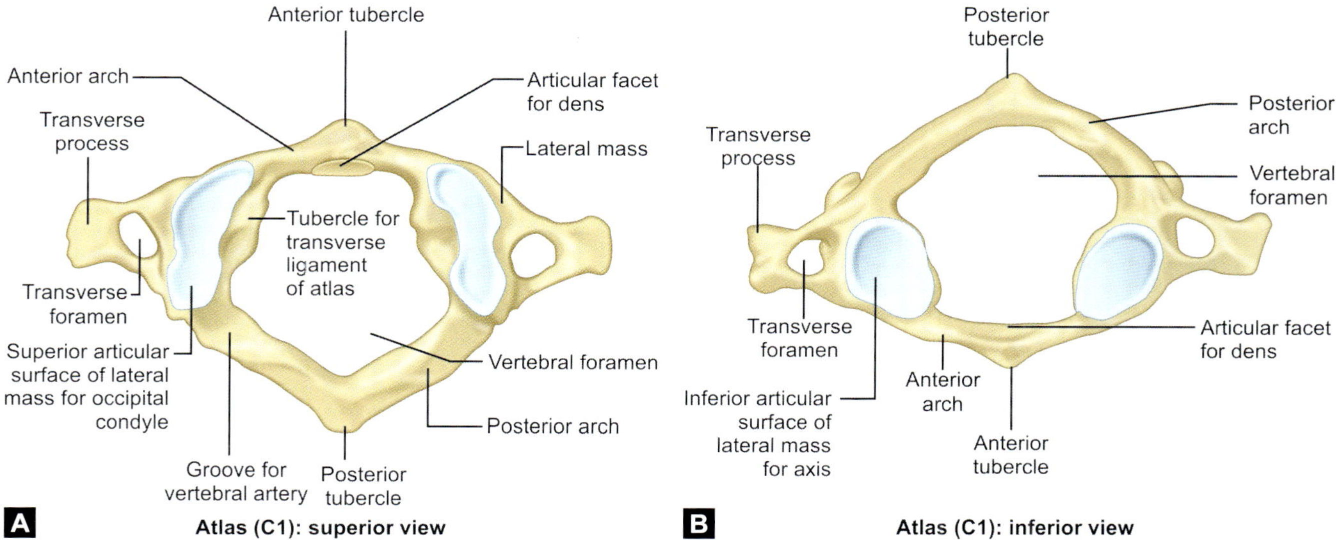


**Figs. 1.6A and B:** Superior and inferior views of C1.

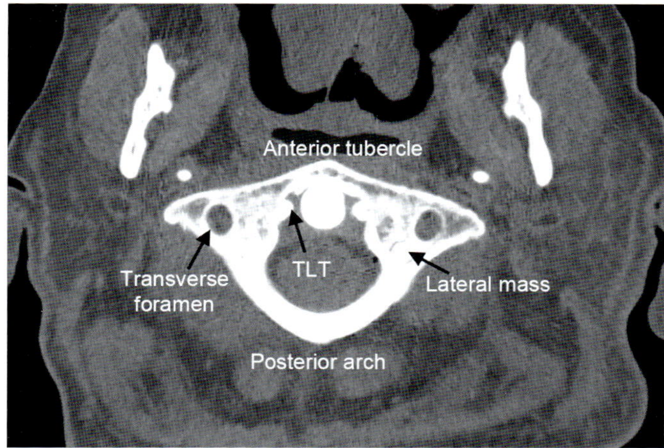


**Fig. 1.7:** Axial noncontrast computed tomography image of C1 demonstrating prominent transverse ligament tubercle as well as other relevant anatomy.

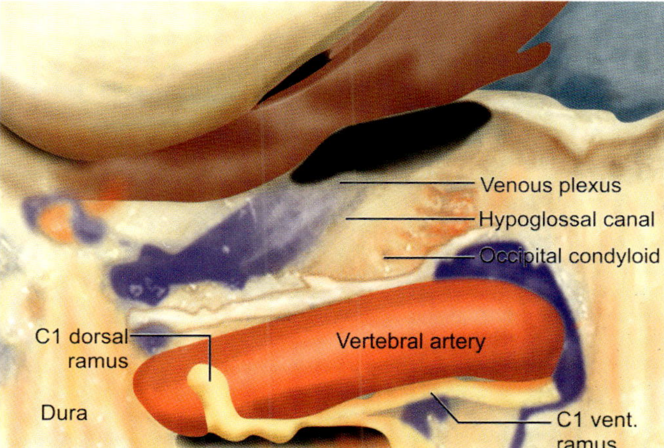


**Fig. 1.8:** Course of C1 nerve root.

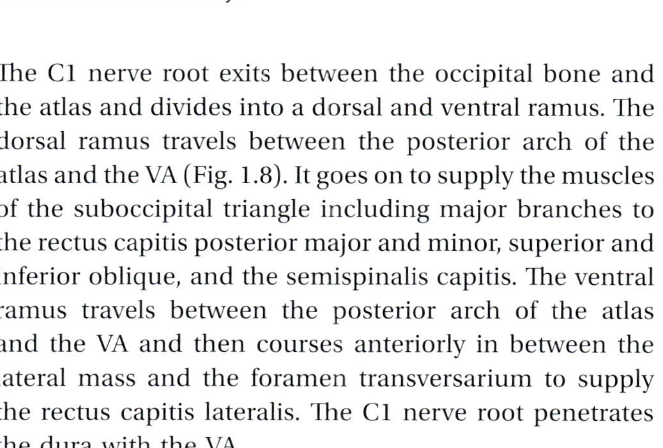

The C1 nerve root exits between the occipital bone and the atlas and divides into a dorsal and ventral ramus. The dorsal ramus travels between the posterior arch of the atlas and the VA (Fig. 1.8). It goes on to supply the muscles of the suboccipital triangle including major branches to the rectus capitis posterior major and minor, superior and inferior oblique, and the semispinalis capitis. The ventral ramus travels between the posterior arch of the atlas and the VA and then courses anteriorly in between the lateral mass and the foramen transversarium to supply the rectus capitis lateralis. The C1 nerve root penetrates the dura with the VA.

## Axis

The axis is the second cervical vertebrae and is a transition between the unique anatomy of the atlas and the characteristic anatomy of the remainder of the cervical vertebrae. The body of the axis serves as the base for the odontoid process, which is also known as the dens. On average, the dens is 1.0–1.5 cm in length and 1 cm wide.[13,16,19] Anteriorly, the dens articulates with the anterior arch of the atlas. Anterolateral to the body and dens are two large, oval-shaped superior facets that articulate with the back of the anterior arch of the atlas. The two

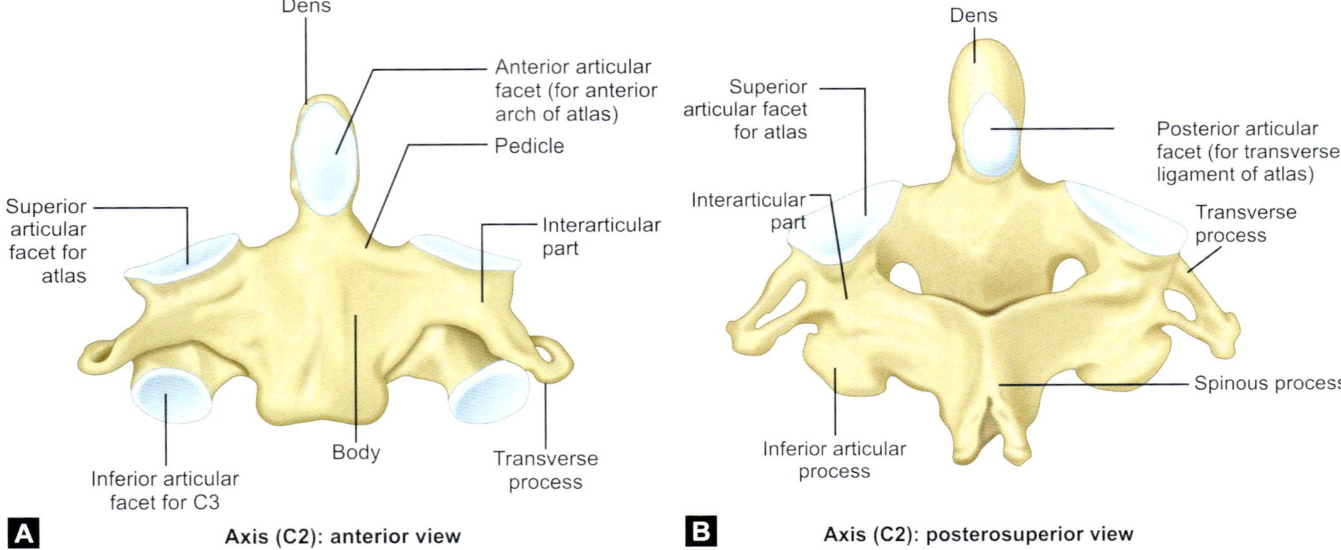


**Figs. 1.9A and B:** Anterior and posterior views of C2.

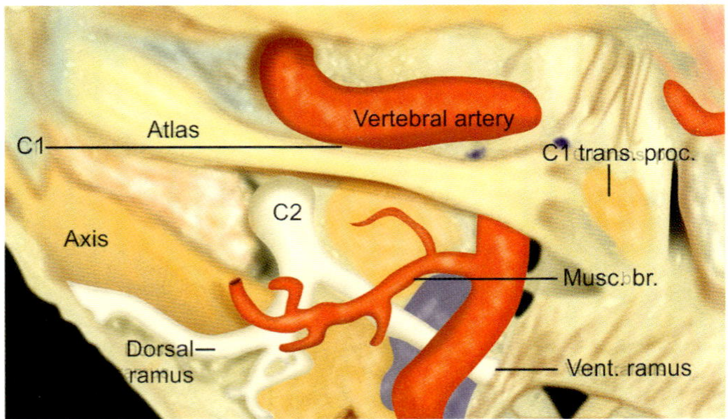


**Fig. 1.10:** Course of C2 nerve root.

inferior facets are also lateral to the body and dens but are situated more posterior than the superior facets. These inferior facets will articulate with the third cervical vertebrae. Lateral to the superior facets are small transverse processes. In between the superior facets and the transverse processes is the foramen transversarium through which the VAs course. The posterior elements of the axis include the pedicle, the lamina, and the spinous process. The laminae of the axis are thicker than that of any other cervical vertebrae. They come together and fuse posteriorly, forming the spinous process (Figs. 1.9A and B).

The C2 nerve arises between the posterior arch of the atlas and the lamina of the axis and then divides into a dorsal and ventral ramus. The ventral ramus travels between the vertebral arches and transverse processes. The dorsal ramus sends a branch to supply the inferior oblique muscle and then further subdivides into medial and lateral branch. The medial branch of the dorsal ramus gives rise to the greater occipital nerve, which supplies the semispinalis capitis and the scalp. The lateral branch of the dorsal ramus supplies the splenius, longissimus, and the semisplenius capitis (Fig. 1.10).

## Joints of the Craniovertebral Junction

### *Occipital-Atlantal Joint*

The oval shape of the occipital condyle that faces inferolaterally allows for articulation with the convex trapezoid-shaped superior articulating process of the atlas. This atlanto-occipital joint is cushioned by an articular capsule and strengthened by anterior and posterior atlanto-occipital membranes. The attachments of the anterior atlanto-occipital membranes are the anterior edge of the foramen magnum superiorly, the superior edge of the anterior arch of the atlas inferiorly, and the articular capsule laterally (Figs. 1.11A and B). The attachments of the posterior atlanto-occipital membranes are the posterior edge of the foramen magnum superiorly and the posterior arch of the atlas inferiorly. The posterior atlanto-occipital membrane does not have any lateral attachments and courses behind the VA and first cervical root (Figs. 1.11A and B). If this membrane ossifies, it creates a partial or complete ring around the VA as will be discussed below.

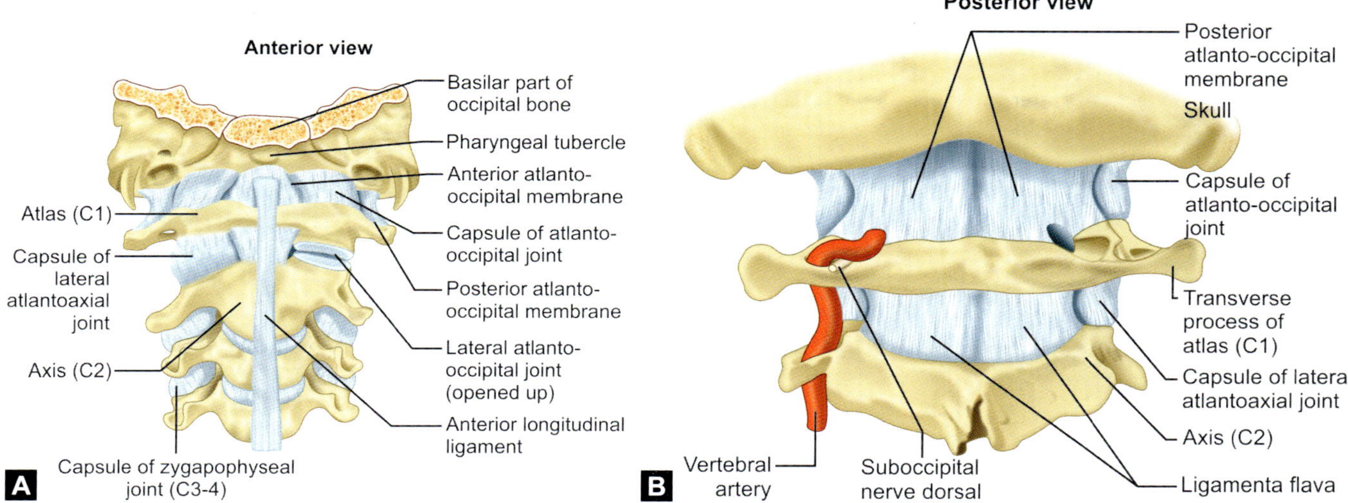


**Figs. 1.11A and B:** Anterior and posterior view of ligaments of the craniovertebral junction.

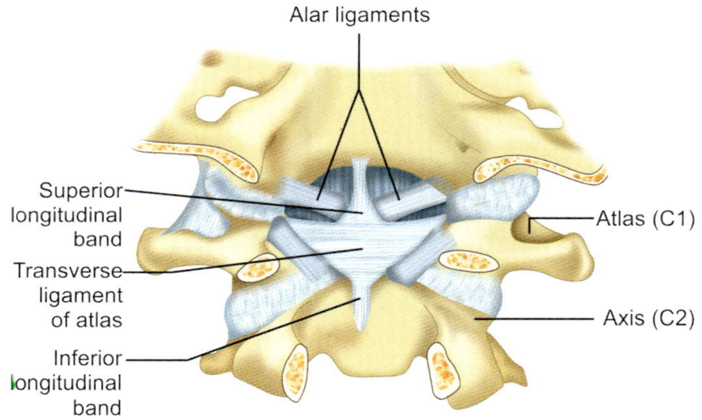


**Fig. 1.12:** Ligaments between C1 and C2.

### *Atlanto-Axial Joint*

The atlanto-axial joint involves four surfaces of articulation. The first articulation is the synovial joint between the anterior surface of the dens and the posterior surface of the anterior arch of the atlas. The second articulation is the synovial joint between the posterior surface of the dens and the anterior surface of the transverse ligament of the atlas. The third and the fourth articulations are the paired lateral ones between the superior facet of C2 and the inferior facet of C1.

In addition to these articular surfaces, there are also ligaments surrounding the C1/2 junction that provide stability while also maintaining range of motion. The cruciform ligament is composed of a transverse portion and a vertical portion that forms a cross behind the dens. The transverse portion, known as the transverse atlantal ligament, attaches to the tubercles that are on the medial border of the lateral masses of C1 (*see* Fig. 1.7). The vertical portions are known as the superior and inferior longitudinal band and attach to the clivus and to the posterior surface of the body of the axis, respectively (Fig. 1.12). On average, the transverse atlantal ligament is 6–7 mm thick. Its tensile strength and relative inelasticity prevents anterior subluxation of C1 and maintains the stability of the craniovertebral junction.[20]

The other ligaments that act in a synergistic fashion to the cruciate ligament are the paired alar ligaments. These ligaments have attachments on the posterior surface of the upper third of the dens, and then each alar ligament is further subdivided into two lateral bands. The occipital-alar band inserts on the occipital bone while the atlanto-alar band inserts to the lateral mass of C1. In addition to the aforementioned ligaments that provide most of the stability to the craniocervical junction, there are other ligaments that also contribute (Table 1.2).

## Subaxial Cervical Spine

The anatomy of the subaxial cervical spine is relatively consistent from C3 to C7 with slight variations and trends in the morphology. Each vertebra is comprised of a vertebral body, which is separated from the adjacent vertebral body by the intervertebral disk. The posterolateral aspect of each vertebral body consists of the uncinate process, which articulates with the superior vertebral body,

**Table 1.2:** Accessory ligaments of the craniovertebral junction.

| *Name* | *Insertions* | *Function* | *Comment* |
|---|---|---|---|
| Arnold ligament | Connects the lateral mass of the atlas to the body of the axis | Rotational stability | Also known as accessory atlanto-axial ligament; extends cephalad and has connection to occipital bone |
| Barkow ligament | Connects the mesial aspect of the two occipital condyles | Rotational stability | Traverses anterior to the superior aspect of the dens and anterior to the alar ligament |
| Lauth ligament | Attaches to the occipital condyles superior to transverse portion of cruciate ligament and posterosuperior to the alar ligament | Unknown | Also known as transverse occipital ligament |
| Suspensory ligament | Connects the tip of the dens to the anterior border of the foramen magnum | None, embryologic remnant | Located between the anterior atlanto-occipital membrane and the cruciate ligament |

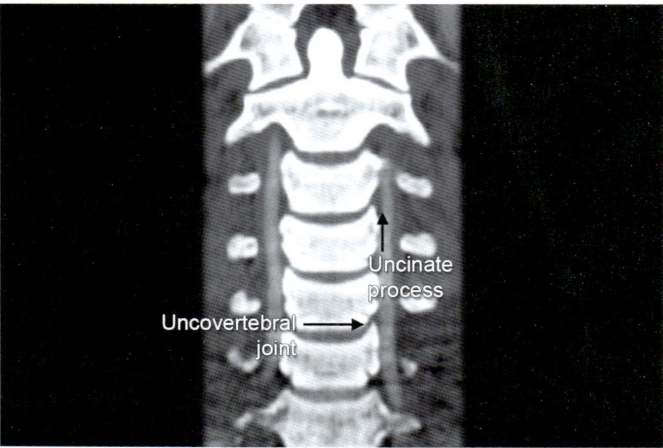


**Fig. 1.13:** Coronal computed tomography angiogram image demonstrating the uncinate process as well as the uncovertebral joint. The vertebral artery is visualized entering the transverse foramen at C6.

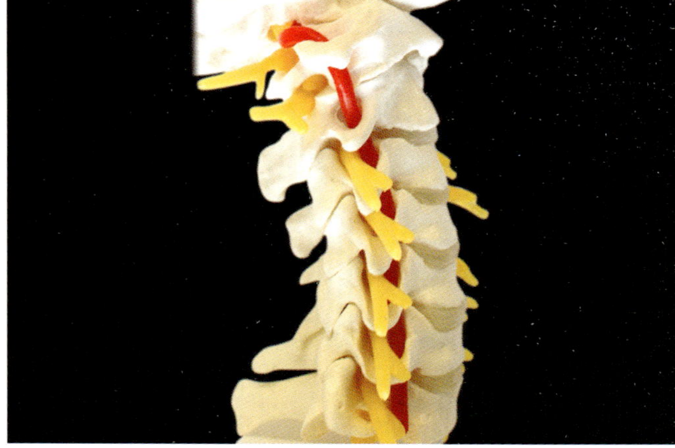

**Fig. 1.14:** Cervical spine from a lateral view. The nerve root (yellow) is visualized traveling out of the neural foramen within the neural groove. It is located posterior to the vertebral artery (red).

forming the uncovertebral joint (Fig. 1.13). Posterior to the uncovertebral joint is the neural foramen and the exiting nerve root. Laterally the vertebral body is connected to the transverse process. The most lateral portions of the transverse process are the anterior and posterior tubercles between which lies the groove for the exiting nerve root (Fig. 1.14). Transitioning from C3 to C7, the posterior tubercle becomes more lateral and posterior such that at C7 is can resemble a true transverse process (Figs. 1.15A and B). Between the tubercles and the vertebral body there is the transverse foramen, which contains the VA. The vertebral body is connected to the posterior elements by the pedicle. Superior to the pedicle is the neural foramen and the exiting nerve root of the corresponding level. The pedicle connects posteriorly with the lateral mass complex, which consists of a superior articular facet and an inferior articular facet. From C3 to C7 there is a trend such that the height (the distance from the superior facet to the inferior facet) increases and the thickness (AP) decreases (Fig. 1.16).[21] The two lateral masses are connected posteriorly by the lamina, which meet to form the spinous process. The spinous process is usually bifid at C3, C4, and C5. At C6, the spinous process is bifid in approximately 50% of patients, whereas C7 is monofid in approximately 99% of patients.[22]

## Vertebral Artery Anatomy

The VA is composed of four segments, of which the first three are extradural. The V1 segment is the portion of the VA from the takeoff of the subclavian artery until the C6 transverse foramen. There is often asymmetry between the VAs, with the left VA being dominant in 40–60% of patients.[23-25] Entrance at the C6 transverse foramen occurs

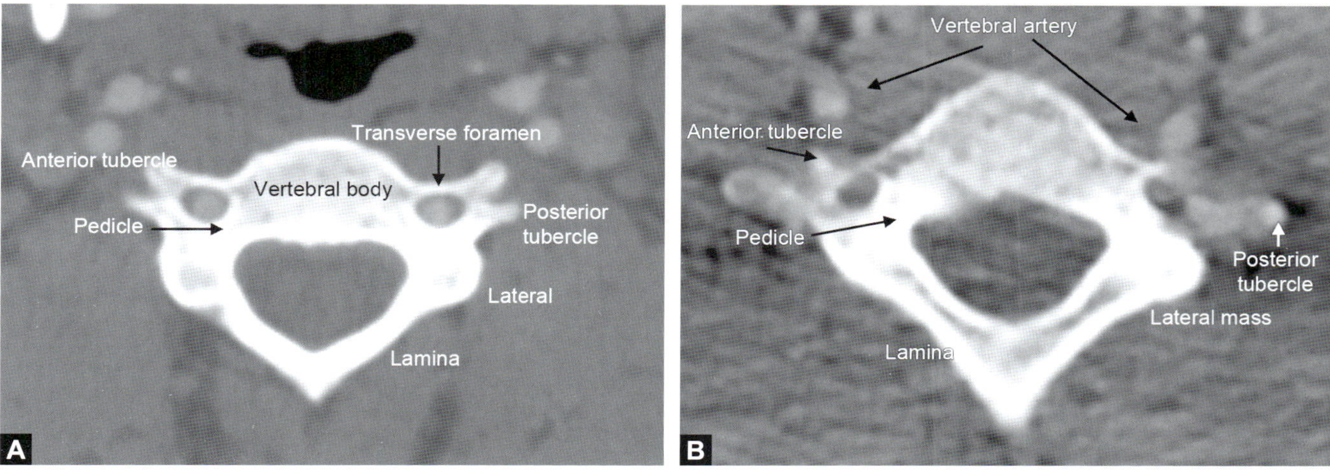


**Figs. 1.15A and B:** (A) Axial noncontrast computed tomography (CT) image of C3 demonstrating the anterior and posterior tubercles as well as surrounding relevant anatomy. (B) Noncontrast CT image of C7 demonstrating the anterior and posterior tubercles as well as surrounding relevant anatomy. Note that the vertebral artery is located anterior to the transverse foramen.

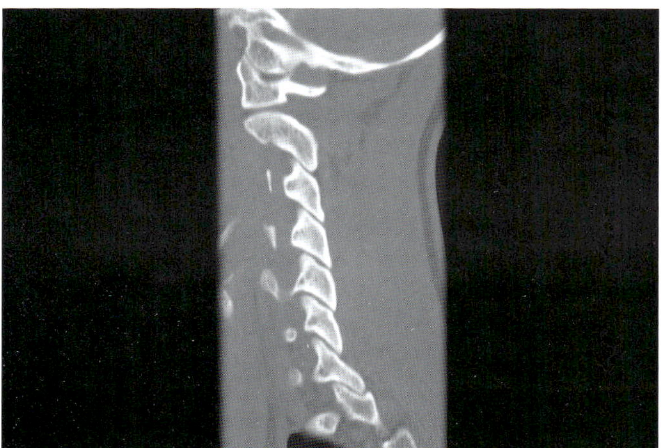

**Fig. 1.16:** Sagittal noncontrast computed tomography demonstrating the lateral masses from C3 to C7. The height of the lateral mass increases and the thickness decreases from C3 to C7.

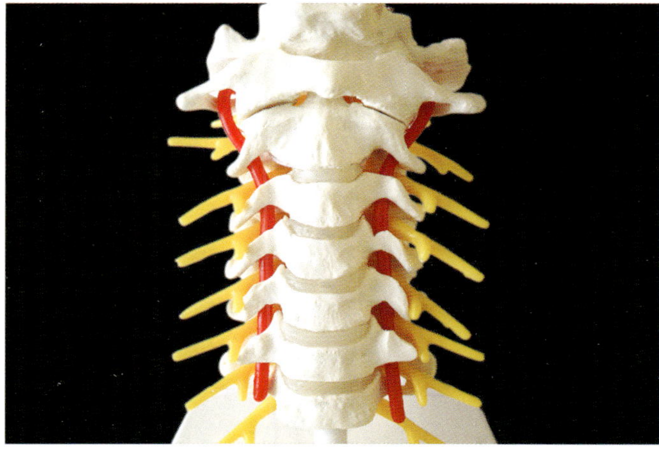

**Fig. 1.17:** Anterior view of model of the cervical spine demonstrating the path of the vertebral artery (red) and its relationship to the nerve root (yellow).

in the majority of patients (90–94%), with a small minority entering at C5, C7, and C4.[26,27] Although C7 has a transverse foramen, the VA is rarely located within it (0.2%) (Fig. 1.15B).[27] The V2 segment begins at the C6 transverse foramen and then the VA travels within each foramen up to C2 (Fig. 1.17). It is located anterior to the nerve root at each interspace lateral to the uncovertebral joint. In anatomic studies, it is found at the posterior one-fourth of the intervertebral disk space (*see* Fig. 1.14).[27] At C2 it makes a turn laterally to enter the C2 transverse foramen. The VA at C2 may be high riding as it loops under the pars interarticularis prior to entering the transverse foramen (Figs. 1.18A and B). The prevalence of a high-riding VA is reported as between 18% and 32%.[28] The V3 segment begins as the VA exits the C2 transverse foramen and extends to the point where it enters the foramen magnum (Figs. 1.19A and B). After exiting the C2 transverse foramen, it courses superiorly and slightly anterior to enter the transverse foramen of C1. Upon exiting the C1 foramen, it travels posteromedially in the sulcus of the posterior arch of C1. In up to 43–50% of patients, the groove for the VA may form a partial ring of bone as a result of ossification of the oblique atlanto-occipital ligament and periosteal sheath (Fig. 1.20).[17,18,28] A complete ossification resulting in an

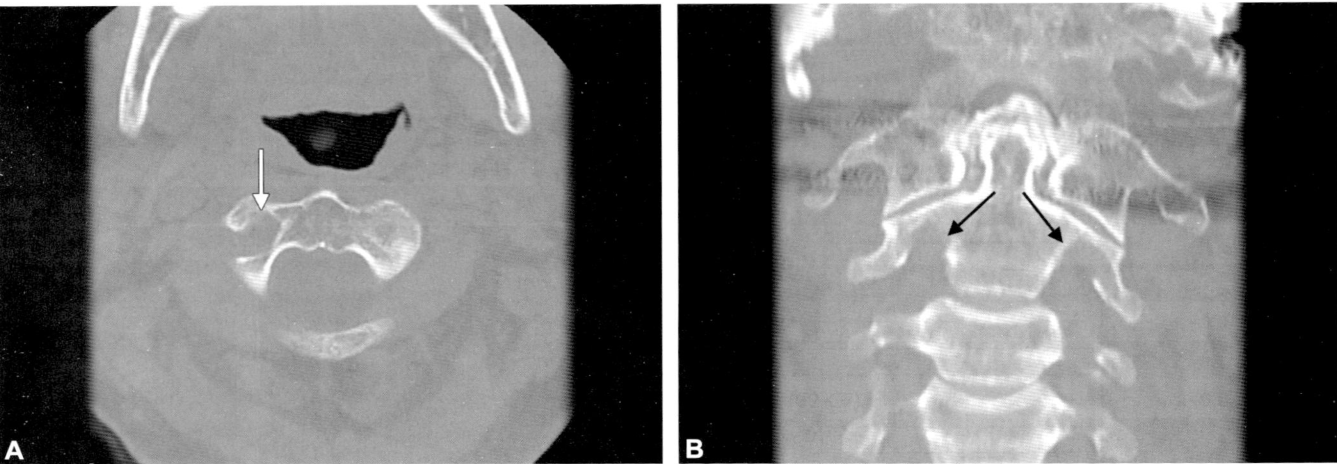

**Figs. 1.18A and B:** (A) Axial noncontrast computed tomography (CT) of C2 demonstrating a high-riding vertebral artery foramen on the right side (white arrow). Note that due to the high-riding vertebral artery, there is a narrow pedicle and thin pars articularis. (B) Coronal non-contrast CT of C2 demonstrating bilateral high-riding vertebral artery (black arrow).

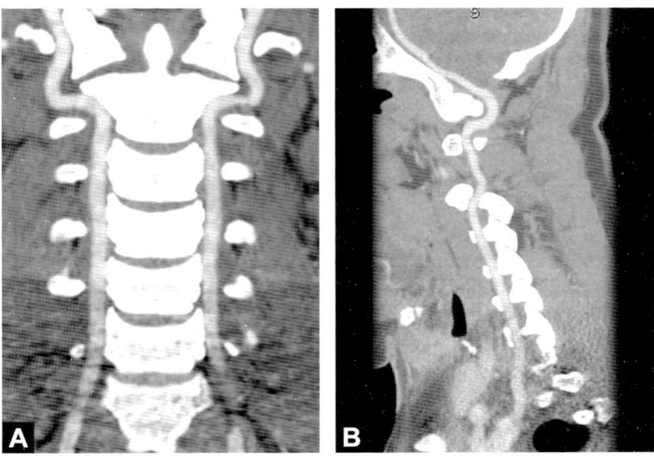

**Figs. 1.19A and B:** (A) Coronal computed tomography (CT) angiogram demonstrating the vertebral artery as it travels within the transverse foramen. It is visualized entering at C6 and then travels cranially to C2. At C2, it turns posterolaterally and then enters the C1 transverse foramen. (B) Sagittal CT angiogram demonstrating the vertebral artery traveling within the transverse foramen. It enters at C6, then travels cranially to C2. At C2, it turns posterolaterally and then enters the C1 transverse foramen.

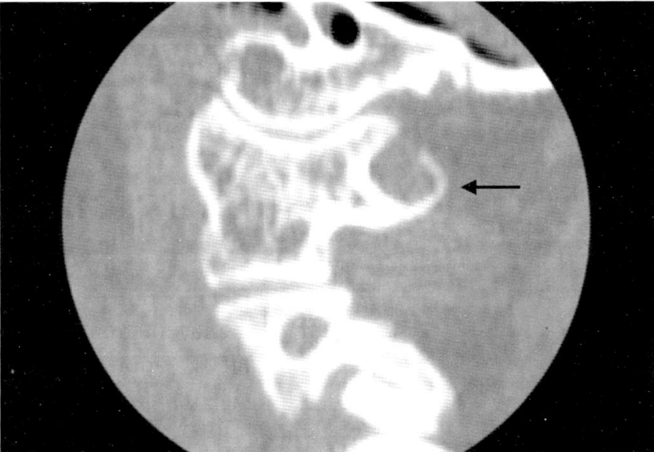

**Fig. 1.20:** Sagittal noncontrast computed tomography of C1 demonstrating a partial ossification of the oblique atlanto-occipital ligament surrounding the sulcus arteriosis.

arcuate foramen is found in 14–26% of patients (Fig. 1.21).[28] The presence of this should be noted on preoperative CT of the upper cervical spine, as this bone will need to be removed in order to access the VA.

The V3 segment ends as the VA pierces the atlanto-occipital membrane at the foramen magnum. This point is located approximately 15–19 mm lateral to the midline posterior tubercle of C1.[29] In order to avoid vertebral injury, surgical exposure should not extend farther than 10–15 mm from the midline of the posterior tubercle. An important variant of the V3 segment is the presence of an extradural origin of the posterior inferior cerebellar

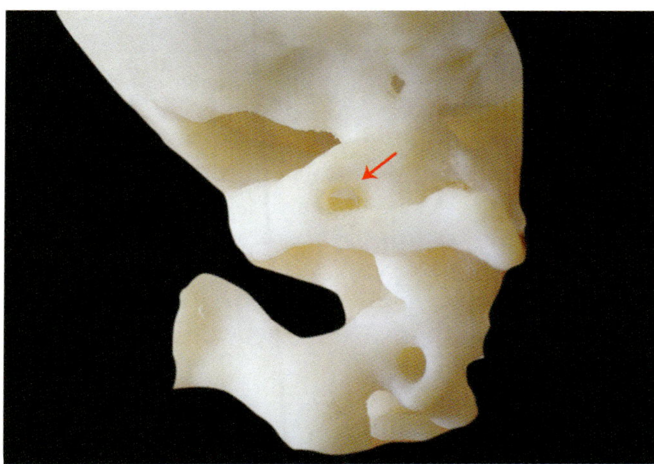

**Fig. 1.21:** Lateral image of model of C1. There is complete ossification of the oblique atlanto-occipital ligament surrounding the vertebral artery creating an arcuate foramen (red arrow).

artery (PICA). Although rare, occurring in 5% of cases, inadvertent injury can result in significant neurologic deficit.[30,31] If surgical access to or around the V3 segment is necessary, a CT angiogram or conventional angiogram should be performed to identify the possible presence of an extradural PICA origin.

## REFERENCES


1. Pang D, Thompson DN. Embryology and bony malformations of the craniovertebral junction. Childs Nerv Syst. 2011;27(4):523-64.
2. Christ B, Wilting J. From somites to vertebral column. Ann Anat. 1992;174(1):23-32.
3. Gruber DP, Brockmeyer D. Pediatric skull base surgery. 1. Embryology and developmental anatomy. Pediatr Neurosurg. 2003;38(1):2-8.
4. Hita-Contreras F, Roda O, Martinez-Amat A, et al. Embryonic and early fetal period development and morphogenesis of human craniovertebral junction. Clin Anat. 2014;27(3): 337-45.
5. Kim HJ. Cervical spine anomalies in children and adolescents. Curr Opin Pediatr. 2013;25(1):72-7.
6. Menezes AH. Craniocervical developmental anatomy and its implications. Childs Nerv Syst. 2008;24(10):1109-22.
7. Skorzewska A, Grzymislawska M, Bruska M, et al. Ossification of the vertebral column in human foetuses: histological and computed tomography studies. Folia Morphol (Warsz). 2013;72(3):230-8.
8. Steinmetz MP, Mroz TE, Benzel EC. Craniovertebral junction: biomechanical considerations. Neurosurgery. 2010; 66(3 Suppl):7-12.
9. Martin MD, Bruner HJ, Maiman DJ. Anatomic and biomechanical considerations of the craniovertebral junction. Neurosurgery. 2010;66(3 Suppl):2-6.
10. Prescher A. The craniocervical junction in man, the osseous variations, their significance and differential diagnosis. Ann Anat. 1997;179(1):1-19.
11. Pang D, Thompson DN. Embryology, classification, and surgical management of bony malformations of the craniovertebral junction. Adv Tech Stand Neurosurg. 2014;40: 19-109.
12. Rhoton AL Jr. The foramen magnum. Neurosurgery. 2000; 47(3 Suppl):S155-93.
13. Rhoton AL Jr. The far-lateral approach and its transcondylar, supracondylar, and paracondylar extensions. Neurosurgery. 2000;47(3 Suppl):S195-209.
14. Naderi S, Korman E, Citak G, et al. Morphometric analysis of human occipital condyle. Clin Neurol Neurosurg. 2005;107(3):191-9.
15. Le TV, Dakwar E, Hann S, et al. Computed tomography-based morphometric analysis of the human occipital condyle for occipital condyle-cervical fusion. J Neurosurg Spine. 2011;15(3):328-31.
16. Dowd GC, Zeiller S, Awasthi D. Far lateral transcondylar approach: dimensional anatomy. Neurosurgery. 1999;45(1):95-9; discussion 99-100.
17. de Oliveira E, Rhoton AL Jr, Peace D. Microsurgical anatomy of the region of the foramen magnum. Surg Neurol. 1985; 24(3):293-352.
18. Sen CN, Sekhar LN. An extreme lateral approach to intradural lesions of the cervical spine and foramen magnum. Neurosurgery. 1990;27(2):197-204.
19. Smoker WR. Craniovertebral junction: normal anatomy, craniometry, and congenital anomalies. Radiographics. 1994;14(2):255-77.
20. Debernardi A, D'Aliberti G, Talamonti G, et al. The craniovertebral junction area and the role of the ligaments and membranes. Neurosurgery. 2011;68(2):291-301.
21. Barrey C, Mertens P, Jund J, et al. Quantitative anatomic evaluation of cervical lateral mass fixation with a comparison of the Roy-Camille and the Magerl screw techniques. Spine. 2005;30(6):E140-7.
22. Cho W, Maeda T, Park Y, et al. The incidence of bifid C7 spinous processes. Global spine J. 2012;2(2):99-104.
23. Jeng JS, Yip PK. Evaluation of vertebral artery hypoplasia and asymmetry by color-coded duplex ultrasonography. Ultrasound Med Biol. 2004;30(5):605-9.
24. Kazui S, Kuriyama Y, Naritomi H, et al. Estimation of vertebral arterial asymmetry by computed tomography. Neuroradiology. 1989;31(3):237-9.

25. Krayenbuhl H, Yasargil MG. [The vascular diseases in the region of the basilar & vertebral arteries; an anatomopathological, clinical & neuroradiological study]. Fortschr Geb Rontgenstr Nuklearmed. 1957;87(Ergbd. 80):1-170.
26. Kotil K, Kilincer C. Sizes of the transverse foramina correlate with blood flow and dominance of vertebral arteries. Spine J. 2014;14(6):933-7.
27. Russo VM, Graziano F, Peris-Celda M, et al. The V(2) segment of the vertebral artery: anatomical considerations and surgical implications. J Neurosurg Spine. 2011; 15(6):610-9.
28. Elgafy H, Pompo F, Vela R, et al. Ipsilateral arcuate foramen and high-riding vertebral artery: implication on C1-C2 instrumentation. Spine J. 2014;14(7):1351-5.
29. Wanibuchi M, Fukushima T, Zenga F, et al. Simple identification of the third segment of the extracranial vertebral artery by extreme lateral inferior transcondylar-transtubercular exposure (ELITE). Acta Neurochir (Wien). 2009;151(11): 1499-503.
30. Salas E, Ziyal IM, Bank WO, et al. Extradural origin of the posteroinferior cerebellar artery: an anatomic study with histological and radiographic correlation. Neurosurgery. 1998;42(6):1326-31.
31. Lang J. [Extradural origins of the posterior inferior cerebellar artery and their clinical significance]. Neurochirurgia (Stuttg). 1985;28(5):183-7.

# Chapter 2

# Cervical Biomechanics and Clinical Instability

*Shaobai Wang*

## CERVICAL BIOMECHANICS

Biomechanics is a broad topic that focuses on the mechanical laws in living structures. This chapter will focus on cervical biomechanics, specifically the complex three-dimensional (3D) movement of the cervical spine and the clinical definition and diagnosis of motion instability. Cervical biomechanics has important implications for understanding normal and pathological conditions, such as instability and degenerative changes. However, the complicated translation and orientation in 3D space has always represented a challenging topic in research. Researchers started with the understanding of the special cervical morphological structure, proceeded with cadaveric biomechanical testing, and finally obtained in vivo segmental movement data with advanced medical imaging and analysis techniques. The use of biomechanical data to define and diagnose clinical cervical instability is also discussed.

### Basic Definition for Motion in 3D

The definitions of three anatomical planes are fundamental to understanding motion in 3D (Fig. 2.1).

- Sagittal plane (or frontal plane): divides the spine into left and right parts
- Coronal plane (or median plane): divides the spine into front and back parts
- Axial plane (or transverse plane): divides the spine into upper and lower parts.

There are also six degrees of freedom (6 DOF), three translational and three rotational, to fully describe the location and/or motion of the cervical spine in 3D. Each can be positive or negative with respect to a reference, with different terminologies (Fig. 2.2).

Translational DOF:

- Anterior: toward the front or in the front
- Posterior: toward the back or in the back

**Fig. 2.1:** The definition of three anatomical planes in the cervical spine.

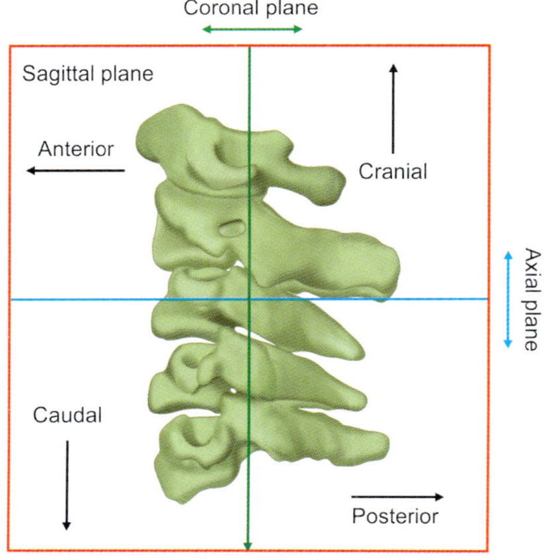


**Fig. 2.2:** The definition of terminologies in the sagittal view.

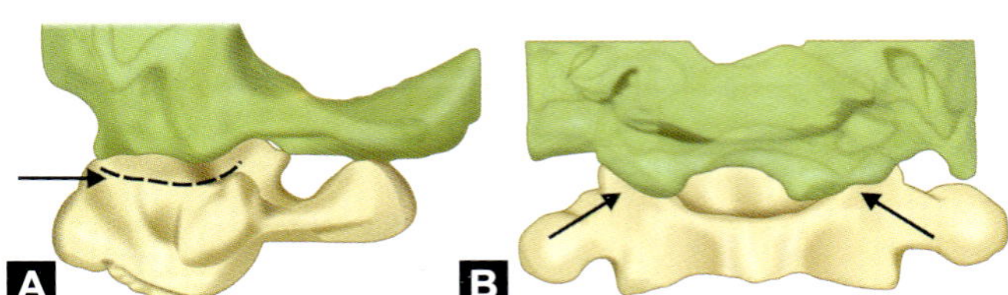


**Figs. 2.3A and B:** (A) Lateral view and (B) Frontal view showing the atlantial socket for nodding movement and limited rotation and translation in other directions.

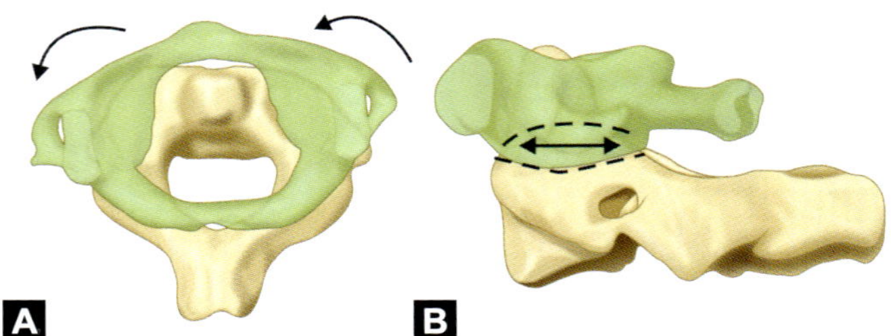


**Figs. 2.4A and B:** (A) Top view showing the rotation of the atlas around the odontoid process. (B) Lateral view showing the biconcave structure of the atlanto-axial joint to facilitate translation.

- Medial: closer to or toward the midline
- Lateral: away from the midline
- Cranial (or cephalad, proximal): close to or toward head, means "up"
- Caudal (or caudad, distal): close to or toward foot, means "down"
- Superior: the upper part of a structure or above a specific location
- Inferior: the lower part of a structure or below a specific location.

Rotational DOF:

- Flexion: forward bending
- Extension: backward bending
- Left/Right lateral bending: left/right side bending
- Left/Right torsion: left/right twisting (or rotation).

Body motion and spinal motion are usually different and should not be confused. When the neck rotates in a primary direction, there are corresponding primary rotation and complex combined motion in the cervical segments. The corresponding rotational DOF is defined as the primary (or principal) DOF and the other five DOFs are defined as coupled motion. For example, during flexion/extension of the neck, flexion/extension of the cervical segments is the primary motion and the rest translations; bending and twisting of the cervical spine are the coupled motion.

## Morphological Consideration and Normal Kinematics

The cervical spine can be divided into four units with unique anatomy and thus unique contribution to the functions of the complete cervical spine. The units are the atlas, the axis, the C2-3 junction and the remaining subaxial cervical vertebrae. These are also called the cradle, the axis, the root, and the column.

### *The Atlas*

The atlanto-occipital joints, which unite between the head and atlas, allow flexion-extension motion (e.g. nodding) while limiting the translational and rotational motion in all other DOFs. The atlanto-occipital joint consists of the occiput situated in the deep atlantial socket (Fig. 2.3A). The flexion-extension movement is achieved by the condyles rolling and sliding in a socket in the sagittal plane. The side walls of the sockets prevent the occiput from translations sideways in the medial-lateral direction (Fig. 2.3B). Separation, i.e. cranial-caudal motion, is resisted by tension in the joint capsules. For the joint to rotate in the axial rotation and lateral bending, the condyles must rise up their respective walls, which are resisted by the tension in the joint capsule. In addition, the axial and lateral rotations are also limited by impaction of the condyles against the socket walls.

### *The Axis*

The atlanto sits on the atlas to form the atlanto-axial joint to carry the weight of the head and perform primary axial rotation (Fig. 2.4A). The anterior arch of the atlas can pivot on the odontoid process and the lateral mass (transverse) slides back and forth to allow significant range of axial rotation. The cartilages of both the atlantial and the axial facets are convex, resulting in a biconvex contact[1] that facilitates the sliding motion of the bilateral facets and causes drop of the atlas during rotation (Fig. 2.4B). No ligaments have been explicitly pointed to restrict flexion-extension of the joint and there are no restrictions from the biconvex joint surface. The atlanto-atlas joint is free to flex or extend until the posterior arch hits the occiput or the arch of C2, respectively. The other motion patterns of the atlanto-axial joints, such as axial rotation, lateral bending, anterior-posterial translation, and lateral

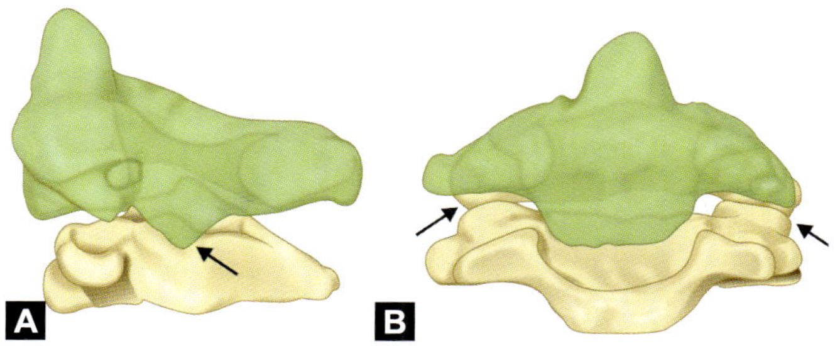


**Figs. 2.5A and B:** (A) Lateral view and (B) Frontal view showing the medial orientation of the zygapophysial joint and the low superior articular process that cause different motion of C2-3 than the subaxial segments.

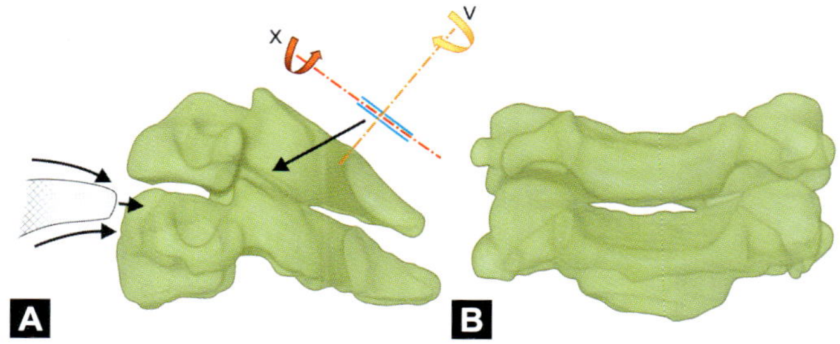


**Figs. 2.6A and B:** (A) Lateral view showing the orientation of the zygapophysial joint that allows coupled axial and bending rotation. A taper-shaped disk allows gliding in all directions. (B) Frontal view showing the ellipsoid joint formed by the convex superior and concaved inferior disk endplate.

translation are mainly limited by multiple ligaments, and ultimately limited by bony obstruction in the corresponding directions.

### *C2-3*

From the C2-3 joint, the remaining joints share similar morphological features. However, the kinematics and thus clinical relevance of the C2-3 joint is unique as transitional vertebrae. This is partly caused by the unique orientation of the more medially oriented zygapophysial joint[2] and lower superior articular processes of C3 than the cranial segments (Figs. 2.5A and B).[3] Together, various different motion patterns are expected but they are yet to be explored. For example, during lateral bending the coupled axial rotations are reported to the opposite direction of the primary bending, which is different from the lower cranial levels.[4]

### *Subaxial*

From C3 to C7, the vertebral bodies sit on one another and are separated by the intervertebral disks to form the subaxial cervical spine. In the sagittal plane, the corresponding superior and inferior endplates of a cervical joint are curved, which facilitates flexion-extension. The inferior surface of the vertebral body is convex and the superior surface of the opposing vertebral body is concave, forming an ellipsoid joint for rotation (Fig. 2.6B). Therefore, the motion of the cervical motion is essentially affected by the structure of the zygapophysial joint. Along the direction perpendicular to the zygapophysial joint surface, rotational motion is limited by the impact of the facets (Fig. 2.6A). Along the direction parallel to the zygapophysial joint surface, rotational motion is free. In other words, rotations are not limited in the principal body axis (i.e. coronal and transverse planes) but in the plane perpendicular to the zygapophysial joint surface. Therefore, coupled twisting and bending are always observed and studied. The zygapophysial joint surface orients approximately 45° to the transvers plane and at various angles at different levels,[3] which may explain the different ranges of motion of different levels detailed below.

Rather than flat in the lumbar spine, the cervical intervertebral disks taper laterally and posteriorly (*see* Fig. 2.6A). The posterior part of the disks is thin and lacking annulus fibers. Therefore, the posterior part of the vertebral body is free to move laterally. As it moves, the cervical disk also translates up and down when gliding in the concaved uncinated processes. In an intact cervical spine, the ligaments, the disks, and the zygapophysial joints maintain the stability and allow a few millimeters of translations in all directions.

## Quantitative Measurements

### *Atlanto-Occipital Joint*

Cadaveric studies reported about 15° flexion-extension of the atlanto-occipital joint (Table 2.1).[5,6] A couple also reported mean side-to-side axial rotations (SD) to be 9.9° (3.0°) and mean lateral bending to be 9.1° (1.5°) (Tables 2.2 and 2.3).[7] It should be noted that the results depend largely where force and torque were applied to the cadavers. No muscular activity and control existed in cadaveric testing. In vivo radiographic studies have reported an average of about 15° flexion-extension. However, the standard deviations were relatively large, indicating a large variation between normal individuals. Lind et al.[8] reported >100% coefficient of variation between normal individuals.

**Table 2.1:** Results of studies of normal range of cervical flexion-extension.

| Author | Approach | Number of subjects | *Range of motion mean (SD) (in degree)* | | | | | | |
|---|---|---|---|---|---|---|---|---|---|
| | | | Occ-C1 | C1-C2 | C2-C3 | C3-C4 | C4-C5 | C5-C6 | C6-C7 |
| Panjabi et al.[7*] | In vitro flexion | 16 | 7.2 (2.5) | 12.3 (2.0) | 3.5 (1.3) | 4.3 (2.9) | 5.3 (3.0) | 5.5 (2.6) | 3.7 (2.1) |
| Panjabi et al.[7†] | In vitro extension | 16 | 20.2 (4.6) | 12.1 (6.5) | 2.1 (1.0) | 3.4 (2.1) | 4.8 (1.9) | 4.4 (2.8) | 3.4 (1.9) |
| Lind et al.[8] | Functional radiograph | 70 | | | 10 (4) | 14 (6) | 16 (6) | 15 (8) | 11 (7) |
| Dvorak et al.[12] | Functional radiograph | 28 | | | 10 (3) | 15 (3) | 19 (4) | 20 (4) | 19 (4) |
| Anderst et al.[22] | Biplanar X-ray | 20 | | | 10.2 (2.4) | 14.2 (2.6) | 15.9 (2.1) | 14.6 (4.7) | 12.5 (4.6) |

*Reported range of flexion.
†Reported range of extension.

**Table 2.2:** Results of studies of normal range of cervical axial rotation.

| Author | Approach | Number of subjects | Side* | *Range of motion mean (SD) (in degree)* | | | | | | | |
|---|---|---|---|---|---|---|---|---|---|---|---|
| | | | | Occ-C1 | C1-C2 | C2-C3 | C3-C4 | C4-C5 | C5-C6 | C6-C7 | C7-T1 |
| Panjabi et al.[7] | In vitro | 16 | 2 | 9.9 (3.0) | 56.7 (4.8) | 3.3 (0.8) | 5.1 (1.2) | 6.8 (1.3) | 5.0 (1.0) | 2.9 (0.8) | |
| Penning and Wilmink[18] range† | Functional computed tomography (CT) | 26 | 1 | 1 | 40.5 | 3 | 6.5 | 6.8 | 6.9 | 2.1 | 2.1 |
| | | | | – 2–5 | 29–46 | 0–10 | 3–10 | 1–12 | 2–12 | 2–10 | – 2–7 |
| Mimura et al.[10] | Biplanar X-ray | | 1 | 75 (12)‡ | | 7 (6) | 6 (5) | 4 (6) | 5 (4) | 6 (3) | |
| Lin CC et al.[17] | Biplanar fluoroscopy | 10 | 1 | | | | 4.2 (1.3) | 4.6 (1.3) | 3.0 (1.0) | 1.3 (0.8) | |
| Salem et al.[21] | Functional CT | 20 | 1 | 2.5 (1.0) | 37.5 (6.0) | 1.5 (2.0) | 5.0 (2.0) | 5.5 (1.0) | 5.0 (2.0) | 4.0 (2.0) | |
| Ishii et al.[20] | Functional magnetic resonance imaging | 10 | 1 | | | 3.6 (1.5) | 5.4 (1.3) | 5.0 (1.3) | 5.3 (1.3) | 4.9 (2.1) | 1.2 (1.2) |

*Side: 1, rotation range from neutral to one side, 2, rotation range from one side to the other side.
†Penning and Wilmink reported mean and range of subjects' range of rotation.
‡Combined Occ-C1 and C1-C2 rotation range.

### *Atlanto-Axial Joint*

Cadaveric studies reported about 50° of axial rotation,[9] 10° of flexion-extension[5] and 5° of lateral bending.[6] From plain radiographs, most investigators reported only flexion-extension of the joint of about 10°–20°, mainly due to obscuring of the bone structure and limitation in imaging directions (Table 2.1). Alternative technologies such as biplanar X-ray imaging and positional computed tomography (CT) scans were used to study atlanto-axial joint rotation. In the biplanar radiography measurement,[10] the total range of rotation was reported to be 75.2° (SD 11.8°). However, the accuracy of this technique largely depends on accurately allocating the corresponding vertebrae corner points. Coupled extension of 14° (SD 6°) and contralateral lateral bending of 24° (SD 6°) were also reported.

**Table 2.3:** Results of studies of normal range of cervical lateral bending.

| Author | Approach | Number of subjects | Side* | Range of motion mean (SD) (in degree) | | | | | | | |
|---|---|---|---|---|---|---|---|---|---|---|---|
| | | | | Occ-C1 | C1-C2 | C2-C3 | C3-C4 | C4-C5 | C5-C6 | C6-C7 | C7-T1 |
| Panjabi et al.[7] | In vitro | 16 | 2 | 9.1 (1.5) | 6.5 (2.3) | 9.6 (1.8) | 9.0 (1.9) | 9.3 (1.7) | 6.5 (1.5) | 5.4 (1.5) | |
| Lin CC et al.[17] | Biplanar fluoroscopy | 10 | 1 | | | | 6.4 (2.3) | 5.2 (1.4) | 6.1 (1.8) | 6.1 (1.8) | |
| Ishii et al.[19] | Functional magnetic resonance imaging | 12 | 1 | 1.9 (0.9) | 1.6 (1.3) | 3.7 (2.0) | 3.5 (1.4) | 3.3 (1.0) | 4.3 (1.4) | 5.7 (1.9) | 4.1 (2.7) |

*Side: 1, rotation range from neutral to one side, 2, rotation range from one side to the other side.

Functional CT utilizes multiple CT scans at the end range of motion. Dvorak found 43° (SD 5.5°) of axial rotation to each side, within minimal 3° of asymmetry (Table 2.2).[11]

### *Subaxial Cervical Spine*

Early studies of the lower cervical spine reported range of flexion-extension using functional plain radiographs (Table 2.1).[8,12-16] Radiographs were taken in the lateral projection at maximal flexion and extension and analyzed to obtain segmental vertebral range of flexion-extension. Similarly, radiographs were taken in the frontal projection at maximal bending to the left and right to quantify range of lateral bending (Table 2.3). This technique was not suitable for quantifying range of axial rotation due to the difficulty of projection in the transverse plane and substantial bone overlapping in this direction. However, functional radiographs only provide perspective in the two-dimensional (2D) projection plane. More recently, with the assistance of modern imaging technique such as functional magnetic resonance imaging (MRI)/CT and biplanar radiography, in vivo segmental ranges of lateral and axial rotations have been reported by several studies (Tables 2.1 to 2.3).[10,17-22] A typical biplanar system consists of two X-rays or fluoroscopes positioned with their image intensifiers perpendicular to each other.[23] Orthogonal images of the spine segments along the motion path are captured from two perpendicular views (Fig. 2.7A). The geometry of the biplanar system is reproduced in the computer environment. Three-dimensional vertebral models, from CT or MRI scans, were introduced into the virtual environment. The 3D models of the vertebrae were independently translated and rotated in until their outlines matched the osseous outlines of the corresponding vertebrae captured on the biplanar images (Fig. 2.7B). Such a procedure can usually reach sub-degree and sub-millimeter accuracy in rotation and translation, respectively.[23] Functional MRI/CT takes scans from several end-range positions of rotation. Three-dimensional volumetric information of the vertebral segments was obtained from the scans and registered between different positions to calculate relative segmental motion. As explained in the previous section, the structure of the subaxial cervical spine allows motion in all directions, and substantial motions were found in all directions. On average, flexion-extension ranged from 10° to 20° (*see* Table 2.1). Segmental ranges of lateral bending and axial rotation were about 5° to one side (Tables 2.2 and 2.3). Most studies reported non-significant difference at different vertebral levels. Only Lin[17] reported a decrease in axial rotation from 4.2° degree at C3-4 to 1.3° degree at C6-7.

### *Coupled Motions*

In addition to quantifying range of primary rotations, the 3D techniques allow exploration of coupled rotations and translations. Coupled motion is the rotation or translation about or along axes that are different than the primary rotation axis. Reported by several studies,[17,19,21,22] the normal segmental translations were usually < 1 mm in all anterior-posterior, medial-lateral, and superior-inferior directions. However, the accuracy in determination of translations of these techniques was also about 1 mm, which might eliminate further meaningful discussion of coupled translations. As noted in the previous anatomic considerations, coupled twisting and bending were common due to the oblique orientation of the zygapophysial

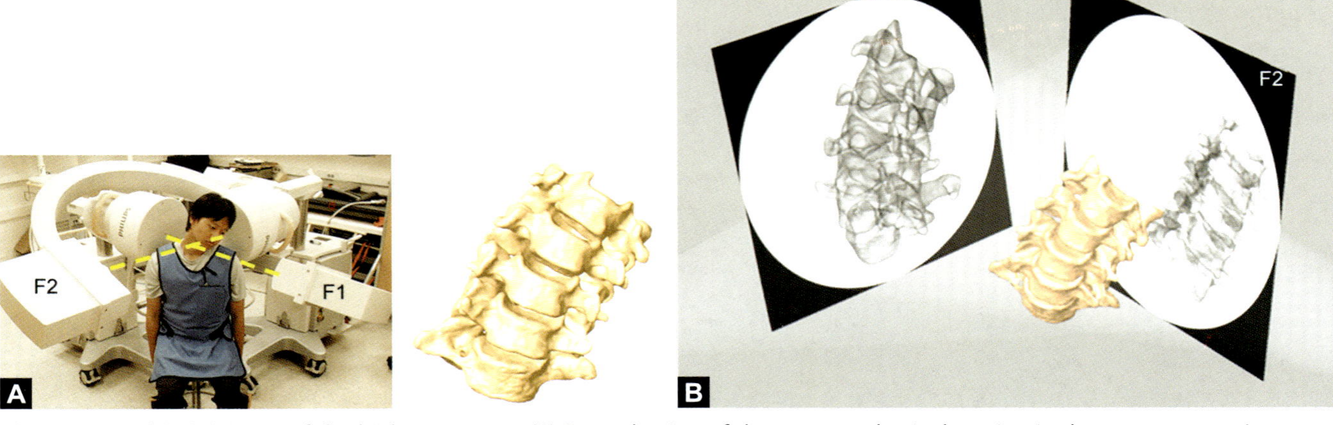


**Figs. 2.7A and B:** (A) Setup of the biplanar system. (B) Reproduction of the segmental spinal motion in the computer environment.

**Table 2.4:** Direction of coupled lateral bending with primary axial rotation.

| *Author* | *Approach* | *Occ-C1* | *C1-C2* | *C2-C3* | *C3-C4* | *C4-C5* | *C5-C6* | *C6-C7* | *C7-T1* |
|---|---|---|---|---|---|---|---|---|---|
| Panjabi et al.[4] | In vitro | O | O | | | | | | |
| Panjabi et al.[7] | In vitro | O | O | S | S | S | S | S | S |
| Penning et al.[24] | In vitro | O | O | S | S | S | S | S | S |
| Mimura et al.[10] | In vivo | | | | | S | S | S | S |
| Iai et al.[25] | In vivo | S | O | S | S | S | S | S | S |
| Ishii et al.[19] | In vivo | O | O | | | | | | |
| Ishii et al.[20] | In vivo | | | S | S | S | S | S | S |
| Lin CC et al.[17] | In vivo | | | | S | S | S | S | |

(S: Bending and rotation to the same side, ipsilateral; O: Bending and rotation to the opposite side, contralateral).

**Table 2.5:** Direction of coupled axial rotation with primary lateral bending.

| *Author* | *Approach* | *Occ-C1* | *C1-C2* | *C2-C3* | *C3-C4* | *C4-C5* | *C5-C6* | *C6-C7* | *C7-T1* |
|---|---|---|---|---|---|---|---|---|---|
| Panjabi et al.[4] | In vitro | S | O | | | | | | |
| Panjabi et al.[7] | In vitro | S | S | S | S | S | S | S | S |
| Penning et al.[24] | In vitro | S | S | S | S | S | S | S | S |
| Ishii et al.[19] | In vivo | O | O | S | S | S | S | S | O |
| Lin et al.[17] | In vivo | | | | S | S | S | S | |

(S: Bending and rotation to the same side, ipsilateral; O: Bending and rotation to the opposite side, contralateral).

joint surface. High agreement in the coupling directions was reported by most in vitro and in vivo studies.[4,7,10,17,19,20,24,25] When axial rotation is the primary motion, studies reported contralateral (lateral bending and axial rotation to the opposite side) in upper cervical segments occiput-C1 and C1-2, and ipsilateral (lateral bending and axial rotation to the same side) in subaxial cervical spines C3-T1 (Table 2.4). When lateral bending is the primary motion, studies reported ipsilateral in subaxial cervical spine C3-T1 as well, but no consensus in the upper cervical spine (Table 2.5). In addition, the coupled lateral bending and axial rotation were usually similar in magnitude, which agreed with the approximately 45° oblique orientation of the zygapophysial joint surface.

### *Center of Rotation*

In addition to range-of-motion studies, centers of rotation, sometimes called instantaneous centers of rotation (ICR), have also been explored by some investigators to describe cervical biomechanics. The ICRs were usually obtained between full extension and full flexion planar X-ray images and represent a 2D sagittal measurement of the motion pattern of the superior vertebra with respect to the immediate adjacent inferior one. The location of the ICR is the point where the superior vertebra rotates around between the two X-ray positions with fixed inferior vertebra (Fig. 2.8). The location can be determined by the intersection of perpendicular bisection lines of the corresponding points in the two X-ray images. Several studies have shown that in normal subjects, ICRs distribute consistently and concordantly in the inferior segments.[16,26-28] Van Mameren et al.[29] have rigorously showed that a given ICR can be reliably and consistently calculated within a small margin of technical error. Moreover, in contrast to range of motion, the location of the ICR is independent of the motion path, whether it is calculated on the basis of anteflexion or retroflexion films. Also, the ICR is stable over time, with no significant differences in location occurring after recalculation in 2 weeks or 10 weeks after the initial observation. In addition, abnormal ICRs were shown to be statistically significantly related with cervical pathology.[30,31] Amevo et al.[31] studied 109 patients with post-traumatic neck pain and reported that 77% exhibited an abnormally located ICR at least at one level. Modern digital images and computer-assisted software (ICR Tracer, Innomotion Inc.) (Figs. 2.9A to D) have further improved the accuracy, reliability, and convenience of ICR measurements while normalizing for vertebral size. The computer-assisted environment may utilize machine learning to accumulate a large database for normative and abnormal data to improve statistical power and serve as a promising clinical tool.

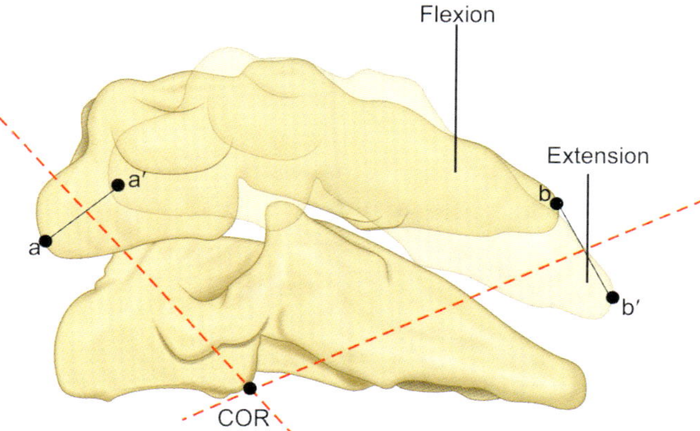


**Fig. 2.8:** Calculation of center of rotation (COR) from the intersection of perpendicular bisection lines of the corresponding points.

## CLINICAL INSTABILITY

### Definition

As described above, the cervical spine is designed for a great deal of mobility in all directions; thus stability is necessary for proper function of the cervical spine. Spine instability is a major cause of neck pain.[32] Panjabi[33] conceptualized the common components of spinal stability into passive, active, and neural control functional subsystems. The passive subsystem consists of the vertebral bodies, facet joints, and capsules, spinal ligaments, and passive tension from spinal muscles and tendons to provide

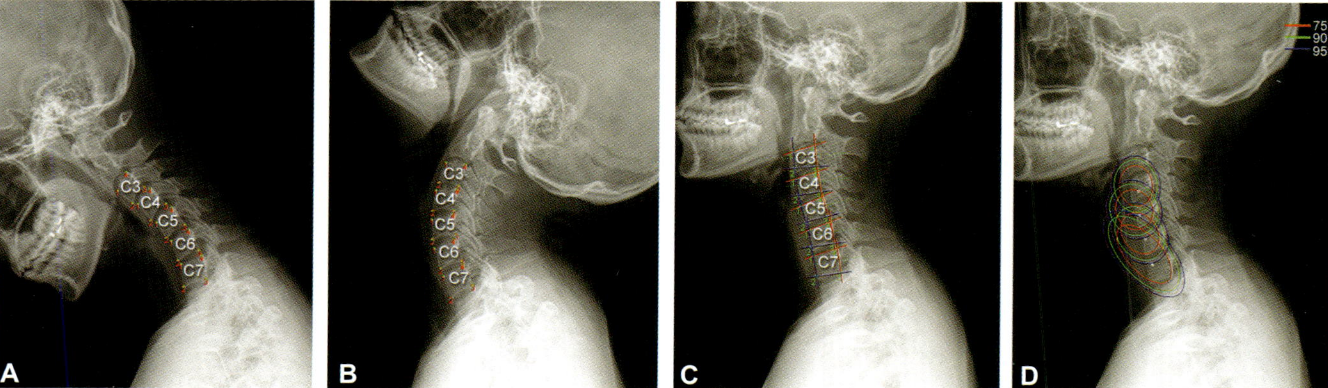


**Figs. 2.9A to D:** Digitization of the corresponding vertebral points in (A) Flexion and (B) Extension functional radiographs. (C) Local coordinate systems for normalization. (D) Accumulation and statistical analysis of the cervical center of rotation.

basic stiffness and resistance of the motion segment unit. The active subsystem consists of the spinal muscles and tendons to actively generate the forces required to stabilize the spine in response to changing loads. Through peripheral nerves and the central nervous system, the neural control subsystem receives information from the passive and active subsystems about vertebral position, vertebral motion, and forces generated by spinal muscles. The neural control subsystem then determines the requirements for spinal stability and acts on the spinal muscles to produce the required forces.

An accurate diagnosis of the spinal "instability" is important for the surgical management of this condition.[34] A clear definition would help to measure "instability" of the spine objectively. Despite variations in definition, the general agreement on instability follows the keywords of "altered motion pattern" and "increased range of motion." Panjabi[35] proposed that clinical instability of the spine is "the loss of the ability of the spine under physiological loads to maintain its patterns of displacement so that there is no initial or additional neurological deficit, no major deformity, and no incapacitating pain." Dupuis et al.[36] described instability in anatomic terms and used kinematic verification. They proposed a progressive degenerative process of dysfunction, instability, and restabilization. The unstable phase results in a reduction in disk height, laxity of the ligaments and facet capsules, and degeneration of the facet joints. This results in an increased and abnormal range of movement. A workable definition[37] is that instability is synonymous with a loss of motion segment stiffness, such that force application to that motion segment produces greater displacement than would be seen in a normal structure. To that definition, Pope[38] also added the following clinical qualifying criteria: the condition will cause pain, has the potential to result in progressive deformity, and will place neurologic structures at risk. Alternatively, researchers have also divided the total range of motion of the segments into the neutral zone and elastic zone[33,35] and defined instability as the increase of neutral zone relative to the total range of motion.

## Clinical Assessment

Cadaveric studies have confirmed altered motion pattern and increased translations and rotations in 6 DOF by sequentially sectioned structures of the functional spinal unit.[39,40] In vivo studies also found flexion and extension of the cervical spine in patients with "instability" to be significantly different from those of normal subjects.[41] It is hypothesized that this might be caused by a combination of an "unstable" segment and its adjacent motion segments, which form a "hypermobile and hypomobile segments complex." During flexion and extension, the unstable segments might compensate for the hypomobile segments and provide abnormal intervertebral motion. Consequently, it might cause a change in the flexion and extension of the cervical spine.

**Table 2.6:** Checklist for the diagnosis of clinical instability in the lower cervical spine.

| *Element* | *Point value* |
|---|---|
| Anterior elements destroyed or unable to function | 2 |
| Posterior elements destroyed or unable to function | 2 |
| Relative sagittal plane translation > 3.5 mm | 2 |
| Relative sagittal plane rotation > 11° | 2 |
| Positive stretch test | 2 |
| Spinal cord damage | 2 |
| Nerve root damage | 1 |
| Abnormal disk narrowing | 1 |
| Dangerous loading anticipated | 1 |
| Total of 5 or more = unstable | |

*Source*: Adapted from White AA 3rd, Panjabi MM.[34]

White and Panjabi[34] have proposed a scoring method for what they describe as "clinical instability" (Table 2.6). Specifically, the spine can be considered unstable if a vertebral body has translation >3.5 mm and rotation >11° between flexion and extension, in relation to the adjacent vertebrae. This can be measured from flexion and extension (or so-called functional) radiographs of the cervical spine in the lateral view, and this method was followed by many investigators.[8,12-16]

Passive intervertebral motion manual examination may reveal hypermobility and decreased passive restraints to motion at end-range of passive spinal segmental motion (i.e. a loose end feel). Through such a testing procedure, an increase of the "neutral zone" with compromise of the passive component of the spinal stabilizing system may be felt by an experienced operator. Manual examination and sequential physical therapy intervention require high skill and may be affected by inter-observer reliability. The purpose of the manual therapy followed Panjabi's model[35] by using exercises that enhance the active and neurological subsystems' abilities to effectively compensate for the

**Table 2.7:** Rating system for evaluating passive intervertebral motion of the spine and passive accessory motion of the temporomandibular and extremity joints.

| *Grade* | *Description* | *Criteria* |
|---|---|---|
| 0 | Ankylosed | No detectable movement. Requires stress film radiology for confirmation. |
| 1 | Considerable restriction (hypomobility) | Significant decrease in expected range. Significant resistance to movement. |
| 2 | Slight restriction (hypomobility) | Limitation expected in range. Some resistance to movement. |
| 3 | Normal | Expected range for body type. Uniform movement throughout range. |
| 4 | Slight increase (hypermobility) | Some increase expected in range. Less than normal resistance to movement. |
| 5 | Considerable increase (hypermobility) | Excessive range but eventually restricted by capsular and ligament structures. |
| 6 | Unstable | Excessive range (as in Grade 5) but without the restraint of capsular and ligament structures. |

*Source*: Adapted from Gonnella C, Paris SV, Kutner M.[42]

impaired passive component of the stabilizing system in an attempt to restore function and reduce pain. A rating system for the evaluation of cervical passive motion for manual examination and physical therapy has been proposed (Table 2.7).[42]

## Concerns and Future Perspectives

Many investigators have used lateral functional radiographs to determine whether there is instability. However, most functional radiographs are not interpreted so easily, especially with patients who do not have a history of injury. The alignment of the cervical spine in the two plain X-rays can be difficult and subjective. The distortion and bony overlap can introduce error in measurements. Therefore, the reliability of this method is questionable, and comparison of the results between patients is difficult. Reports of failure to diagnose "instability" of the cervical spine are common.[43-46]

Currently, investigations of cervical spine biomechanics attempt analysis of end-range flexion and extension to diagnose cervical spine instability through functional 3D CT or MRI scans and biplanar radiographs.[17-22] These novel means have the potential for yielding highly accurate data with little disruption of normal motion patterns. Such data, it is hoped, will enable the establishment of new, objective, kinematic-based criteria to define instability. Usually, advanced image processing skills and a long processing time are required with these novel methods. Only a few commercial software programs are available to perform 3D kinematic analysis tasks (Fluo-Motion, Innomotion, Inc.) (*see* Figs. 2.7A and B), and they have yet to be integrated into routine clinical practice.

## REFERENCES


1. Koebke J, Brade H. Morphological and functional studies on the lateral joints of the first and second cervical vertebrae in man. Anat Embryol (Berl). 1982;164 (2):265-75.
2. Mestdagh H. Morphological aspects and biomechanical properties of the vertebroaxial joint (C2-C3). Acta Morphol Neerl Scand. 1976;14(1):19-30.
3. Nowitzke A, Westaway M, Bogduk N. Cervical zygapophyseal joints: geometrical parameters and relationship to cervical kinematics. Clin Biomech (Bristol, Avon). 1994;9(6):342-8.
4. Panjabi MM, Oda T, Crisco JJ, et al. Posture affects motion coupling patterns of the upper cervical spine. J Orthop Res. 1993;11(4):525-36.
5. Werne S. The possibilities of movement in the craniovertebral joints. Acta Orthop Scand. 1959;28(3):165-73.
6. Worth DR. Movements of the craniovertebral joints. Modern manual therapy of the vertebral column. Vol. 53. Edinburgh: Churchill Livingstone; 1986.
7. Panjabi MM, Crisco JJ, Vasavada A, et al. Mechanical properties of the human cervical spine as shown by three-dimensional load-displacement curves. Spine (Phila Pa 1976). 2001;26 (24):2692-700.
8. Lind B, Sihlbom H, Nordwall A, et al. Normal range of motion of the cervical spine. Arch Phys Med Rehabil. 1989;70(9):692-5.
9. Dvorak J, Panjabi M, Gerber M, et al. CT-functional diagnostics of the rotatory instability of upper cervical spine. 1. An experimental study on cadavers. Spine (Phila Pa 1976). 1987;12 (3):197-205.
10. Mimura M, Moriya H, Watanabe T, et al. Three-dimensional motion analysis of the cervical spine with special reference to the axial rotation. Spine (Phila Pa 1976). 1989;14(11):1135-9.
11. Dvorak J, Hayek J, Zehnder R. CT-functional diagnostics of the rotatory instability of the upper cervical spine. Part 2. An evaluation on healthy adults and patients with suspected instability. Spine (Phila Pa 1976). 1987;12(8):726-31.
12. Dvorak J, Froehlich D, Penning L, et al. Functional radiographic diagnosis of the cervical spine: flexion/extension. Spine (Phila Pa 1976). 1988;13(7):748-55.

13. Bhalla SK, Simmons EH. Normal ranges of intervertebral-joint motion of the cervical spine. Can J Surg. 1969;12(2):181-7.
14. Bohrer SP, Chen YM, Sayers DG. Cervical spine flexion patterns. Skeletal Radiol. 1990;19(7):521-5.
15. Good CJ, Mikkelsen GB. Intersegmental sagittal motion in the lower cervical spine and discogenic spondylosis: a preliminary study. J Manipulative Physiol Ther. 1992;15(9):556-64.
16. Pearcy MJ, Bogduk N. Instantaneous axes of rotation of the lumbar intervertebral joints. Spine (Phila Pa 1976). 1988;13(9):1033-41.
17. Lin CC, Lu TW, Wang TM, et al. In vivo three-dimensional intervertebral kinematics of the subaxial cervical spine during seated axial rotation and lateral bending via a fluoroscopy-to-CT registration approach. J Biomech. 2014;47(13): 3310-7.
18. Penning L, Wilmink JT. Rotation of the cervical spine. A CT study in normal subjects. Spine (Phila Pa 1976). 1987; 12(8):732-8.
19. Ishii T, Mukai Y, Hosono N, et al. Kinematics of the cervical spine in lateral bending: in vivo three-dimensional analysis. Spine (Phila Pa 1976). 2006;31(2):155-60.
20. Ishii T, Mukai Y, Hosono N, et al. Kinematics of the subaxial cervical spine in rotation in vivo three-dimensional analysis. Spine (Phila Pa 1976). 2004;29(24): 2826-31.
21. Salem W, Lenders C, Mathieu J, et al. In vivo three-dimensional kinematics of the cervical spine during maximal axial rotation. Man Ther. 2013;18(4):339-44.
22. Anderst WJ, Lee JY, Donaldson WF 3rd, et al. Six-degrees-of-freedom cervical spine range of motion during dynamic flexion-extension after single-level anterior arthrodesis: comparison with asymptomatic control subjects. J Bone Joint Surg Am. 2013;95(6):497-506.
23. Wang S, Passias P, Li G, et al. Measurement of vertebral kinematics using noninvasive image matching method-validation and application. Spine (Phila Pa 1976). 2008;33 (11):E355-61.
24. Penning L. Normal movements of the cervical spine. AJR Am J Roentgenol. 1978;130(2):317-26.
25. Iai H, Moriya H, Goto S, et al. Three-dimensional motion analysis of the upper cervical spine during axial rotation. Spine (Phila Pa 1976). 1993;18(16):2388-92.
26. Penning L. Differences in anatomy, motion, development and aging of the upper and lower cervical disk segments. Clin Biomech (Bristol, Avon). 1988;3(1):37-47.
27. Penning L. Nonpathologic and pathologic relationships between the lower cervical vertebrae. Am J Roentgenol Radium Ther Nucl Med. 1964;91:1036-50.
28. Amevo B, Worth D, Bogduk N. Instantaneous axes of rotation of the typical cervical motion segments: a study in normal volunteers. Clin Biomech (Bristol, Avon). 1991;6(2):111-7.
29. van Mameren H, Sanches H, Beursgens J, et al. Cervical spine motion in the sagittal plane. II. Position of segmental averaged instantaneous centers of rotation–a cineradiographic study. Spine (Phila Pa 1976). 1992;17(5):467-74.
30. Dimnet J, Pasquet A, Krag MH, et al. Cervical spine motion in the sagittal plane: kinematic and geometric parameters. J Biomech. 1982;15(12):959-69.
31. Amevo B, Aprill C, Bogduk N. Abnormal instantaneous axes of rotation in patients with neck pain. Spine (Phila Pa 1976). 1992;17(7):748-56.
32. Olson KA, Joder D. Diagnosis and treatment of cervical spine clinical instability. J Orthop Sports Phys Ther. 2001;31(4):194-206.
33. Panjabi MM. The stabilizing system of the spine. Part I. Function, dysfunction, adaptation, and enhancement. J Spinal Disord. 1992;5(4):383-9; discussion 397.
34. White AA 3rd, Panjabi MM. The role of stabilization in the treatment of cervical spine injuries. Spine (Phila Pa 1976). 1984;9(5):512-22.
35. Panjabi MM. The stabilizing system of the spine. Part II. Neutral zone and instability hypothesis. J Spinal Disord. 1992;5(4):390-6; discussion 397.
36. Dupuis PR, Yong-Hing K, Cassidy JD, et al. Radiologic diagnosis of degenerative lumbar spinal instability. Spine (Phila Pa 1976). 1985;10(3):262-76.
37. Pope MH, Panjabi M. Biomechanical definitions of spinal instability. Spine (Phila Pa 1976). 1985;10(3):255-6.
38. Pope MH, Frymoyer JW, Krag MH. Diagnosing instability. Clin Orthop Relat Res. 1992;(279):60-7.
39. Panjabi MM, Krag MH, White AA 3rd, et al. Effects of preload on load displacement curves of the lumbar spine. Orthop Clin North Am. 1977;8(1):181-92.
40. Tanz SS. Motion of the lumbar spine; a roentgenologic study. Am J Roentgenol Radium Ther Nucl Med. 1953;69(3):399-412.
41. Mofidi A, Tansey C, Mahapatra SR, et al. Cervical spondylolysis, radiologic pointers of stability and acute traumatic as opposed to chronic spondylolysis. J Spinal Disord Tech. 2007;20 (6): 473-9.
42. Gonnella C, Paris SV, Kutner M. Reliability in evaluating passive intervertebral motion. Phys Ther. 1982;62(4):436-44.
43. Evans DK. Anterior cervical subluxation. J Bone Joint Surg Br. 1976;58(3):318-21.
44. Nash CL Jr. Acute cervical soft-tissue injury and late deformity. A case report. J Bone Joint Surg Am. 1979;61(2):305-7.
45. Phillipson A, Cogley D, Lynch M. Hidden dangers in apparently stable neck injuries. Injury. 1993;24(5):353-5.
46. Webb JK, Broughton RB, McSweeney T, et al. Hidden flexion injury of the cervical spine. J Bone Joint Surg Br. 1976; 58(3):322-7.

Chapter 3

# Cervical Alignment

*Shaleen Vira, Matthew A Spiegel, Virginie Lafage, Frank Schwab*

## INTRODUCTION

The history of spinal deformity dates back to Hippocrates, the father of medicine, who described spinal curves in his book, "On Bones and Joints."[1] In the times of antiquity, understanding alignment of the spinal column was limited to gross qualitative descriptions based on cadavers and prone patient positioning. Since then, cervical alignment, as a discipline that informs the diagnosis and treatment of myelopathy, has grown to a robust subspecialty within cervical spine surgery.

More recently, a great revolution in spinal deformity examination occurred after Roentgen discovered radiographic imaging, X-rays.[2] Consequently, health care providers are now able to visualize spinal deformities first documented by Hippocrates in two dimensions, and without direct visualization through dissection. X-rays remain the primary modality used to evaluate cervical alignment in myelopathic patients.

## SIGNIFICANCE OF SPINAL ALIGNMENT

Humans require an erect stance for locomotion. During hominid evolution, the pivotal landmark that afforded bipedalism was the acquisition of sagittal balance of the trunk on the lower limbs.[3] Specifically, an ideal compromise between mobility and stability was reached by the evolution towards the double S shape of the vertebral column.[4] *Homo sapiens* is the only species to have both a lumbar and cervical curvature. The pelvic vertebra, the keystone of equilibrium, participated in this evolution by progressive widening and retroversion; this enabled the acquisition of erect posture. The alignment of the spinal column allows humans to carry food, hunt, use tools, and participate in parenting.

The vertebral column serves to provide support and balance to the human body. Specifically, the spine is the primary means by which the body can maintain an upright posture and a horizontal gaze. Dubousset asserted that there exists a conus within which the whole body can maintain an upright posture. His conus ranges from the "cone of economy," representing minimal exertion, to the "cone of maximum work," which is the upper limit of energy expenditure.[5] Specifically, he visualized a conus of balance for the standing position, in which the feet are located within a zone called the "polygon of sustentation", and the body, under the influence of muscle function and ligamentous support, can move in a conical fashion without moving the feet.[5] He further expanded his concept of "conus of economy", where the body can stay balanced with minimal muscle action.[5]

The body adapts to changes in balance in order to regulate the center of gravity (COG) over as narrow a perimeter as possible.[6] This fundamental tendency towards equilibrium is what drives compensatory changes in the spine as it attempts to adapt to pathological processes that are global, regional, or focal. To maintain a center of mass over the feet, the body recruits truncal rotation or translation, thoracolumbar curvature, and pelvic and lower limb compensatory mechanisms. While the cervical spine may play less of a role in this capacity, it likely plays a greater role in maintaining horizontal gaze due to its proximity to the cranium. Furthermore, changes in cervical alignment, in turn, contribute towards the development of pathologic conditions that can eventually contribute to myelopathy.

## RADIOGRAPHIC PARAMETERS

The cervical spine is the most mobile part of the spinal column. To fully evaluate the cervical spine, 3-ft X-rays are recommended. With this modality, most radiographic parameters for sagittal alignment can be measured.

### Craniocervical Region

One of the first attempts to quantify alignment was in 1885 describing the Frankfurt horizontal line, defined as

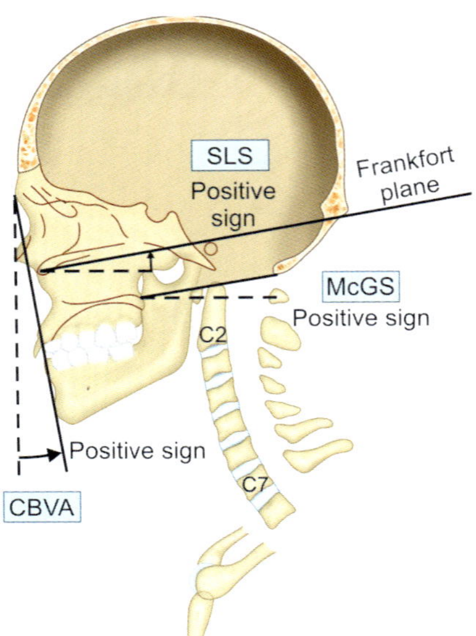


**Fig. 3.1:** Chin-brow vertical angle (CBVA), and CBVA surrogates: slope of line of sight and McGregor slope.

an extended line connecting the lower border of the orbit and the external auditory meatus.[7] Since then, a plethora of parameters to quantify alignment in the cervical and thoracolumbar spine have been developed.

The chin-brow vertical angle (CBVA) is a useful parameter for understanding a patient's ability to maintain horizontal gaze. Loss of the ability to maintain horizontal gaze has a significant negative impact on activities of daily living and quality of life (QOL).[8] Chin-brow vertical angle is defined as the angle subtended between a line drawn from the patient's chin to brow, and a vertical line (Fig. 3.1).[8]

A limitation of CBVA is that it is not readily measured on most standing lateral spine radiographs. Slope of line of sight (SLS) and McGregor slope (McGS) (Fig. 3.1) are two surrogate measures of horizontal gaze that are more readily available and have been found to be strongly correlated with CBVA.[9] Slope of line of sight, also known as the slope of Frankfort line, is subtended by the anteroinferior margin of orbit to the top of the external auditory meatus.[7] McGregor slope is a line subtended by the posterior margin of the hard palate and the most caudal part of the occiput.[10]

The maintenance of horizontal gaze is an important goal of craniocervical alignment. Normal CBVA values have not been specifically studied in asymptomatic volunteers, but in the postoperative settings patients appear to tolerate values of –10° to +10°.[11,12] Recently, the following CBVA range of values were found to be correlated with low disability: CBVA = [-4.7°; 17.7°]. Similarly, the following range of values for SLS and McGS has been elucidated: SLS = [-4.1°; 18.5°]; McGS = [-5.7°; 14.3°].[9]

## Cervical Region

There are several methods to assess cervical lordosis (CL), each with its benefits and limitations. The Cobb angle method, most widely used, measures lordosis from either C1-C7 or C2-C7. The first line is drawn either parallel to the inferior endplate of C2, or extending from the anterior tubercle of C1 to the posterior margin of the spinous process. The second line is drawn parallel to the inferior endplate of C7. Orthogonal lines are then drawn from each of the two lines noted in the earlier text. The angle subtended between the crossings of the perpendicular lines is the cervical curvature angle.[13,14] Less commonly used, the Harrison posterior tangent method, involves drawing parallel lines to the posterior surfaces of cervical vertebral bodies, C2-C7, and summing segmental angles for the total angle.[13] Finally, the Jackson physiological stress lines method requires drawing parallel lines from posterior surfaces of C2 and C7 vertebral bodies, and measuring the angle between them.[14]

Every radiographic parameter has its benefits and limitations. The C2-C7 lordosis is easily measured, is widely accepted, and has reference values (5–20°). However, age-related degenerative changes affect what is considered a "normal" value. Furthermore, individual variation and morphotypes of the human body make it challenging to adapt to all patients. As Faline et al. described, only 29% of asymptomatic patients had lordotic alignment above 10°.[15] Indeed, distinguishing between normal variants and pathology remains a challenge. Finally, in comparison to other parameters, as Ames et al. summarized, it has been suggested that the Cobb, C1-C7 angle, overestimates CL, the Cobb C2-C7 underestimates CL, while the Harrison method provides the best estimate of lordosis.[13,14] Despite this finding, the Cobb method remains the clinical mainstay of CL measurements due to its ease of use, as well as its robust intra- and inter-rater reliability.

The C2-C7 sagittal vertical axis (cSVA) is defined as the offset from C2 plumbline (PL) to the posterosuperior corner of C7. It is a measure of regional alignment of the cervical spine and normative values have been established at 1.5 cm +/- 1 cm.[16] The benefits of this measure are that it correlates with health-related QoL and it is easy to measure. Approximately 4 cm of C2-C7 SVA corresponds to a Neck

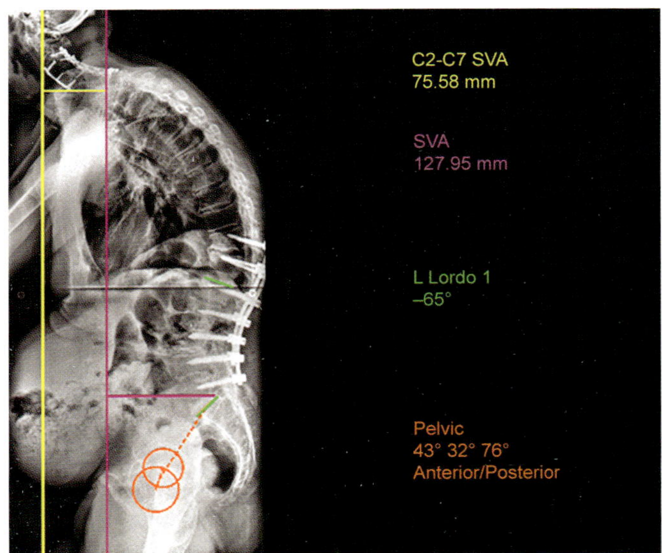


**Fig. 3.2:** Film emphasizing the sagittal vertical axis measurements.

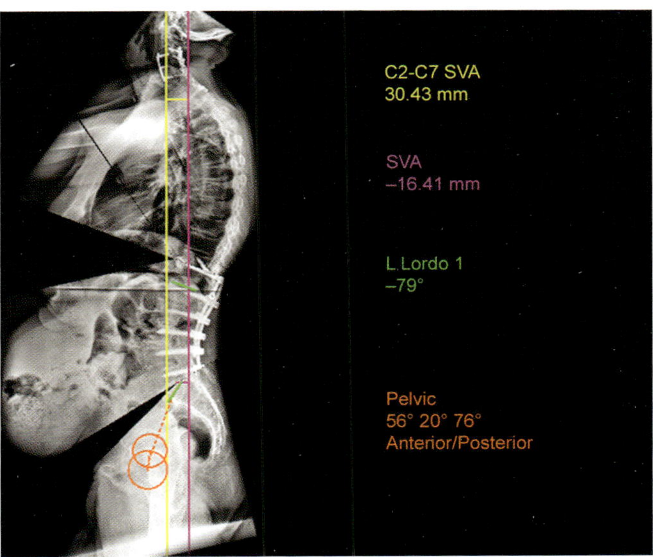


**Fig. 3.3:** Note the decreased cervical sagittal vertical axis as compared with Figure 3.2, secondary to compensatory changes.

Disability Index (NDI) of 25.[6] However, it requires calibrated images. Moreover, it can be affected by thoracolumbar deformity. For example, in Figure 3.2, C2-C7 PL is 7.5 cm. Is this a driver or consequence of deformity outside the cervical spine? The patient has global malalignment and pelvic retroversion and thoracolumbar kyphosis, due to proximal junctional kyphosis, may be the true driver of the cervical deformity. This illustration emphasizes the need to remove thoracolumbar compensatory mechanisms to evaluate the cervical spine. Figure 3.3 shows that when the compensatory mechanisms are accounted for, C2-C7 SVA is decreased. Indeed, there is a limit to the utility of any PL and one requires a global vision of the patient with a bottom to top analysis for truly understanding cervical alignment pathology.

## Cervicothoracic Junction

In recent years, there has been a proliferation of novel parameters that have facilitated our understanding of cervical alignment, with their complex relations to QOL and surgical outcomes. For example, investigators have focused attention on the cervicothoracic junction as an important contributor to cervical alignment. The basis of this relationship goes back to the primary role of the spine: maintenance of horizontal gaze.

The shape and orientation of the thoracic inlet helps maintain a balanced upright posture.[17] Accordingly, Lee et al. introduced neck tilt (NT) and thoracic inlet angle (TIA), as radiographic parameters.[17] Neck tilt as they defined it is an angle between two lines, both originating from the upper end of the sternum, with one being a vertical line and the other connecting to the center of the T1 endplate. Thoracic inlet angle, as they defined it, is the angle between an orthogonal line through the center of the T1 endplate, and a line drawn from center of the T1 endplate to the upper end of the sternum. Subsequent to this, Lee et al. discovered the fundamental relation that TIA is equal to the T1 slope (T1S) (angle between the horizontal plane and T1 endplate), plus NT.[17] This is analogous to the established relationship of the lumbar spine, in which pelvic incidence (PI) equals the sacral slope, plus pelvic tilt.

The TIA is clinically relevant because it has been found to be significantly correlated with cranial offset and craniocervical alignment.[17] A small TIA creates a small T1S and a small CL angle, for which to maintain physiological neck tilting, and vice versa.[14] Lee et al. explained that the TIA and T1S may be used for evaluation of sagittal balance, prediction of physiological alignment, and guidance of deformity correction in the cervical spine.[17] The T1S determines the amount of subaxial lordosis required to maintain COG of the head in a balanced position, and varies depending on global spinal alignment, as measured by SVA and by the inherent upper thoracic kyphosis (TK). In patients with scoliosis, the T1S has been shown to correlate directly with SVA (as measured from

**Table 3.1:** Correlations between T1 slope, C2-C7 sagittal vertical axis (SVA), C2-C7 lordosis, and T1 slope, C2-C7 lordosis.

| *Parameter* | *Parameter* | *Pearson (r)* |
|---|---|---|
| C2-C7 SVA | C2-C7 lordosis | 0.45 |
| C2-C7 SVA | T1 slope | 0.44 |
| C2-C7 lordosis | T1 slope | 0.38 |

*Source*: Ames CP, Blondel B, Scheer JK, et al. Cervical radiographical alignment: comprehensive assessment techniques and potential importance in cervical myelopathy. Spine (Phila Pa 1976). 2013;38:S149-60.

**Table 3.2:** Normal segmental cervical angles in asymptomatic adults from literature.

| *Level* | *Angle (°)* |
|---|---|
| C0-C1 | 2.1 ± 5.0 |
| C1-C2 | −32.2 ± 7.0 |
| C2-C3 | −1.9 ± 5.2 |
| C3-C4 | −1.5 ± 5.0 |
| C4-C5 | −0.6 ± 4.4 |
| C5-C6 | −1.1 ± 5.1 |
| C6-C7 | −4.5 ± 4.3 |
| Subtotal (C2-C7) | −9.6 |
| Total (C1-C7) | −41.8 |

*Source*: Ames CP, Blondel B, Scheer JK, et al. Cervical radiographical alignment: comprehensive assessment techniques and potential importance in cervical myelopathy. Spine (Phila Pa 1976). 2013;38: S149-60. Values presented as the means ± SD and the negative sign indicates lordosis in the segmental values.

**Table 3.3:** Normal cervical lordosis values for men and women in different age groups in asymptomatic adults from literature.

| *Age* | *Male (°)* | *Female (°)* |
|---|---|---|
| 20–25 | 16 ± 16 | 15 ± 10 |
| 30–35 | 21 ± 14 | 16 ± 16 |
| 40–45 | 27 ± 14 | 23 ± 17 |
| 50–55 | 22 ± 15 | 25 ± 11 |
| 60–65 | 22 ± 13 | 25 ± 16 |

*Source*: Ames CP, Blondel B, Scheer JK, et al. Cervical radiographical alignment: comprehensive assessment techniques and potential importance in cervical myelopathy. Spine (Phila Pa 1976). 2013;38:S149-60. Values presented as the means ± SD.

a C2 odontoid PL), to provide a measure of overall sagittal alignment.[18] The significant correlations between T1S and C2-C7 lordosis, T1S and C2-C7 SVA, as well as C2-C7 SVA and the difference between T1S and C2-7 lordosis, are well illustrated in Table 3.1. Generally, C2-C7 lordosis should be proportional to T1S.[19,15]

Recently, an objective target of how much CL is required was developed as follows: T1S minus C2-C7 lordosis (TS-L) of 17° correlates with a C2-C7 SVA of 4 cm.[20] This can provide an objective target of how much lordosis is required based on T1S, thus underscoring the importance of cervicothoracic junctional radiographic parameters on understanding cervical alignment.

### *Normal Cervical Alignment*

The cervical spine affords neck mobility, and there exists significant normal variation to the extent each level contributes to this versatility. Table 3.2 depicts the normal segmental cervical angles in asymptomatic adults.[16] In addition, there are slight gender- and age-related differences in CL (Table 3.3).[21] In asymptomatic normal volunteers, the mean total CL is approximately -40°.[16] The C1-C2 articulation is responsible for the largest percentage, 75–80%, of cervical standing lordosis.[16,22] This can be explained by the idea that the COG of the head sits directly above the centers of the C1 and C2 vertebral bodies.[23] The lower cervical levels are responsible for the remaining lesser portion of lordosis. C4-C7 is only responsible for approximately 6°, or 15%, of lordosis.[16] The mean C2-C7 sagittal Cobb angles for those in their 20s and those older than 60 years are reported to be –8.98° (standard deviation = 10.98°) and –13.70° (standard deviation = 10.48°), respectively (Table 3.4).[24] Finally, with respect to the odontoid-C7 PL distance, average values range from 15 to 17 +/–11.2 mm (Table 3.5).[16]

## Thoracic and Lumbar Regions

The simple concept that the cervical spine is connected to the thoracolumbar spine implies that the cervical spine cannot be studied in isolation. The long-established thoracic, lumbar, and pelvic parameters all play a role in determining cervical alignment.

For example, there is a known regional parameter chain of correlation, such that PI correlates with lumbar lordosis (LL), which correlates with TK, which finally correlates with CL (Figs. 3.4 and 3.5). Conversely, there is a lack of direct correlation found between PI and TK, making this chain of correlation, from pelvis to cervical spine, more complicated. The current view is that LL is proportional to PI and TK. Pelvic incidence is a fixed

**Table 3.4:** Comparison of sagittal alignment and angle parameters between the younger and older groups.

| | *Young* | | *Old* | |
|---|---|---|---|---|
| | *Mean* | *SD* | *Mean* | *SD* |
| C2-C7 (mm) | +13.21 | 7.22 | +13.68 | 9.86 |
| S1-C2 (mm) | +11.81 | 30.49 | +32.60 | 40.88 |
| S1-C7 (mm) | +1.27 | 31.92 | +20.54 | 41.63 |
| T apex to C2 (mm) | +62.14 | 16.70 | +78.25 | 31.40 |
| T apex to C7 (mm) | +49.36 | 16.12 | +66.87 | 26.97 |
| L apex to C2 (mm) | -33.28 | 28.62 | -12.33 | 40.75 |
| L apex to C7 (mm) | -44.95 | 30.56 | -23.92 | 41.41 |
| C0-C2 (°) | -16.44 | 7.89 | -14.44 | 8.79 |
| C2-C7 (°) | -8.98 | 10.98 | -13.70 | 10.48 |
| T1-T12 (°) | +39.00 | 11.52 | +33.37 | 17.94 |
| L1-S1 (°) | -49.46 | 11.45 | -45.59 | 19.63 |
| T1 slope (°) | +23.76 | 7.06 | +19.96 | 6.77 |

*Source*: Park MS, Moon S-H, Lee H-M, et al. The effect of age on cervical sagittal alignment: normative data on 100 asymptomatic subjects. Spine (Phila Pa 1976). 2013;38:E458-63.

**Table 3.5:** Normal cervical sagittal vertical axis (cSVA) values in asymptomatic adults from literature.

| *cSVA in Asymptomatic Adults (mm)* | |
|---|---|
| Odontoid marker at C7 | 15.6 ± 11.2 |
| Odontoid marker at sacrum | 13.2 ± 29.5 |

*Source*: Ames CP, Blondel B, Scheer JK, et al. Cervical radiographical alignment: comprehensive assessment techniques and potential importance in cervical myelopathy. Spine (Phila Pa 1976). 2013;38:S149-60. Values presented as the means ± SD.

parameter and TK has little flexibility. Subjects with a small PI or a small TK are shown to have smaller LL than subjects with small PI and large TK. This demonstrates that TK is not a result of LL, but rather LL is a result of TK and PI. The increase in CL as TK increases is not large enough to maintain the head over the pelvis, but it does provide adequate maintenance of horizontal gaze.[25,26] Understanding thoracolumbar alignment is important because surgical correction of global balance at the thoracolumbar area can, in some cases, spontaneously improve cervical alignment.[27]

## Sagittal Plane Translation

Sagittal plane translation of the cervical spine can be measured in different ways but the common theme among these methods is the concept of the already described above, the cervical SVA. Sagittal vertical axis in general measures a horizontal distance between a PL dropped from a defined point and another defined point, commonly the posterior superior corner of the sacrum. Again, in terms of cervical regional alignment, a cervical SVA can be defined as the distance between a PL dropped from the centroid of C2 (or odontoid) and the posterior superior aspect of C7. This is known as the C2-C7 SVA (Fig. 3.6).[14] Meanwhile, global sagittal alignment can be defined using either the C2 SVA or the C7 SVA. These parameters are used to measure the distance from the respective C2/C7 PLs to the posterior superior corner of the sacrum.[14] Another parameter used in global sagittal alignment analysis is the gravity line. The gravity line is similar to the C7 SVA, in that a PL is again dropped, but this time, from the head's COG.[28,29] The COG can be approximated on lateral radiographs using the anterior portion of the external auditory canal as an initial point for the PL (Fig. 3.7).[23]

# RADIOGRAPHIC PARAMETERS AND MYELOPATHY ASSOCIATION

The true value of the cervical parameters discussed above lies in how they correlate with clinical measures of pain and disability. There has been a plethora of studies regarding this topic and they center on the theme of how sagittal malalignment leads to disability. However, depending on the patients studied and the methods used, there is some

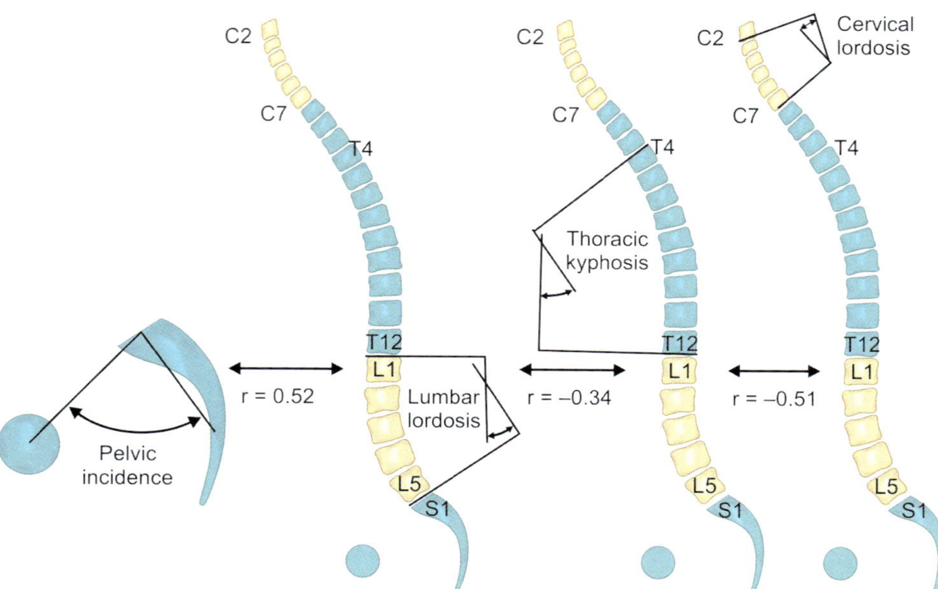


**Fig. 3.4:** Chain of correlation between pelvic incidence (PI) and regional sagittal parameters with the corresponding Pearson coefficient r values. A large PI requires a large lumbar lordosis (LL). An increase of LL is correlated with an increased TK, which is correlated with an increased cervical lordosis.

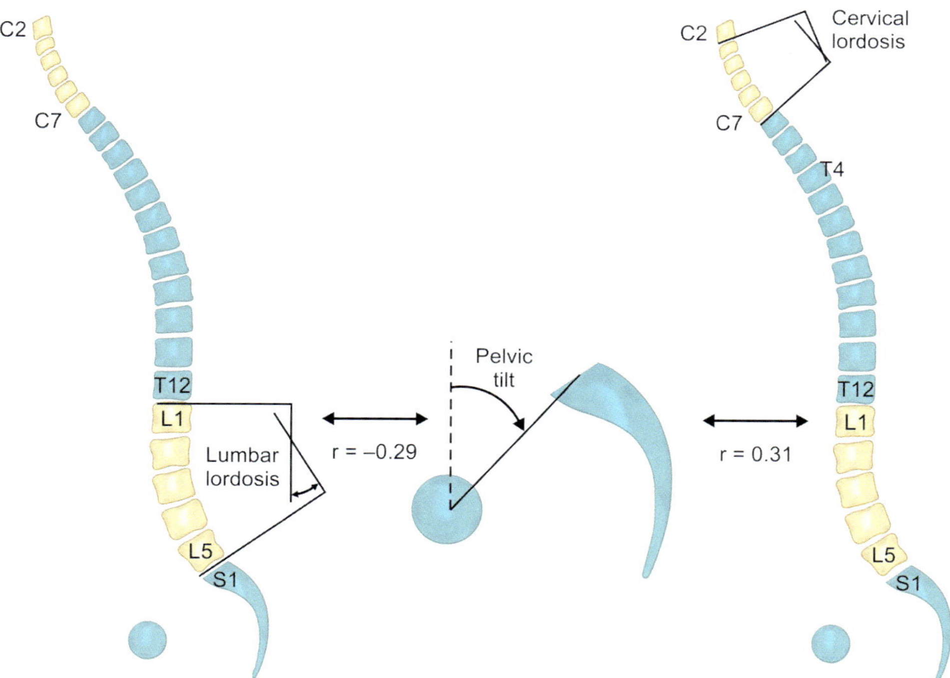


**Fig. 3.5:** Correlation between pelvic tilt and lumbar/cervical lordosis (CL). A loss of lumbar lordosis is correlated with a pelvic retroversion acting as compensatory mechanisms. Pelvic retroversion is also correlated with an increased CL.

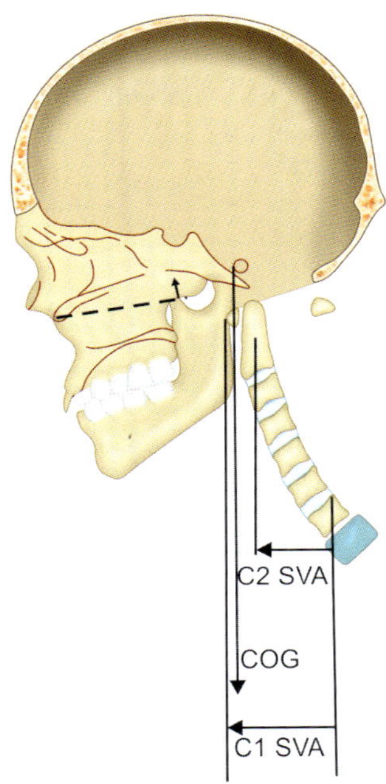


**Fig. 3.6:** Visual representation of the technique used to measure cervical sagittal vertical axis (SVA). C1 SVA is the distance between plumbline (PL) dropped from anterior tubercle of C1 and posterior superior corner of C7, C2 SVA is the distance between PL dropped from centroid of C2 and posterior superior corner of C7, and COG (center of gravity) is the distance between PL dropped from anterior margin of external auditory canal and posterior superior corner of C7.

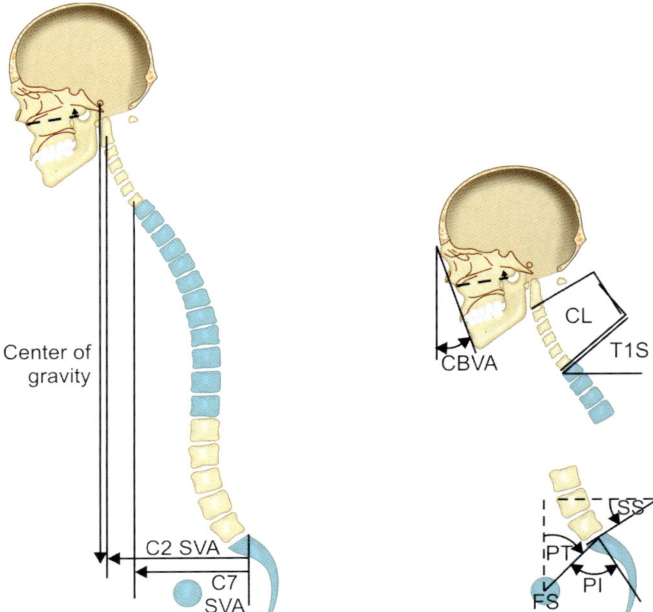


**Fig. 3.7:** The spine functions as a global unit so that cervical alignment parameters influence and are influenced by parameters in the lower regions. (CBVA: Chin-brow vertical axis; CL: Cervical lordosis; T1S: T1 slope; COG: Center of gravity; FS: Femoral shaft; PI: Pelvic incidence; PT: Pelvic tilt; SVA: Sagittal vertical axis).

controversy in the literature as to the exact role of how derangements in cervical alignment, as measured by cervical parameters, amount to disability. A full discussion of these issues is presented in Chapter 21.

## CONCLUSION

This introductory chapter emphasizes the importance of understanding spondylotic myelopathy as a pathological process intimately dependent on cervical alignment. The reported normative data on cervical alignment and correlations between key parameters related to standing posture offer critical reference values as well as a foundation for the analysis and treatment of spinal malalignment conditions. Visualizing myelopathy from a "lens" of alignment considerations affords a richer awareness as to why there are large differences in outcomes among various treatments, and promotes acuity in critical evaluation of proposed surgical interventions developed for the future.

## REFERENCES

1. Hippocrates. De Prisca Medicina.In: Littre PE (Ed.). Oeuvres Completes d'Hippocrate, Vol. 9. Amsterdam: AM Hakkert; 1982.
2. Keevil G. The Roentgen rays. Br Med J. 1896;1:433-4.
3. Tardieu C, Bonneau N, Hecquet JJ, et al. How is sagittal balance acquired during bipedal gait acquisition? Comparison of neonatal and adult pelves in three dimensions. Evolutionary implications. J Hum Evol. 2013;2013:209-22.
4. Schmitt D. Insights into the evolution of human bipedalism from experimental studies of humans and other primates. J Exp Biol. 2003;206:1437-48.
5. Dubousset J. Three-dimensional analysis of the scoliotic deformity. In: Weinstein SL (Ed.). The Pediatric Spine. New York: Raven Press; 1994, pp. 479-96.
6. Tang JA, Scheer JK, Smith JS, et al. The impact of standing regional cervical sagittal alignment on outcomes in posterior cervical fusion surgery. Neurosurgery. 2012;71:662-9; discussion 669.
7. Garson J. The Frankfort Craniometric Agreement, with Critical Remarks Thereon. J Anthropol Inst Gt Britain 1885.

8. Suk K, Kim K, Lee S, et al. Significance of chin-brow vertical angle in correction of kyphotic deformity of ankylosing spondylitis patients. Spine (Phila Pa 1976). 2003;28:2001-5.
9. Lafage R, Challier V, Ferrero E, et al. Validation of correlation between CBVA, SLS and McGregor's Slope. Scoliosis Res. Soc. (SRS); Sept. 10-13, Anchorage, Alaska: 2014.
10. McGregor M. The significance of certain measurements of the skull in the diagnosis of basilar impression. Br J Radiol 1948;21(244):171-81.
11. Pigge RR, Scheerder FJ, Smit TH, et al. Effectiveness of preoperative planning in the restoration of balance and view in ankylosing spondylitis. Neurosurg Focus. 2008;24:E7.
12. Kim K-T, Suk K-S, Cho Y-J, et al. Clinical outcome results of pedicle subtraction osteotomy in ankylosing spondylitis with kyphotic deformity. Spine (Phila Pa 1976). 2002;27:612-8.
13. Harrison DE, Harrison DD, Cailliet R, et al. Cobb method or Harrison posterior tangent method: which to choose for lateral cervical radiographic analysis. Spine (Phila Pa 1976). 2000;25:2072-8.
14. Ames CP, Blondel B, Scheer JK, et al. Cervical radiographical alignment: comprehensive assessment techniques and potential importance in cervical myelopathy. Spine (Phila Pa 1976). 2013;38:S149-60.
15. Faline A, Szadkowski S, Berthonnaud E, et al. Morphological study of the lower cervical curvature: results of 230 asymptomatic subjects. EuroSpine, Brussels, Belgium: 2007.
16. Hardacker JW, Shuford RF, Capicotto PN, et al. Radiographic standing cervical segmental alignment in adult volunteers without neck symptoms. Spine (Phila Pa 1976). 1997;22:1472-80; discussion 1480.
17. Lee S, Kim K, Seo E, et al. The influence of thoracic inlet alignment on the craniocervical sagittal balance in asymptomatic adults. J Spinal Disord Tech. 2012;25:E41-7.
18. Knott PT, Mardjetko SM, Techy F. The use of the T1 sagittal angle in predicting overall sagittal balance of the spine. Spine J. 2010;10:994-8.
19. Marnay T. Equilibre du rachis et du bassin. Cah D'enseignement La SOFCOT Elsevier, Paris 1988.
20. Protopsaltis TS, Terran J, Bronsard N, et al. T1 slope minus cervical lordosis (TS-CL), the cervical answer to PI-LL, defines cervical sagittal deformity in patients undergoing thoracolumbar osteotomy. Cerv Spine Res Soc Annu Meet. December 5-7, 2013.
21. Gore DR, Sepic SB, Gardner GM. Roentgenographic findings of the cervical spine in asymptomatic people. Spine (Phila Pa 1976). n.d.;11:521-4.
22. Jackson RP, McManus AC. Radiographic analysis of sagittal plane alignment and balance in standing volunteers and patients with low back pain matched for age, sex, and size. A prospective controlled clinical study. Spine (Phila Pa 1976). 1994;19:1611-8.
23. Beier G, Schuck M, Schuller E, et al. Determination of physical data of the head. I. Center of gravity and moments of inertia of human heads. Munich: University of Munich;1979.
24. Park MS, Moon S-H, Lee H-M et al. The effect of age on cervical sagittal alignment: normative data on 100 asymptomatic subjects. Spine (Phila Pa 1976). 2013;38:E458-63.
25. Lafage V, Ferrero E, Lafage R, et al. Chain of compensation related to PI-LL mismatch: a complete standing axis investigation including lower extremities. Scoliosis Res Soc (SRS); Sept. 10-13, Anchorage, Alaska: 2014.
26. Lafage VC, Ferrero E, Lafage R, et al. Maintaining chin brow vertical angle (CBVA) and horizontal gaze in lumbar fatback deformity: full body analysis of the chain of compensation from the cervical spine to the feet 2014.
27. Smith JS, Shaffrey CI, Lafage V, et al. Spontaneous improvement of cervical alignment after correction of global sagittal balance following pedicle subtraction osteotomy. J Neurosurg Spine. 2012;17:300-7.
28. El Fegoun AB, Schwab FJ, Gamez L, et al. Center of gravity and radiographic posture analysis: a preliminary review of adult volunteers and adult patients affected by scoliosis. Spine (Phila Pa 1976). 2005;30:1535-40.
29. Gangnet N, Pomero V, Dumas R, et al. Variability of the spine and pelvis location with respect to the gravity line: a three-dimensional stereoradiographic study using a force platform. Surg Radiol Anat. 2003;25:424-33.

Chapter 4

# Clinical Diagnosis of Cervical Myelopathy

*Brett M Walker, Krister Radcliff*

## INTRODUCTION

Cervical spondylotic myelopathy (CSM) is recognized as the most common cause of acquired adult spinal cord dysfunction.[1] Other causes include trauma, tumors, ischemia, and ossification of the posterior longitudinal ligament. Male patients are most often affected and are frequently over the age of 50.

The full constellation of symptoms of CSM was not well described until 1952, when Brain et al. reported the first large series of patients.[2] Soon after, Clarke and Robinson described the natural history in their series of 120 patients with cervical spondylosis. In this large retrospective case series, 75% of cases appeared episodic, experiencing periods of new symptoms; 20% of patients experienced a slow, steady decline; and 5% of patients suffered from a rapid onset followed by a long period of no new symptoms.[3] In a similar series, Lees and Turner reported that the majority of patients experience a prolonged disease course with several periods of non-progressive disability.[4] The indolent clinical course of CSM frequently leads to delayed diagnosis and therefore delays in therapeutic intervention. One study reported an average of 6.3 years from initial symptoms to diagnosis. Prolonged time to diagnosis was frequently associated with poorer patient outcomes.[5]

The pathogenesis of CSM is multifactorial. Canal stenosis and decreased sagittal diameter are strongly related to development of this condition. This process is due to a collection of degenerative events, typically occurring over a long period of time. It is widely accepted that the initial event is degeneration of the intervertebral disk, which slowly progresses and is often asymptomatic.[6] A cascade of events then ensues that may include osteophyte formation, uncovertebral and facet joint hypertrophy, spondylotic bar formation, ligamentum flavum hypertrophy, or even ossification of the posterior longitudinal ligament.[1,7] All of these processes collectively decrease the sagittal diameter of the spinal canal. There is no single measurement of spinal canal dimension that is universally considered to represent stenosis, although $<13$ mm is the commonly reported measurement, likely due to radiographic magnification differences.[8,9] This inconsistency prompted Pavlov et al. to evaluate the ratio of spinal canal to vertebral body sagittal diameter. The authors reported 92% accuracy in diagnosis of stenosis if the ratio is $<0.82$. The normal is $>1.0$.[10] Patients with congenitally narrow canals are at particular risk for developing spinal cord compression.[11-14]

The variability in pathogenesis associated with CSM prompted Crandall and Batzdorf to divide cervical myelopathy into five categories based on neurologic symptoms. *Transverse lesion syndrome* represents involvement of the corticospinal, spinothalamic, and posterior columns in equal severity below the level of the lesion. This was the most frequent presentation, and the authors hypothesized that this represented end-stage disease. *Motor system syndrome* is characterized by deficit in the corticospinal tracts. Sensory tracts are only mildly affected, if at all. Spasticity is common in this category. *Central cord syndrome* is marked by sensory and motor dysfunction, which affects the upper extremities more severely than the lower extremities. *Brown-Séquard syndrome* affects the spinal cord unilaterally. It is marked by ipsilateral loss of corticospinal tract function and contralateral analgesia below the level of the lesion. *Brachialgia and cord syndrome* occurs with upper extremity pain and long tract symptoms. Unlike the other categories, patients frequently experience associated radicular symptoms.[15] Ferguson and Caplan proposed an alternative and simplified classification. *Medial syndrome* consists primarily of long tract signs. *Lateral syndrome* primarily produces radicular symptoms. *Combined syndrome* is observed most frequently and includes both spinal cord and root involvement. *Vascular syndrome* is characterized by ischemia of the spinal cord and has a rapid, variable presentation.[16]

Accurate diagnosis of CSM requires a complete patient history and physical examination. Correlation with imaging studies helps to solidify a diagnosis; however, the clinician must have a high index of suspicion and a keen understanding of similarly presenting conditions in the differential diagnosis.

## HISTORY

A thorough history is an essential tool to guide clinicians toward an accurate diagnosis. A history should begin with the patient's chief complaint. Several studies have demonstrated that the earliest patient complaint is a sense of clumsiness in the hands or gait abnormality.[17-19] The onset and duration of symptoms should be recorded, as well as whether any periods of stability or improvement have occurred. Enlisting the help of family members or close friends may be valuable to assist in forming accurate timelines as symptoms are often subtle and slowly progress over a period of years.

Next, the location of neurologic symptoms should be established. Are the patient's symptoms bilateral or unilateral? Are the upper extremities or lower extremities affected more severely? Loss of dexterity and nonspecific weakness of the upper extremities typically occurs. The history should include any difficulties in handwriting, buttoning shirts, and grasping or identifying small objects as well as the use of computers, cell phones or remote controls.[20-22] A wide-based, jerky gait may be present, which results in frequent falls.[21] Careful attention should be paid to a history of falls, as well as the use of assistive devices for ambulation. Patients may report subtle changes such as having to use handrails while climbing stairs.[22] Changes in gait frequently lead to early fatigue, and patients should be questioned regarding stamina. Patients should be asked about their ability to complete activities of daily living. A history of numbness and tingling in the extremities should be documented. Paresthesias that are non-specific and non-dermatomal are often reported by patients.[23] Reports of axial neck pain in CSM are highly variable, with some reports being as low as 34%, making its diagnostic value questionable.[24] The history should also include questions regarding bowel and bladder habits as severe cases of CSM may cause dysfunction. Finally, any provocative or alleviating measures should be documented. Past medical, surgical, social, and family histories should also be thoroughly reviewed. Valuable information regarding acute and chronic conditions, previous diagnosis of cervical or cranial pathology or hereditary conditions may be obtained. Special attention should be paid to any history of previous cervical operations as it may affect future surgical planning. Table 4.1 summarizes common history elements found with myelopathy.

**Table 4.1:** History findings consistent with myelopathy.

| | | | |
|---|---|---|---|
| Feeling "unsteady" | Inability to button shirts | Difficulty grasping small objects | Slow progression of symptoms |
| Frequent falls | Decline in quality of handwriting | Numbness in the hands | Steady decline of function |

## PHYSICAL EXAMINATION

Physical examination findings in CSM are highly variable, and its diagnosis requires a high index of suspicion. There is no one pathognomonic sign or symptom associated with myelopathy, making its diagnosis extremely difficult.[20] Additionally, many of the physical examination findings may be subtle and will vary depending on the level (s) of compression.[1,25]

As previously mentioned, gait abnormalities are often among the most common signs of CSM. Often, a sense of unsteadiness is the first sign noticed by the patient. Several studies have demonstrated a prevalence of gait changes in 90–100% of patients with myelopathy.[5,19] Therefore, careful observation of a patient's gait should be included in the physical examination. The patient should be asked to ambulate down a hallway both toward and away from the clinician while he or she observes the gait pattern for abnormalities. The patient should also be asked to attempt toe-walking, heel walking, and heel-toe walking. Even in subtle cases, the myelopathic patient will have difficulty performing these tasks, which require more balance and proprioception. Traditionally, the gait associated with myelopathy is described as broad-based and hesitant with difficulty in heel-toe walking. Patients often appear "jerky" and spastic.[26] Patients may also have difficulty with turning, using walls or handrails for assistance. Maezawa et al. performed a detailed gait analysis of patients with CSM. Patients demonstrated decreased walking speed, increased time in stance phase, decreased time in single stance phase, decreased stance length and increased stance width.[27]

The *Romberg test* is provocative of positional sense and may provide additional diagnostic information. By

**Table 4.2:** The Nurick classification.

| *Grade* | *Clinical findings* |
|---|---|
| 0 | Root symptoms only or normal |
| 1 | Physical signs of cord compression, normal gait |
| 2 | Difficulty with gait. Fully employed |
| 3 | Gait difficulties prevent employment. Able to walk unassisted |
| 4 | Unable to walk without assistance |
| 5 | Wheelchair or bed bound |

having the patient close his/her eyes and stand on one leg with arms extended, the examiner can evaluate the patient's posterior column function.[28] Findlay et al. reported a positive Romberg test in just 34% of the myelopathic patients in their series. A modified "walking Romberg" test was proposed in the same study, improving the positive value to 74%.[29] In this test, the patient was asked to ambulate for a distance of 5 meters with his or her eyes open. The patient was then asked to walk the same distance with the eyes closed. Patients were closely escorted by the clinician to avoid potential falls. A positive result was any indication of swaying, falling or failure to complete the distance due to instability. In 1972, Nurick published a case series of 160 patients with myelopathy. The *Nurick classification* was developed to grade the severity of myelopathy based on the patient's gait abnormalities.[30] Six grades of CSM range from 0 to 5, each with increasing severity of dysfunction. Evaluation of the Nurick classification has demonstrated its validity and sensitivity as a measure of CSM.[31] The Nurick classification is detailed in Table 4.2.

Cervical range of motion should be evaluated in all planes. This includes flexion, extension, side bending, and rotation. The clinician should pay particular attention to limitations of extension, which may be painful in patients with stenosis or root compression. Lack of cervical extension may also be important for future surgical planning, as special care must be taken during positioning and intubation.[28] The *Lhermitte sign* is positive when flexion or extension of the cervical spine produces shock-like sensations in the torso or the extremities.[32] Crandall and Batzdorf reported a positive Lhermitte sign in 28% of myelopathic patients in their series.[15]

The cranial nerves (II–XII) should also be examined in order to rule out lesions that originate in the brain or brainstem. Many conditions may present with similar motor and sensory examinations to myelopathy. In patients with CSM, however, cranial nerve testing should be normal.

A complete neurological evaluation of the upper and lower extremities including motor, sensory and reflex testing is crucial. Additionally, vibratory testing should be completed to test dorsal (posterior) column function. We recommend using the American Spinal Injury Association impairment scale for grading of motor and sensory function (Fig. 4.1).[33,34] Motor function is graded from 0 to 5. Light touch and pinprick sensation are graded from 0 to 3 based on dermatomal distribution. This method allows for consistency across examinations.

Next, deep tendon reflexes (DTRs) should be tested and recorded. Traditionally, DTRs are graded from 0 to 4.[35] Generally, lower motor neuron involvement (weakness, hyporeflexia) is found at the level of compression, and upper motor neuron involvement (spasticity, hyperreflexia) is found caudal to compression.[17] Given that compression can occur at multiple levels, mixed upper and lower motor neuron findings are typically observed in the upper extremities, depending on the level of compression. For example, a patient with cord compression at C4-C5 may present with lower motor neuron symptoms of weakness in the deltoid or biceps with hyporeflexia of the biceps. Below the level of compression, hyperreflexia of the brachioradialis and triceps may also be present. The patient's lower extremities would exhibit symptoms of upper motor neuron lesions.[21] Generally, upper extremity symptoms tend to be unilateral, while lower extremity symptoms are usually bilateral.[18] Hyperreflexia and spasticity are common clinical findings in CSM, especially in the lower extremities.[17,19,36] It should be noted that in addition to cervical spinal stenosis, many patients concurrently suffer from lumbar spinal stenosis. This may present with symptoms of lower motor neuron dysfunction in one or both lower extremities, complicating the clinical picture.

A sensory examination should be completed, including light touch and pinprick. In patients with CSM, sensory deficits will also depend on the location of spinal cord compression. Spinothalamic tract disruption will result in decreased appreciation of pain and temperature sensation caudally and contralaterally to the site of compression, while light touch is usually preserved. Dorsal root disruption will result in decreased sensation in dermatomal patterns. Compression of the dorsal (posterior) columns leads to decreased vibratory and positional

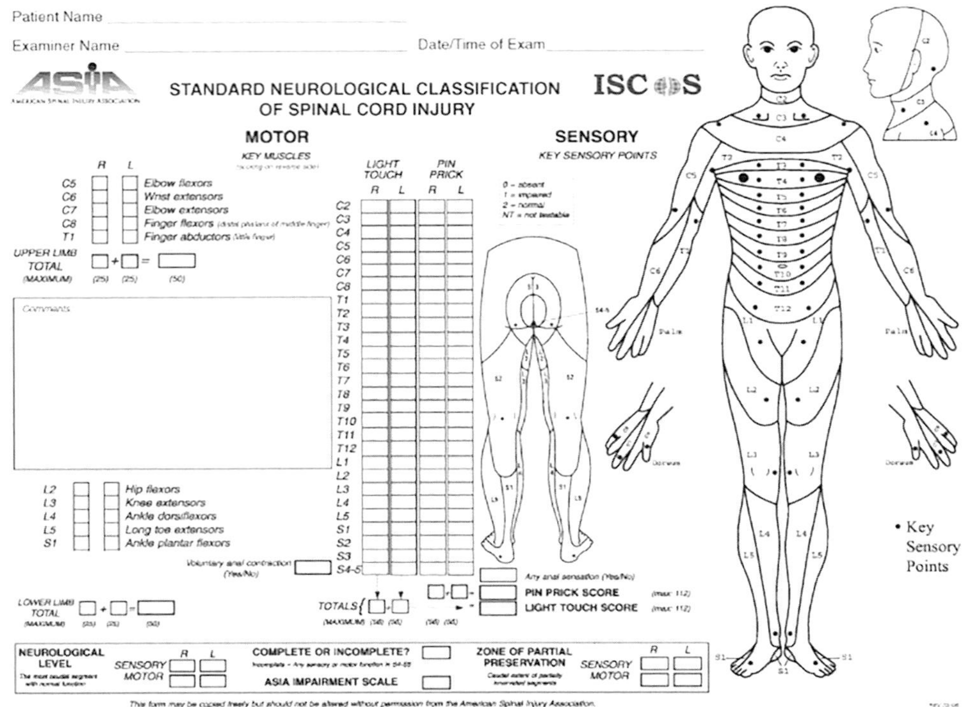


**Fig. 4.1:** The American Spinal Injury Association classification.
*Courtesy*: American Spinal Injury Association.

sensation caudally and ipsilaterally to the lesion, affecting gait and balance. As noted by Crandall, various combinations of ascending tract disruption lead to variability of sensory deficits, which do not follow dermatomal patterns.[15,37] The *Modified Japanese Orthopedic Association scale* was designed to grade severity of cervical myelopathy based on neurologic function (Table 4.3). Motor and sensory functions are individually graded with a maximum score of 17 denoting normal function.[38] One study has demonstrated a high level of intra-observer reliability, making it useful for clinical practice.[30] It is widely used to track the progression of disease or as a postoperative outcome measure.

Several additional reflexes may provide valuable clinical information. For compression occurring cephalad to C4, the *scapulohumeral reflex* may be useful. First described by Shimizu, the reflex is elicited by tapping the tip of the acromion in a caudal direction. Elevation of the scapula or abduction of the humerus is considered a hyperactive reflex.[39] The *jaw-jerk reflex* is elicited by tapping on the chin of a relaxed mandible. When positive, a hyperactive mandible flexion will occur, which may indicate a cranial or brainstem pathology.[40] The *inverted radial reflex* is provoked by tapping the distal brachioradialis tendon. A hypoactive brachioradialis reflex in addition to flexion of the fingers is considered a positive result. Hoffmann, Babinski, and clonus are frequently tested reflexes that represent long tract signs consistent with spinal cord compression.[28] The *Hoffmann reflex* is elicited by flicking the terminal phalanx of the middle finger of a hand at rest. A positive result is when the patient's thumb and index finger simultaneously flex.[41] Reports of the incidence of the Hoffmann reflex in myelopathic patients are variable. Harrop et al. reported a positive Hoffmann in 83.33% of myelopathic patients in one series. The authors cautioned about a high false-positive rate, especially in young patients.[19] A similar prospective, randomized trial demonstrated a positive Hoffman reflex in 59% of myelopathic patients, compared to 16% in the control group. The authors noted 84% specificity for myelopathy.[42] In a series of 50 patients, Findlay et al. found a positive Hoffmann in 78.75% of myelopathic patients.[29] Glaser and colleagues reported a sensitivity of 58% and specificity of 78%.[43] The *Babinski sign* is tested by scratching the lateral plantar aspect of the foot. A normal response is flexion of the great toe, while extension represents a

**Table 4.3:** Modified Japanese Orthopedic Association scale.

| *Score* | *Motor dysfunction upper extremities* |
|---|---|
| 0 | Inability to move hands |
| 1 | Inability to eat with a spoon, but able to move hands |
| 2 | Inability to button shirt, but able to eat with a spoon |
| 3 | Able to button shirt with great difficulty |
| 4 | Able to button shirt with slight difficulty |
| 5 | No dysfunction |
| *Score* | *Motor dysfunction lower extremities* |
| 0 | Complete loss of motor and sensory function |
| 1 | Sensory preservation without ability to move legs |
| 2 | Able to move legs, but unable to walk |
| 3 | Able to walk on a flat floor with an assistive device |
| 4 | Able to walk up and/or down stairs with a hand rail |
| 5 | Moderate to significant lack of stability, but able to walk up and/or down stairs without hand rail |
| 6 | Mild lack of stability but walks with smooth reciprocation unaided |
| 7 | No dysfunction |
| *Score* | *Sensory dysfunction upper extremities* |
| 0 | Complete loss of hand sensation |
| 1 | Severe sensory loss or pain |
| 2 | Mild sensory loss |
| 3 | No sensory loss |
| *Score* | *Sphincter dysfunction* |
| 0 | Inability to micturate voluntarily |
| 1 | Marked difficulty with micturition |
| 2 | Mild to moderate difficulty with micturition |
| 3 | Normal micturition |

pathologic response. The sensitivity of the Babinski sign appears to be low, occurring in only 44%, 13%, and 30.6% of myelopathic patients in the Harrop et al. and Rhee et al. studies, respectively. Some authors note that the specificity for myelopathy was 100% in their series.[19,42] An additional report estimates that an abnormal Babinski sign may be present in 5% of the normal population.[37] *Clonus* is tested by applying a forced dorsiflexion motion on a stationary ankle with the knee flexed. This motion produces an Achilles stretch. Reflexive plantarflexion follows. Sustained clonus (>3 beats) is considered pathologic and may be indicative of cord compression. Rhee et al. reported a low sensitivity (13%) and high specificity (100%) of sustained clonus for myelopathy.[42] Important reflexes are listed in Table 4.4.

**Table 4.4:** Abnormal reflexes found in cervical myelopathy.

| *Reflex* | *Significance* |
|---|---|
| Jaw jerk | Examiner taps on the chin of the relaxed patient. If the patient's jaw clinches, this is considered a hyperactive reflex. Evaluates for cranial or brainstem lesions. |
| Scapulohumeral reflex | Examiner taps the lateral tip of the acromion. Any elevation of the scapula or abduction of the humerus is considered hyperactive. Tests for lesions above the C3 vertebral body. |
| Inverted radial reflex | Finger flexion with hyporeflexia of the brachioradialis reflex is considered an inverted radial reflex and may be pathologic. |
| Hoffmann | With the hand relaxed, the examiner flicks the distal phalanx of the middle finger. Reflexive thumb and index finger flexion represent a positive finding and is found with spinal cord compression. |
| Clonus | The examiner applies a quick and sustained dorsiflexion force to the patient's relaxed foot. Reflexive plantar flexion of >3 beats is considered pathologic. May represent compression of the spinal cord. |

Examination of the hands may provide additional diagnostic clues. The natural history of cervical myelopathy leads to generalized weakness and intrinsic muscle wasting. In 1987, Ono et al. first described several findings suggestive of "myelopathy hand."[44] The *finger escape sign* is defined as a failure of abduction/extension of the ulnar-most two or three fingers. With the palms faced down, the patient is asked to hold the little finger in abduction. A positive test is when the patient cannot do so for >30 seconds. More severe cases may also lead to a lack of metacarpophalangeal joint extension. In addition to abduction, the fingers will maintain a flexed posture. The *rapid grip and release test* is conducted by having the patient grip and release their fingers as quickly and fully as possible. A normal adult should be able to perform this test 20 or more times in 10 seconds. Early intrinsic muscle fatigue is responsible for a patient's inability to complete such tests and is highly suggestive of myelopathy. In this study, these findings were present in 90.3% of patients with CSM.

## DIFFERENTIAL DIAGNOSIS

Several disorders present with symptoms similar to CSM. This tends to a broad differential diagnosis. Conditions that must be considered include multiple sclerosis (MS), amyotrophic lateral sclerosis (ALS), diabetes mellitus, syringomyelia, cerebrovascular accident (CVA), Guillain-Barre syndrome (GBS), normal pressure hydrocephalus (NPH), and central nervous system tumors.[45] In addition to a thorough history and physical examination, magnetic resonance imaging (MRI) of the cervical spine can assist the clinician in making a diagnosis.[5,26]

*Multiple sclerosis* is a disorder caused by demyelination of the central nervous system characterized by both motor and sensory deficits. Unlike cervical myelopathy, pathology also affects the cranial nerves. Patients typically report frequent exacerbations and remissions. During periods of remission, patients often experience a complete resolution of neurologic symptoms.[26,46,47]

*Amyotrophic lateral sclerosis* is a motor neuron disease affecting the spinal cord and lower brain stem. Patients experience progressive muscle weakness affecting the distal musculature more than the proximal, leading to gait abnormalities. Upper motor neuron symptoms will also develop, including Hoffmann, Babinski, and clonus. This combination of symptoms may be confused with cervical myelopathy. A distinguishing factor is that in ALS, sensory function is spared. As mentioned, the disease is progressive, with a mean survival of 3–5 years.[48]

*Diabetes mellitus* affects the small blood vessels and nerves of the body. The most common form of diabetic neuropathy is described as a peripheral, symmetric sensimotor neuropathy.[49] It typically follows a "stocking and glove" distribution, which should be a diagnostic clue. Testing with a Semmes-Weinstein monofilament in this distribution can aid in diagnosis. Lack of sensory feedback from the feet frequently results in an altered gait pattern resembling myelopathy. Unlike CSM, lower extremity reflexes tend to be decreased.[50] *Diabetes mellitus* affects many body systems, and poor glycemic control is associated with disease and symptom progression.[51]

*Syringomyelia* is caused by a fluid collection within the spinal cord and can be the result of multiple etiologies. Its symptoms are nonspecific and may resemble those of cervical myelopathy. A 2011 case series and literature review demonstrated common symptoms of sensory loss, limb weakness, paralysis, and gait abnormalities as well as bowel or bladder dysfunction. In contrast to CSM, the mean age of patients affected by syringomyelia was 39.3.[52] Imaging studies, including MRI or computed tomography (CT) myelography, are especially important for diagnosis as a syrinx will appear bright on T2-weighted images.

*Cerebrovascular accident* is another common cause of motor and sensory deficits. Depending on the area of the brain or brainstem involved, the presentation will vary. Level of consciousness, language, and cranial nerves may also be affected. Motor and sensory symptoms typically follow a hemispherical pattern, affecting one side of the body. Symptoms of a CVA occur rapidly, and resolution depends on the site and extent of damage.

*Guillain-Barré syndrome* was originally described in 1916. About 75% of patients affected report some history of an upper respiratory or gastrointestinal illness before neurologic symptoms appear. A hallmark of GBS is the rapid onset of symptoms. Weakness usually begins in the lower extremities and quickly progresses proximally in an ascending fashion. If untreated, paralysis may progress to the respiratory system, requiring intubation. Weakness typically reaches its worst about 4 weeks after the onset of symptoms, followed by a relative plateau phase and then recovery. Sixty percent of patients are able to return to unaided ambulation by 12 months.[53,54]

*Normal pressure hydrocephalus* may resemble CSM in the early stages of the disease. The most common early presentation of NPH is gait abnormalities. Analysis demonstrates decreased ambulatory speed, decreased step height, and difficulty in turning. Later in the disease course, sphincter dysfunction leads to urinary incontinence. In contrast to myelopathy, signs of dementia frequently develop, including apathy, recall, and inattention.[55]

*Tumors* of the brain or spinal column may present with highly variable symptoms. Mass effect of the spinal cord from a tumor may result in symptoms that are the same as or similar to those found in CSM. Magnetic resonance imaging examination with contrast is valuable to differentiate between myelopathy secondary to spondylosis and tumor.

Table 4.5 highlights diagnostic characteristics of the differential diagnosis.

## DIAGNOSTIC STUDIES

In addition to a thorough history and physical examination, imaging studies assist the clinician in obtaining an accurate diagnosis of CSM as well as assist in future surgical planning. There are several imaging modalities that may be of use, each having benefits and disadvantages.

Plain radiographs are an inexpensive first step and are easily obtained in most clinical settings. Valuable information, including coronal and sagittal cervical alignment, sagittal diameter and Pavlov's ratio, can be obtained from

**Table 4.5:** Distinguishing factors of differential diagnosis.

| *Condition* | *Motor* | *Sensory* | *Cranial nerves* | *Typical course* |
|---|---|---|---|---|
| Cervical myelopathy | Affected | Affected | Spared | Progressive deterioration |
| Multiple sclerosis | Affected | Affected | Affected | Relapse and remit |
| Amyotrophic lateral sclerosis | Affected | Spared | Affected | Progressive deterioration |
| Cerebrovascular accident | Affected | Affected | Affected | Sudden onset with unilateral symptoms |
| Guillain-Barré syndrome | Affected | Rarely affected | Rarely affected | Rapid progression, ascending paralysis, areflexia |

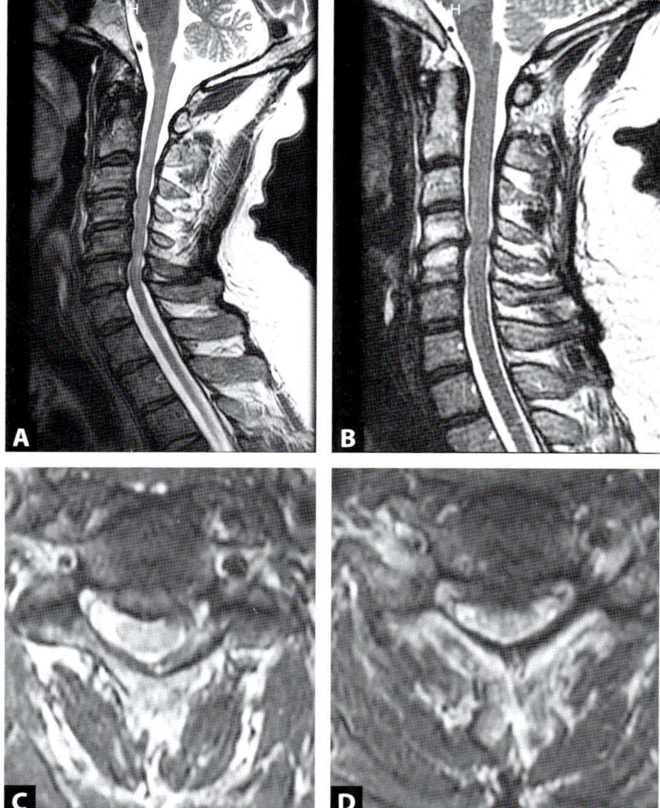

**Figs. 4.2A to D:** Magnetic resonance imaging findings consistent with cervical spondylotic myelopathy.

images. Flexion and extension views may show signs of instability. Plain radiography is unable to evaluate the spinal cord or soft tissues, limiting its diagnostic value.

Computed tomography is superior to plain radiography for the evaluation of osseous anatomy and pathology. The benefit of three-dimensional reconstructions may be helpful for the evaluation of subtle pathologic changes, including ossification of the posterior longitudinal ligament. Additionally, a cross-sectional area of the spinal canal may be measured on axial sequences. One major drawback of CT scans is the increased radiation exposure to the patient. Computed tomography does not provide detailed imaging of soft tissues of spinal cord pathology, but may be a particularly important diagnostic tool in patients who are unable to undergo MRI.

Myelography refers to the addition of intradural dye to plain radiography or CT scanning. This allows for enhanced visualization of areas of spinal cord compression, which will appear as areas of dye constriction. Nerve root compression may also be visualized using this technique. Although compression is visualized, myelography does not provide information about extradural processes.

Magnetic resonance imaging has become the imaging modality of choice for evaluation of the spinal column.[56] Magnetic resonance imaging provides excellent visualization of the spinal cord and surrounding soft tissues, including anatomy and pathology of the intervertebral disks. Additional diagnostic information may be obtained by the addition of intravenous contrast. Like CT scanning, three-dimensional reconstructions allow a cross-sectional area of the spinal canal to be evaluated. Magnetic resonance imaging findings in CSM include intervertebral disk degeneration, canal stenosis, effacement of the cerebrospinal fluid and myelomalacia (hyperintense signal on T2-weighted images or hypointense signal on T1-weighted images).[19] Most patients with MRI signal change develop myelopathy, even if they are asymptomatic initially. Figures 4.2A to D demonstrate MRI findings consistent with myelopathy.

Even in asymptomatic patients, MRI evidence of spinal compression increases with age. One series identified spinal cord compression in 16% of asymptomatic patients under the age of 64 and in 26% of patients over the age of 64.[57] Serial MRI examinations may provide information regarding disease progression. Perioperative MRI has emerged as a method of patient outcome measurement. A 2011 study by Arvin et al. demonstrated that MRI scanning 6 months postoperatively is a valuable tool for prediction of patient functional outcomes at 1 year.[58] Ohshio and colleagues demonstrated that MRI findings correlated with histopathology of various spinal cord lesions.[59]

## SUMMARY

Cervical spondylotic myelopathy is the most common cause of cervical myelopathy. It results from a cascade of degenerative disorders resulting from the aging process. Collectively, these changes slowly begin to cause spinal stenosis and cord compression leading to progressive neurologic dysfunction. There is no one pathognomonic sign or symptom for CSM, making its diagnosis difficult. One study reported an average of 6.3 years from the onset of symptoms to diagnosis, with evidence linking poor patient outcomes to delays in diagnosis.[5] A thorough history and physical examination are critical to diagnosis. Several studies have examined history elements and physical examination findings, reporting on their incidence in myelopathic patients. Harrop et al. reported that the earliest and most common patient complaint is a sense of clumsiness or difficulty with gait, occurring in 90.74% of patients. Any hyperreflexia either in the upper or lower extremities is also extremely common (85.19%). In this series, the majority of patients with radiographically confirmed myelopathy displayed four myelopathic signs.[19] Although no single myelopathic physical examination finding will guarantee a diagnosis, a report by Rhee and colleagues demonstrated that 79% of patients displayed at least one myelopathic sign.[42] Imaging studies are also critical to diagnosis. Today, MRI represents the gold standard and will allow the clinician to rule out conditions in the differential diagnosis. Serial examinations can provide information about disease progression and guide treatment recommendations. Recently, MRI has also been validated as a predictor of patient outcome postoperatively.[58] No matter the specialty of the clinician, a thorough understanding of the history and physical examination findings associated with CSM is critical to early diagnosis and improved patient outcomes.

## REFERENCES


1. Rao R. Neck pain, cervical radiculopathy, and cervical myelopathy: pathophysiology, natural history, and clinical evaluation. J Bone Joint Surg Am. 2002;84-a(10):1872-81.
2. Brain WR, Northfield D, Wilkinson M. The neurological manifestations of cervical spondylosis. Brain. 1952;75(2):187-225.
3. Clarke E, Robinson PK. Cervical myelopathy: a complication of cervical spondylosis. Brain. 1956;79(3):483-510.
4. Lees F, Turner JW. Natural history and prognosis of cervical spondylosis. Br Med J. 1963;2(5373):1607-10.
5. Sadasivan KK, Reddy RP, Albright JA. The natural history of cervical spondylotic myelopathy. Yale J Biol Med. 1993; 66(3):235-42.
6. Parke WW. Correlative anatomy of cervical spondylotic myelopathy. Spine. 1988;13(7):831-7.
7. Singh K, An HS. Anterior cervical fusion: surgical techniques. Semin Spine Surg. 2004;16(4):245-54.
8. Arnold JG Jr. The clinical manifestations of spondylochondrosis (spondylosis) of the cervical spine. Ann Surg. 1955; 141(6):872-89.
9. Park AE. Imaging modalities for cervical myelopathy: Medical decision making and surgical outcomes. Semin Spine Surg. 2004;16(4):241-4.
10. Pavlov H, Torg JS, Robie B, et al. Cervical spinal stenosis: determination with vertebral body ratio method. Radiology. 1987;164(3):771-5.
11. Edwards WC, LaRocca SH. The developmental segmental sagittal diameter in combined cervical and lumbar spondylosis. Spine. 1985;10(1):42-9.
12. Singh A, Tetreault L, Fehlings MG, et al. Risk factors for development of cervical spondylotic myelopathy: results of a systematic review. Evid Based Spine Care J. 2012;3(3):35-42.
13. Matz PG, Anderson PA, Holly LT, et al. The natural history of cervical spondylotic myelopathy. J Neurosurg Spine. 2009;11(2):104-11.
14. Bohlman HH, Emery SE. The pathophysiology of cervical spondylosis and myelopathy. Spine. 1988;13(7):843-6.
15. Crandall PH, Batzdorf U. Cervical spondylotic myelopathy. J Neurosurg. 1966;25(1):57-66.
16. Ferguson RJ, Caplan LR. Cervical spondylitic myelopathy. Neurol Clin. 1985;3(2):373-82.
17. Rumi MN, Yoon ST. Cervical myelopathy history and physical examination. Semin Spine Surg. 2004;16(4):234-40.
18. Clark CR. Cervical spondylotic myelopathy: history and physical findings. Spine. 1988;13(7):847-9.
19. Harrop JS, Naroji S, Maltenfort M, et al. Cervical myelopathy: a clinical and radiographic evaluation and correlation to cervical spondylotic myelopathy. Spine (Phila Pa 1976). 2010;35(6):620-4.
20. Murray MT, Tay BKB. Natural history of cervical myelopathy. Semin Spine Surg. 2004;16(4):222-7.
21. Bernhardt M, Hynes RA, Blume HW, et al. Cervical spondylotic myelopathy. J Bone Joint Surg Am. 1993;75(1): 119-28.
22. Lebl DR, Hughes A, Cammisa FP Jr, et al. Cervical spondylotic myelopathy: pathophysiology, clinical presentation, and treatment. HSS J. 2011;7(2):170-8.
23. Micev AJ, Ivy AD, Aggarwal SK, et al. Cervical radiculopathy and myelopathy: presentations in the hand. J Hand Surg. 2013;38(12):2478-81; quiz 81.
24. Emery SE, Bohlman HH, Bolesta MJ, et al. Anterior cervical decompression and arthrodesis for the treatment of cervical spondylotic myelopathy. Two to seventeen-year follow-up. J Bone Joint Surg Am. 1998;80(7):941-51.
25. Salvi FJ, Jones JC, Weigert BJ. The assessment of cervical myelopathy. Spine J. 2006;6(6 Suppl):182S-9S.
26. Vigna FE, Tortolani PJ. Cervical myelopathy: differential diagnosis. Semin Spine Surg. 2004;16(4):228-33.
27. Maezawa Y, Uchida K, Baba H. Gait analysis of spastic walking in patients with cervical compressive myelopathy. J Orthop Sci. 2001;6(5):378-84.

28. Emery SE. Cervical spondylotic myelopathy: diagnosis and treatment. J Am Acad Orthop Surg. 2001;9(6):376-88.
29. Findlay GF, Balain B, Trivedi JM, et al. Does walking change the Romberg sign? Eur Spine J. 2009;18(10):1528-31.
30. Nurick S. The pathogenesis of the spinal cord disorder associated with cervical spondylosis. Brain. 1972;95(1):87-100.
31. Singh A, Crockard HA. Comparison of seven different scales used to quantify severity of cervical spondylotic myelopathy and post-operative improvement. J Outcome Meas. 2001;5(1):798-818.
32. Kanchandani R, Howe JG. Lhermitte's sign in multiple sclerosis: a clinical survey and review of the literature. J Neurol Neurosurg Psychiatry. 1982;45(4):308-12.
33. Maynard FM Jr, Bracken MB, Creasey G, et al. International standards for neurological and functional classification of spinal cord injury. American Spinal Injury Association. Spinal Cord. 1997;35(5):266-74.
34. Ditunno JF Jr. American spinal injury standards for neurological and functional classification of spinal cord injury: past, present and future. 1992 Heiner Sell Lecture of the American Spinal Injury Association. J Am Paraplegia Soc. 1994;17(1):7-11.
35. Walker HK. Deep tendon reflexes. In: Walker HK, Hall WD, Hurst JW (Eds). Clinical Methods: The History, Physical, and Laboratory Examinations. Boston: Butterworths Publishers;1990.
36. Tetreault LA, Kopjar B, Vaccaro A, et al. A clinical prediction model to determine outcomes in patients with cervical spondylotic myelopathy undergoing surgical treatment: data from the prospective, multi-center AOSpine North America study. J Bone Joint Surg Am. 2013;95(18):1659-66.
37. Lavelle WF, Bell GR. Cervical myelopathy: history and physical examination. Semin Spine Surg. 2007;19(1):6-11.
38. Kalsi-Ryan S, Singh A, Massicotte EM, et al. Ancillary outcome measures for assessment of individuals with cervical spondylotic myelopathy. Spine. 2013;38(22 Suppl 1):S111-22.
39. Shimizu T, Shimada H, Shirakura K. Scapulohumeral reflex (Shimizu). Its clinical significance and testing maneuver. Spine. 1993;18(15):2182-90.
40. Edwards CC 2nd, Riew KD, Anderson PA, et al. Cervical myelopathy. Current diagnostic and treatment strategies. Spine J. 2003;3(1):68-81.
41. Denno JJ, Meadows GR. Early diagnosis of cervical spondylotic myelopathy. A useful clinical sign. Spine. 1991; 16(12):1353-5.
42. Rhee JM, Heflin JA, Hamasaki T, et al. Prevalence of physical signs in cervical myelopathy: a prospective, controlled study. Spine. 2009;34(9):890-5.
43. Glaser JA, Cure JK, Bailey KL, et al. Cervical spinal cord compression and the Hoffmann sign. Iowa Orthop J. 2001; 21:49-52.
44. Ono K, Ebara S, Fuji T, et al. Myelopathy hand. New clinical signs of cervical cord damage. Journal Bone Joint Surg Br. 1987;69(2):215-9.
45. Dvorak J, Sutter M, Herdmann J. Cervical myelopathy: clinical and neurophysiological evaluation. Eur Spine J. 2003;12 (Suppl 2):S181-7.
46. McFarlin DE, McFarland HF. Multiple sclerosis (second of two parts). N Engl J Med. 1982;307(20):1246-51.
47. McFarlin DE, McFarland HF. Multiple sclerosis (first of two parts). N Engl J Med. 1982;307(19):1183-8.
48. Rowland LP, Shneider NA. Amyotrophic lateral sclerosis. N Engl J Med. 2001;344(22):1688-700.
49. Nathan DM. Long-term complications of diabetes mellitus. N Engl J Med. 1993;328(23):1676-85.
50. England JD, Gronseth GS, Franklin G, et al. Distal symmetric polyneuropathy: a definition for clinical research: report of the American Academy of Neurology, the American Association of Electrodiagnostic Medicine, and the American Academy of Physical Medicine and Rehabilitation. Neurology. 2005;64(2):199-207.
51. Partanen J, Niskanen L, Lehtinen J, et al. Natural history of peripheral neuropathy in patients with non-insulin-dependent diabetes mellitus. N Engl J Med. 1995;333(2): 89-94.
52. Roy AK, Slimack NP, Ganju A. Idiopathic syringomyelia: retrospective case series, comprehensive review, and update on management. Neurosurg Focus. 2011;31(6):E15.
53. Winer JB. An update in Guillain-Barré syndrome. Autoimmune Dis. 2014;2014:793024.
54. Winer JB, Hughes RA, Osmond C. A prospective study of acute idiopathic neuropathy. I. Clinical features and their prognostic value. J Neurol Neurosurg Psychiatry. 1988;51(5):605-12.
55. Rosseau G. Normal pressure hydrocephalus. Dis Mon. 2011;57(10):615-24.
56. Tetreault LA, Dettori JR, Wilson JR, et al. Systematic review of magnetic resonance imaging characteristics that affect treatment decision making and predict clinical outcome in patients with cervical spondylotic myelopathy. Spine. 2013;38(22 Suppl 1):S89-110.
57. Sung RD, Wang JC. Correlation between a positive Hoffmann's reflex and cervical pathology in asymptomatic individuals. Spine. 2001;26(1):67-70.
58. Arvin B, Kalsi-Ryan S, Karpova A, et al. Postoperative magnetic resonance imaging can predict neurological recovery after surgery for cervical spondylotic myelopathy: a prospective study with blinded assessments. Neurosurgery. 2011;69(2):362-8.
59. Ohshio I, Hatayama A, Kaneda K, et al. Correlation between histopathologic features and magnetic resonance images of spinal cord lesions. Spine. 1993;18(9):1140-9.

Chapter 5

# Electrodiagnostics

*Athena Lolis, Anna Shor, Aleksandar Beric*

## DIAGNOSTIC AND PROGNOSTIC ROLE OF ELECTRODIAGNOSIS IN CERVICAL MYELOPATHY

The assessment of cervical myelopathy can be challenging. The diagnosis is even more difficult when there is a discrepancy between the clinical findings and imaging findings, or if two or more different disorders affecting the cervical spine are present, ultimately causing both spinal cord and segmental nerve root lesions.

Neurophysiologic assessment plays a major role in such cases, assessing the functional status of both the central and peripheral components of the nervous system. Somatosensory-evoked potentials (SEPs) and motor-evoked potentials (MEPs) assess the integrity of the central nervous system, whereas nerve conduction studies (NCS) with electromyography (EMG) assess the peripheral component. These modalities are the most useful supplemental tests for the evaluation of cervical myelopathy. These investigations help to distinguish between cervical cord, nerve root, brachial plexus, and peripheral nerve lesions. Additionally, they can also help in establishing the underlying mechanism (demyelination vs. axonal loss), severity, and location of the dysfunction. The electrodiagnostic studies can also be used to monitor the disease progression.[1]

The role of testing does not end in the outpatient setting. Once a decision is made to proceed with surgical decompression and spine stabilization in patients with cervical myelopathy, the tools of clinical neurophysiology are also implemented and pertinent throughout the procedure in ensuring that the integrity of the neuroaxis is maintained. Intraoperative neurophysiologic monitoring (IOM) provides the surgeon with immediate feedback and warning before permanent spinal cord or nerve injury has occurred. This has been shown to increase safety and improve outcomes in complex spine surgeries, minimizing any subsequent neurologic deficit.

## EVOKED POTENTIALS IN DIAGNOSIS OF CERVICAL MYELOPATHY

### Somatosensory-Evoked Potentials

Somatosensory-evoked potentials are used to directly assess the function of the posterior spinal cord somatosensory system and indirectly assess the whole spinal cord at a particular level. Somatosensory-evoked potentials are elicited by electrical stimulation applied through the skin to stimulate underlying peripheral nerves. The nerves used in the workup of cervical myelopathy include the posterior tibial from the lower limbs and the median and the ulnar nerves from the upper limbs. The electrical impulses start and propagate through the peripheral nerve, then enter the spinal cord through the cervical roots and travel up the dorsal columns-medial lemniscal system. The potentials are recorded from the contralateral somatosensory cortex in respect to the side of stimulation. Somatosensory-evoked potential components include a series of positive (P) and negative (N) deflections, which are labeled based on their latency and polarity. Depending on latencies and amplitude of the different peaks recorded along the pathway, the localization of the lesion can be made. In radicular and spinal disease, several nerves supplied by different segments must be stimulated to establish an approximate level of cervical spinal cord lesion (Figs. 5.1 and 5.2).[2,3]

The major criteria for abnormality of the SEP test are an absence of main components, abnormal prolongation of latencies, and prolonged interpeak intervals. Additionally, a side-to-side comparison is important, particularly to establish any amplitude asymmetry. Somatosensory-evoked potential abnormalities seen in myelopathy typically will consist of poorly formed responses with prolonged latencies or a complete absence of responses in more severe lesions.[2]

Somatosensory-evoked potentials have also a value in the differential diagnosis of cervical myelopathy,

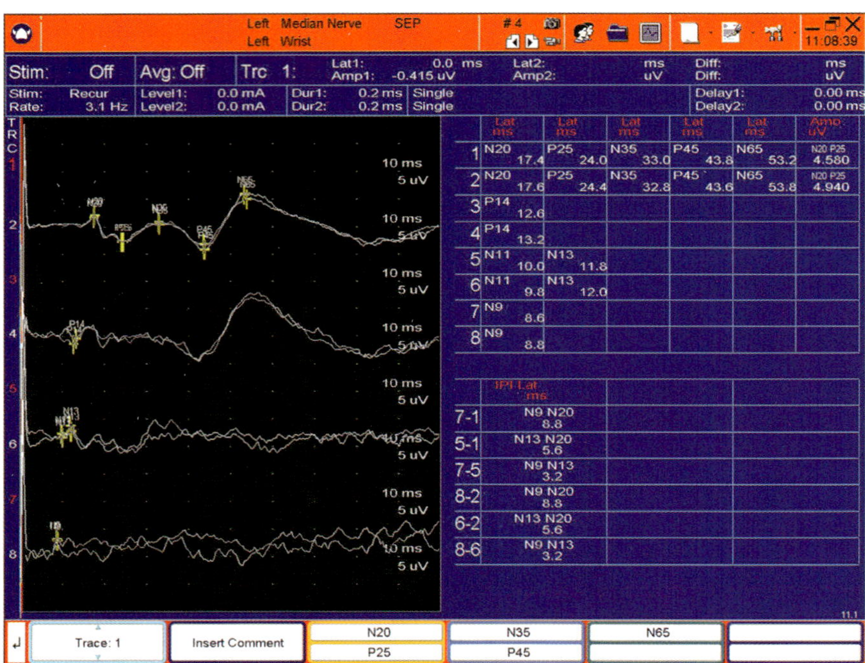


**Fig. 5.1:** Median nerve somatosensory-evoked potential. The top trace is the primary somatosensory cortex recording showing the typical complex waveform of several peaks with the initial negative peak N20. The second trace from the top is the subcortical recording. The third trace from the top is the cervical recording showing N11 and N13 cervical components. The bottom trace is the brachial plexus recording showing N9 negative peak. The right side shows peak latencies and amplitudes for two repetitions including inter-peak latencies.

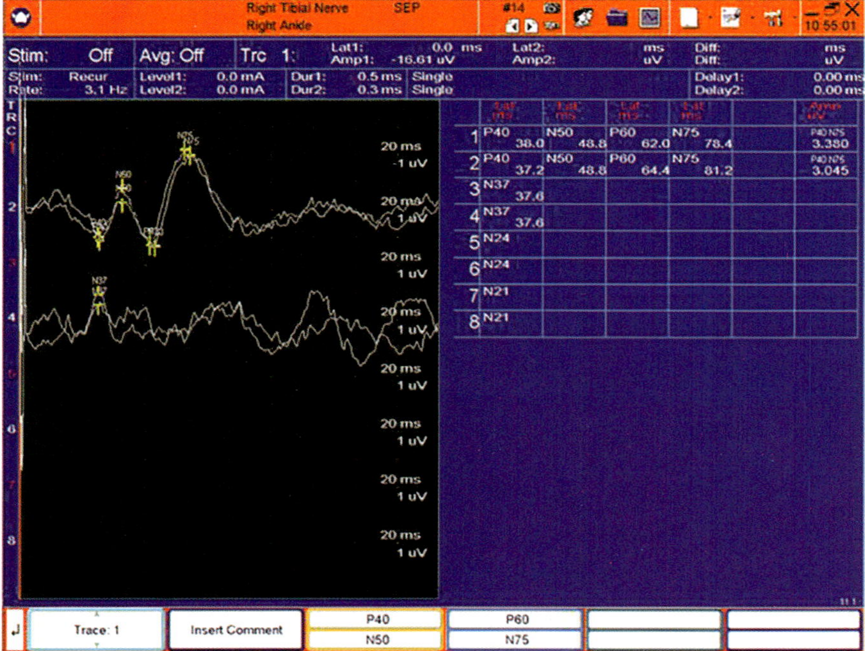


**Fig. 5.2:** Tibial nerve somatosensory-evoked potential. The top trace is the primary somatosensory cortex recording showing the typical "W" waveform with the initial P40 positive peak. The second trace is the primary somatosensory cortex from a different montage.

particularly with motor neuron disorders. Severe SEP abnormalities in patients with spastic weakness are consistent with cervical myelopathy rather than motor neuron disease.

There are many limitations of SEPs. Since SEPs only assess the posterior part of the spinal cord, they could be entirely normal in anterolateral spinal cord lesions. Also, SEPs are not a sensitive test and can be normal despite significant sensory deficits, since many parallel afferent somatosensory pathways such as the anterior spinothalamic tract in addition to dorsal column tracts can carry signals to the brain. Furthermore, there are technical limitations since the recorded signals are very small, requiring multiple stimulations and averaging process in order to extract the SEPs from the other brain electrical activity and external noise. The success of SEP recording also depends on the patient's cooperation as poor relaxation increases scalp EMG activity, which in turn interferes with SEP activity recognition.

### Motor-Evoked Potentials

Motor-evoked potentials are used to assess the integrity and function of the corticospinal tract. A method of transcranial high-voltage electrical stimulation of the cerebral cortex was introduced in 1980 by Merton and Morton,[4] followed by the introduction of practically painless magnetic stimulation for the same purpose of obtaining MEPs by Barker et al. in 1985.[5] They applied short magnetic pulses to the scalp over the motor cortex and recorded muscle action potentials from upper and lower limb muscles, resulting from propagation of electrical impulses through the descending corticospinal pathway and corresponding peripheral nerves. Motor-evoked potentials used in cervical myelopathy are generally recorded at the following muscles: deltoid, biceps brachii, triceps brachii, abductor pollicis, and tibialis anterior muscles. The same principle of segmental innervation of these muscles as in afferent nerves stimulated for the SEPs is applied in order to establish the level of spinal cord lesion.

Motor-evoked potentials are frequently abnormal in patients with cervical myelopathy. The prolongation of latency, configuration changes between two sites of recording, and decreased amplitude of the MEP, as well as absence of response in the more severe conditions, establish the level and degree of the spinal cord compromise.[2,6]

Considering the current availability of high-resolution magnetic imaging, the use of MEPs in the outpatient setting has become more limited in the evaluation of cervical myelopathy. Motor-evoked potentials are still a useful and important tool in cases of equivocal neuroimaging, providing neurophysiological evidence of a corticospinal conduction defect. It is also important in situations when multiple lesions present on magnetic resonance imaging, helping to determine the particular lesion causing dysfunction, or in demonstrating that the level of corticospinal conduction defect is above a suspected lesion on spinal imaging, thus ruling out the relevance of the lesion to the patient's condition.

There are many limitations of MEPs as a diagnostic tool. These limitations include lack of normative data for MEP amplitude and latencies values (due to significant variability); stimulation that elicits painful involuntary contraction of the muscles of the body, making it hard to tolerate for the patient; and the variety of potential (even though rare) adverse effects, including seizures, cardiac arrhythmia, adverse neuropsychologic effects, headaches, endocrine disturbance, and tongue lacerations. In summary, this is a modality that is rarely used in the outpatient setting today.

## NERVE CONDUCTION STUDIES AND EMG

Nerve conduction studies and EMG can be helpful in clarifying the diagnosis of cervical myelopathy as well as detecting the presence of other pathology, such as superimposed nerve root (or multiple roots) or nerve entrapment, plexus disorder, or motor neuron disease.

### Nerve Conduction Study

The NCS consists of the following components: motor NCS, sensory NCS and F-wave study.[3] Motor NCS is performed by electrical stimulation of a peripheral nerve with recording from a muscle supplied by this nerve. The elicited response recorded from the muscle is called the compound muscle action potential (CMAP). It provides a physiologic assessment of the descending motor axons in the pathway below the level of stimulation, the neuromuscular junction, and the muscle fibers activated by the stimulus. Compound muscle action potentials are useful in providing objective measurements of the extent and type of weakness, as well as establishing the site of the lesion, distinguishing between peripheral nerve disease, neuromuscular junction disease, and disease of the muscle. Even though the motor NCS assess the distal portion of the motor pathway, it is important to note that in cases of spinal cord lesion, like cervical myelopathy, where the

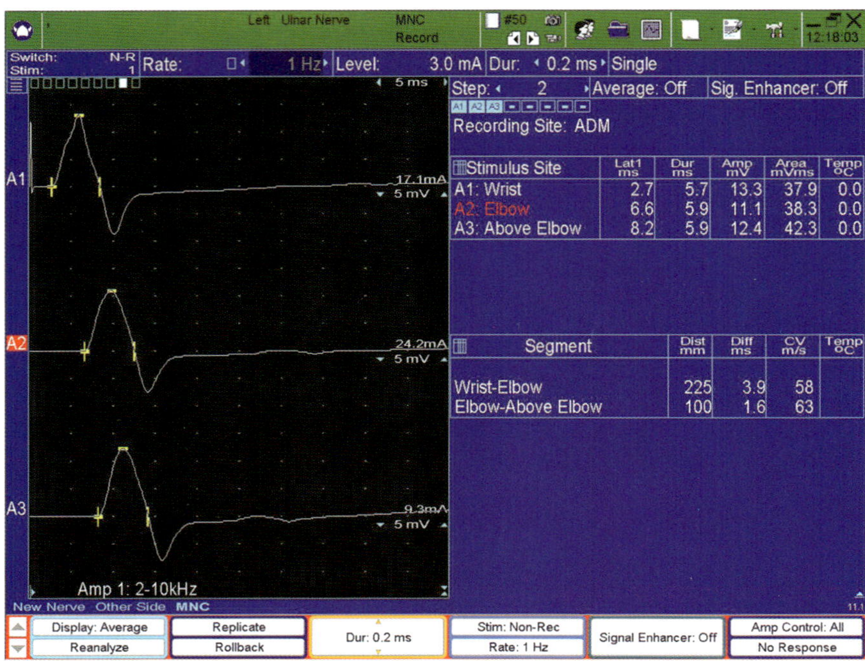


**Fig. 5.3:** Ulnar nerve motor conduction study with stimulation at three different points along the arm. The top trace depicts the compound muscle action potential from the most distal stimulation at the wrist. The middle trace shows stimulation below the elbow. The bottom trace is the stimulation above the elbow. The latencies of the onset, amplitudes of the responses, and conduction velocities are shown.

anterior horn cell are affected, the motor NCS may demonstrate low amplitude proportional to the degree of muscle atrophy and loss of motor neurons (Fig. 5.3).

Sensory NCS is performed by electrical stimulation of a peripheral nerve and recording from a purely sensory portion of the nerve. It is important to pointout that in contrast to motor conduction studies, in which CMAP reflects conduction along motor nerve, neuromuscular junction, and muscle fibers, only nerve fibers are assessed in sensory conduction studies, hence the synonym electroneurography. Since the bodies of the sensory nerves located outside the spinal cord, in the dorsal root ganglia, any lesion of the nerve root leaves the dorsal root ganglion and its peripheral axon intact. Consequently, the sensory NCS will be normal despite the patient's sensory symptoms in the corresponding dermatome, if the lesion is proximal to the dorsal root ganglia. In cases of cervical myelopathy, the sensory NCS will be normal, unless there is a concomitant compression in the periphery such as one from the carpal tunnel or cubital tunnel, the most common compressive neuropathies that exist in the population (Fig. 5.4).

The F-response is elicited by propagation of an electrical impulse antidromically up to the spinal cord, to the anterior horn cell, and subsequently activating small population of anterior horn cells. The activated anterior horn cells in turn fire an action potential that travels orthodromically down the same nerve past the stimulation site to the muscle. Distinct delay of the F-waves or a reduced number of clearly distinguishable F-waves in association with normal distal motor conduction is a sign of a proximal lesion. F-responses are mostly useful for identifying acute polyradiculopathy such as in Guillain-Barré syndrome and are usually normal in mild cases of radiculopathy, because almost all muscles are supplied by at least two, if not three, nerve roots. In the case of cervical myelopathy, there should be no difference in the F-wave latencies when compared to normal subjects unless there is underlying cervical radiculopathy, which could impair peripheral conduction.

## Needle EMG

Electromyography is a diagnostic tool that evaluates the integrity and condition of the muscle and the nerve that supplies that muscle.[3] It is performed by inserting a needle containing a recording electrode into the muscle. The electrical activity picked up by the electrode is then

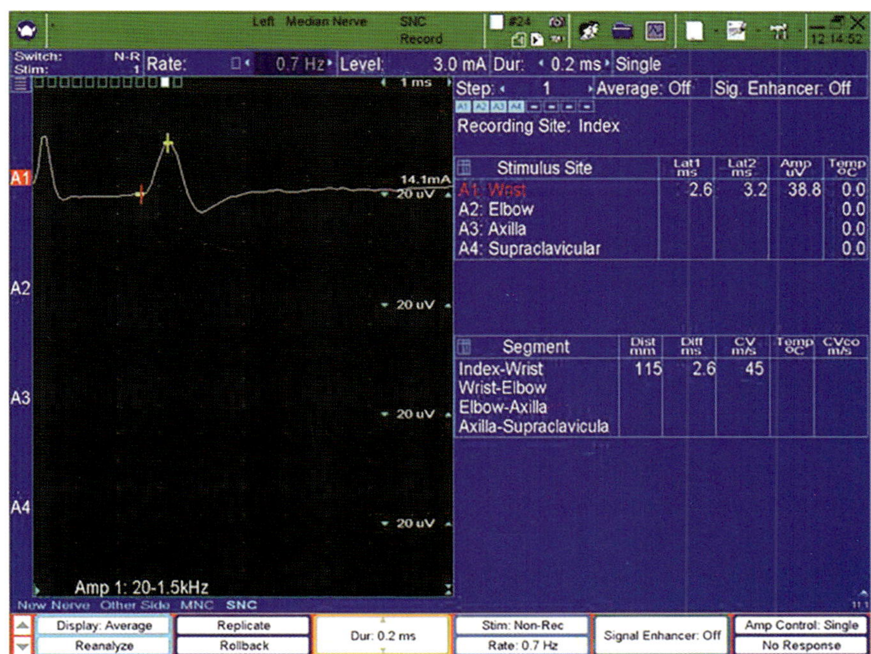


**Fig. 5.4:** Median nerve sensory conduction study. The trace depicts the sensory nerve action potential (SNAP) with the latency and amplitude of the response with stimulation at the wrist. The second table on the lower right depicts the calculated conduction velocity of the median nerve across the hand.

displayed on an oscilloscope. An audio-amplifier is used so the activity can be heard. Electromyography measures the electrical activity of a muscle during rest, slight contraction, and forceful contraction. Interpretation of the EMG involves evaluating the muscle at rest, where any abnormal insertional activity and abnormal spontaneous activity is first assessed (Fig. 5.5). Abnormalities include the presence of fibrillation, positive sharp waves, and fasciculation. Then the motor unit action potentials (MUAP) are evaluated, specifically looking at their duration, shape, and amplitude. Finally, the recruitment pattern is assessed, looking for any loss of motor units (Fig. 5.6).

In pure cervical myelopathy, the only EMG abnormality should be the upper motor neuron type of recruitment pattern. This consists of "loss" of MUAP due to irregular and decreased firing rate. The clinical utility of performing an EMG in the evaluation of cervical myelopathy is really in differential diagnosis and to evaluate for possible concurrent motor neuron disease, radiculopathy, or neuropathy. The findings of increased insertional activity, positive sharp waves, fibrillations, fasciculation, and diminished motor unit recruitment, which are all signs of denervation, can be seen in any of these lesions. The EMG is also helpful in prognostication by establishing the presence of reinnervation process, its degree, and its extent.

Since degenerative processes like spondylosis and intervertebral disk herniation are the most common causes of cervical myelopathy, they can also frequently cause an impingement of the cervical nerve roots. In such circumstances, the clinical presentation may be very similar to amyotrophic lateral sclerosis, with both lower motor neuron signs in arms (atrophy, wasting, loss of reflexes) and upper motor neuron signs distally (leg hyper-reflexia, spastic gait and weakness, urinary frequency, etc.). The role of electrodiagnostics and especially EMG is invaluable in such cases, helping to differentiate between cervical radiculomyelopathy, where surgical decompression is a treatment of choice, and motor neuron disease, in which surgery should be avoided and if done, usually causes further deterioration with respiratory complications including precipitous demise.

## INTRAOPERATIVE NEUROPHYSIOLOGIC MONITORING IN CERVICAL MYELOPATHY

Serious neurologic injuries can be frequently encountered no matter how carefully surgery involving the spinal cord is performed. In addition to congenital and acquired deformities of the spine and relatively rare spinal tumors, common degenerative spine diseases within the aging general population contribute to a growing number of pathologies with myelopathies. This is important because antecedent myelopathy increases spinal cord risk during surgical treatment.[7]

Intraoperative neurophysiologic monitoring was born when SEPs were first used to monitor the spinal cord during scoliosis surgery in 1970s, as reported by Nash et al. in 1977 and Engler et al. in 1978. Since then IOM has become an integral part of spinal surgery, as it helps in preventing intraoperative injuries as well as identifying potential injuries as information is obtained quickly for assessment and immediate mitigating efforts such as administering steroids and increasing blood pressure. Intraoperative monitoring plays a role in many aspects of surgery to the spine, including cervical, thoracic, lumbar, and scoliosis surgeries. For surgeries involving the cervical spine, where the most serious complication is quadriplegia, the commonly used modalities are SEPs, MEPs, and free-running EMG. Sutter et al. concluded that in contrast to any single modality, multimodal intraoperative monitoring is an effective method of monitoring the spinal cord functional integrity during spine surgery and can, therefore, lead to a reduction of neurological deficits and consequently improve postoperative results.[8] This is especially important in surgeries involving treatment of cervical myelopathy where the chronic compression may cause hypoperfusion and subsequent decompression may result in stretching of the spinal cord, and even reperfusion-related negative events can occur as a result.

It is important to note that intraoperative monitoring used in the operating room is not used for diagnostic purposes. Instead of comparing the information obtained to normative data, each patient essentially serves as his or her own control. Depending on which modality is requested by the surgeon, the results are taken and then an effective baseline is set. Repeated real time data are then collected at appropriate time intervals and certain alarm criteria are followed. Any changes from the baseline are then reported to the surgeon.

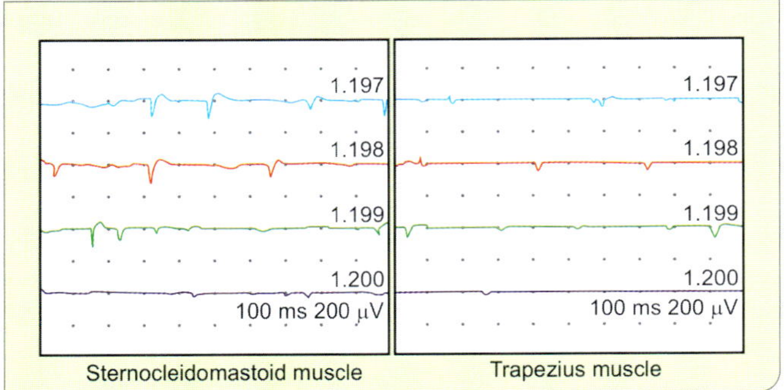


**Fig. 5.5:** Electromyography activity at rest. The traces show positive sharp wave activity, which are signs of an active denervation process.

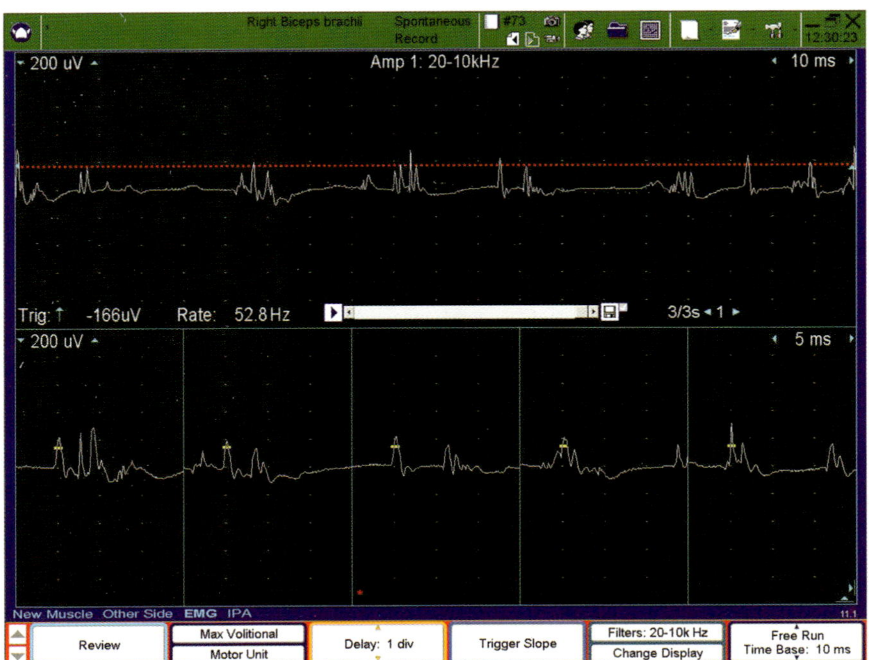


**Fig. 5.6:** Electromyography activity during voluntary activation-contraction.

## Somatosensory-Evoked Potentials

Somatosensory-evoked potentials are the most frequently used intraoperative method for monitoring the integrity of the dorsal column medial lemniscal pathway, which is the sensory pathway of the central nervous system. Monitoring of SEPs during cervical spine surgery has been found to be sensitive for detecting possible neurological insult caused by mechanical stress, surgical manipulation, hypotension, and ischemia.[9] The use of SEPs is of special clinical significance while performing surgery for cervical myelopathy. Typically, the posterior portion of the spinal cord, or the dorsal columns, are indirectly compressed from anterior compression or directly compressed from ligamentum flavum hypertrophy. This will typically result in prolongation of the conduction in the recordings from the upper extremities. If the myelopathy is severe enough, there will often be no response or a poorly formed and poorly repeatable response from the lower extremity stimulation.

### *Anatomy*

The first-order neurons are large, myelinated, and rapidly conducting, whose cells are located in the dorsal root ganglia and receive information from touch or joint position receptors. Their axons ascend ipsilaterally to the medulla where they synapse with second-order neurons, which are located in the caudal medulla. Their axons decussate and form the medial leminscus, which then ascends along the contralateral brainstem projecting to the ventral posterolateral (VPL) nucleus of the thalamus. The third-order neurons are in the VPL where the axons are then sent through the posterior limb of the internal capsule to the somatosensory cortex areas 3, 1, and 2.

### *Technique*

For cervical spine surgeries, the nerves that are stimulated to obtain SEPs are the tibial nerve, median nerve, and ulnar nerve. A pair of electrodes that is used for stimulation is typically stick-on pads that have a diameter of 2 cm with the cathode placed proximal to the anode. For the median nerve stimulation, the pads are placed over the median nerve at the wrist, 2 cm proximal to the wrist crease. Ulnar nerve pads are placed 2 cm proximal to the wrist crease and along the ulnar side. For tibial nerve stimulation, the cathode is typically placed at the ankle behind the medial malleolus. For the upper extremities, constant current stimulation with rectangular pulses of 300 ms and a frequency of 3.1 Hz and a time base of 50 ms is used. For the lower extremity SEP stimulation, constant current stimulation with rectangular pulses of 500 ms and a frequency of 2 Hz and a time base of 100 ms is used. In both upper and lower stimulation, the intensity is adjusted until a moderate twitch of hand intrinsic or foot intrinsic muscles, respectively, is achieved.

Recording electrodes that capture the SEP response as it reaches the post-central gyrus of the somatosensory cortex are corkscrew or subdermal needles. Somatosensory-evoked potentials are recorded using multichannel derivation-montages of cortical and subcortical responses. The recording sites are based on positions of the 10–20 International System of EEG electrode placement. All the wires are connected to neurophysiologic intraoperative monitoring machine, which has a 16–32 channel amplifier where the filtered and averaged EEG activity is being displayed using IOM software onto a PC.

For cervical surgery, the standard SEP setup consists of bilateral median and ulnar nerve stimulation for the upper extremities and bilateral tibial nerve stimulation that monitors neural integrity of the fibers from the lower extremities.

### *Interpretation*

For the upper extremity SEP recordings (Figs. 5.7 to 5.9), N13 is the potential seen as the fibers synapse in the dorsal horn of the cervical spinal cord. Other large fibers cross and travel in the medial lemniscus to the thalamus. N20 and P25, which is the subsequent negativity-positivity, is generated in the primary somatosensory cortex. Tibial nerve SEPs travel in the peripheral nerve through the lumbosacral plexus to the cauda equina and conus medullaris where they generate the negative potential. After that, they enter the dorsal columns of spinal cord and, when traversing the cervical spinal cord, generate a travelling negative wave that can be recorded over the neck, and ultimately cross to the opposite side at the caudal medullary level and travel to VPL and generate P40 wave when the ascending volley reaches the primary somatosensory foot cortex.

Alarm criteria that are concerning for possible neurologic injury include a >10% prolongation in the latency and a >50% reduction in the amplitude.[10]

In patients with severe and chronic myelopathy, often SEPs are not measurable. When they are present, they are not well formed in the upper extremities and can be absent altogether in the lower extremities. Another

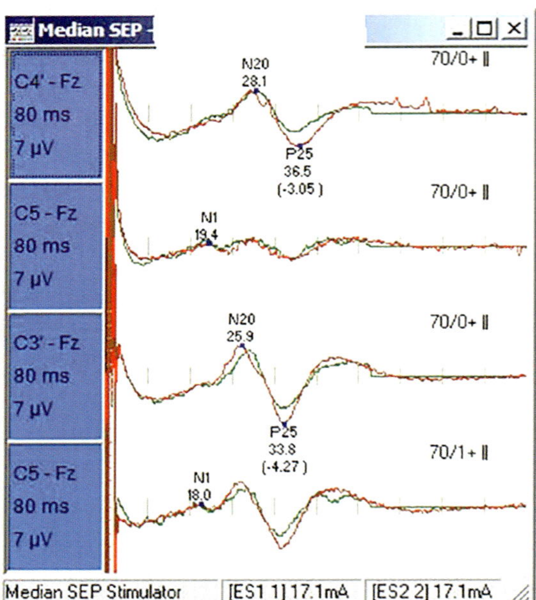


**Fig. 5.7:** Median nerve somatosensory-evoked potential during intraoperative neurophysiologic monitoring. The top trace is the left median nerve primary somatosensory cortex recording. The second trace is the left median nerve cervical recording. The third trace is the right median nerve primary somatosensory cortex recording. The last trace is the right median nerve cervical recording. Two repetitions are shown; the baseline and superimposed is the active recording. The N20 latency on the cortical recording is the response that is followed throughout the procedure, while N1 is used as the control response for the appropriate spinal cord and brain input.

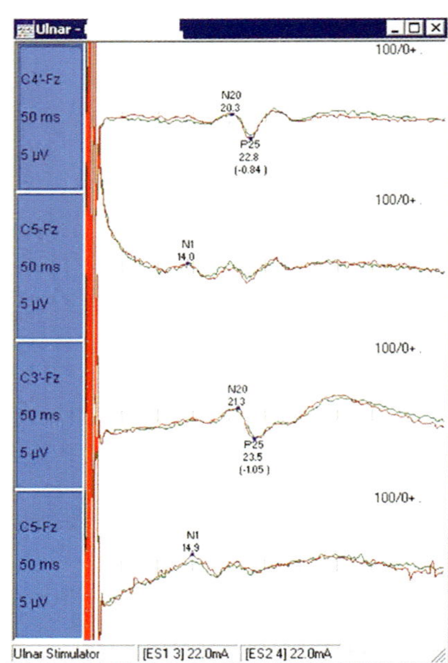


**Fig. 5.8:** Ulnar nerve somatosensory-evoked potential during intraoperative neurophysiologic monitoring. The traces and the waveforms are similar as described in Figure 5.7; however, the input is through different cervical spine roots.

frequent condition that can also affect the SEPs is polyneuropathy. Using this modality alone during surgery on a myelopathic cervical spine can often be inefficient. Additionally, the lack of specificity of SEP monitoring has prompted the additional use of MEP monitoring during cervical decompression.

## Motor-Evoked Potentials

Motor-evoked potentials are generated by motor cortex stimulation through the scalp with recording compound MUAP from the peripheral muscle groups, allowing assessment of the entire motor axis. Motor-evoked potentials were Food and Drug Administration-approved in 2002 and are used to monitor the integrity of the corticospinal tracts. They serve a complementary role to conventional SEPs, especially in the case of cervical myelopathy, where the incidence of having abnormal SEPs is high. The use of MEPs in monitoring for cervical myelopathy is also important as they are a reflection of the neural integrity of the anterior portion of the spinal cord. Anterior spinal cord compression in cervical myelopathy typically comes from direct compression by the ossification of the posterior longitudinal ligament. The presence or absence of MEPs in cervical myelopathy will depend on the degree of compromise of the spinal cord.

### *Anatomy*

The nerve fibers that make up the corticospinal tract arise from the cell bodies of the pyramidal cells in layer V of the motor cortex. Their axons make up the fibers that travel through the internal capsule and the cerebral peduncle as they make their way to the medulla where they cross over to form the spinal portion of the corticospinal tract. These upper motor neurons will then travel through the white matter of the spinal cord and reach the corresponding vertebral level of the muscles that they innervate. At this point they will depolarize alpha motor neurons, which in turn propagate action potential through their corresponding motor axon to the corresponding muscles and generate the muscle MEP.

### *Technique*

Stimulating transcranial electrodes usually consist of corkscrews that are placed in the scalp according to the 10–20 EEG classification system over the motor cortex

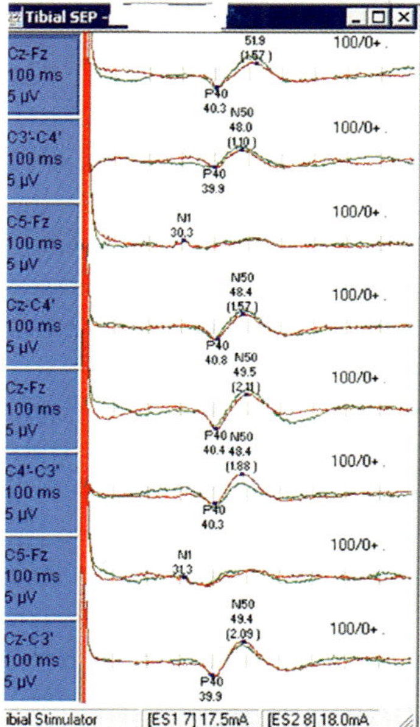


**Fig. 5.9:** Tibial nerve somatosensory-evoked potential during intraoperative neurophysiologic monitoring. The top two traces are from the left tibial nerve primary somatosensory cortex recording. The third trace is the left tibial nerve cervical recording. The fourth and fifth traces are from the right tibial nerve primary somatosensory cortex recording. The last trace is the right tibial nerve cervical recording. Two repetitions are again shown; the baseline and superimposed is the active recording. The P40 latency on the cortical recording is the response that is followed throughout the procedure, while N1 is used as the control response for the appropriate spinal cord and brain input.

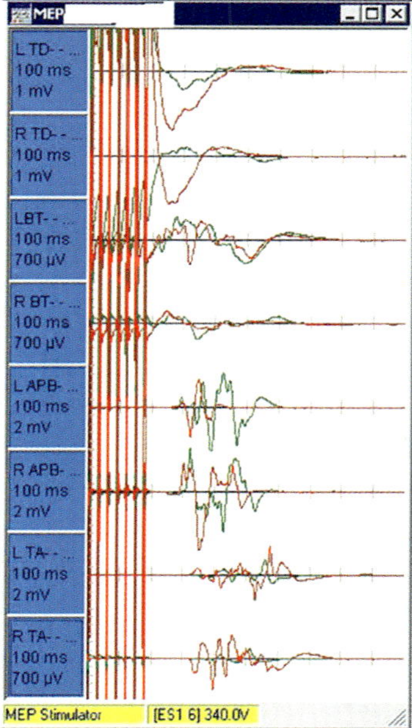


**Fig. 5.10:** Motor-evoked potential response during intraoperative neurophysiologic monitoring. The top two traces show the left and right trapezius and deltoid responses. The next two traces show the left and right biceps brachii and triceps brachii responses. The fifth and sixth traces show the left and right abductor pollicis brevis responses. The last two traces depict the left and right tibialis anterior responses. There are well-formed muscle responses present from the bilateral abductor pollicis brevis and tibialis anterior muscles.

areas. A stimulus is then delivered to the motor cortex via a short train of 5–7 stimuli that are spaced about 4 ms apart. Typically the single pulse duration in the train is anywhere from 0.3 to 0.5 ms and the maximum voltage delivered is not >400 V for most commercial IOM machines, unless a separate transcranial electrical stimulator is used that can deliver very short pulses in trains with up to 1500 V. The motor cortex is stimulated and the descending responses traverse the cortical spinal tract, where a measurable response is generated in the form of muscle activity recorded from the straight subdermal needles that are placed in the bellies of the abductor pollicis brevis, triceps brachii, biceps brachii, deltoid, trapezius, and tibialis anterior muscles. This ultimately provides information about the upper and lower extremity motor function.

### *Interpretation*

The presence of MEP responses (Fig. 5.10) is best described by the "all or none" criterion. What this means is that MEP responses are documented as being present or absent independent of what the stimulation voltage is. Of note, when the MEPs at the start of the procedure have very high thresholds in order to be obtained, their presence should be documented to the surgeon as unreliable. Often, after exposure is completed and the surgery is under way, any change such as a slight drop in blood pressure, blood loss, and/or accumulation of anesthetic will result in more voltage necessary in order to elicit the MEP response, thus quickly surpassing the allowable amount of voltage that can be safely delivered, and eventually the MEP will be unable to be obtained. If the surgeon is informed from the baseline that MEPs are not reliable, then an IOM plan (e.g. the need for a wake-up test) can be discussed and avoided in the event that the MEP response is no longer present.

In patients with cervical myelopathy, often there are no muscle responses able to be elicited with direct cortical stimulation. One theory is that the chronic compression that is producing the myelopathy has already caused irreversible ischemia to the spinal cord.

## Electromyography

Spontaneous EMG monitors the integrity of the nerve root of a particular level of the spinal cord. Electromyography of the cervical roots typically is not affected by cervical myelopathy, unless the etiology of the myelopathy is related to severe central canal stenosis. If the stenosis is severe enough, it may by way of foraminal stenosis cause a multilevel radiculopathy distal to the compression. Obtaining NCS and EMG prior to the operative setting in these cases is important as they will delineate the presence of any peripheral involvement in addition to the central cord dysfunction.

### *Technique*

The muscles that are selected have the innervation of the levels that are part of the surgical plan. For cervical surgery, this should include the trapezius (XI and C4), deltoid (C5 and C6), biceps brachii (C5 and C6), triceps brachii (C6 and C7), and abductor pollicis brevis (C8 and/or T1). There is always some overlap in the spinal segments chosen. Sterile recording needles are placed in the bellies of the above-mentioned muscles. They are then connected to an amplifier, which can be on any commercial intraoperative monitoring machine. Alarm criteria include detection of any spikes, bursts or trains of EMG activity in corresponding muscles.

In cervical myelopathy, there should be no abnormalities seen in the baseline EMG recordings. As the surgery proceeds, firing may be seen as a result of manipulation, distraction, or decompression. The use of cautery can also interfere with the recordings.

## Anesthesia Requirements

Reliable interpretation of SEP and MEP responses during cervical spine surgery is dependent on suitable anesthetic protocols. Volatile anesthetic agents such as isoflurane suppress both SEP and especially MEP potentials. Neuromuscular depolarizing agents will effectively paralyze the patient and suppress any motor unit activation, ultimately leading to the absence of any evoked MEP response as well as giving a false-negative response for any EMG activity. The most favorable anesthetic regimen for intraoperative recordings is total intravenous anesthesia consisting of constant infusion of propofol and fentanyl.

## Intraoperative Monitoring Changes

As previously mentioned, during IOM, depending on which modalities are chosen, a baseline recording is obtained at the start of the procedure and subsequent traces are then compared to the original one. If alarm criteria are met, a series of questions should be asked and investigated in a time-critical manner prior to alarming the surgeon. There are many factors that can influence IOM monitoring modalities.

The first question to be raised should be what the patient's blood pressure is. Changes in blood pressure can result in an alteration of the waveform, including lowering of the amplitude, which can be reversed when perfusion is restored. Additionally, a lower blood pressure will also affect cerebral perfusion pressure, and can result in an increased threshold for obtaining an MEP response, or may result in a temporary loss of the MEP as well. Careful attention to the amount of blood loss sustained during the procedures is necessary, as blood loss can inadvertently affect the overall blood pressure and oxygenation of neurons.

The patient's core body temperature should also be checked. A lower temperature will cause the SEP latency to be prolonged. Inadvertently, it may also limit the metabolism of certain anesthetic agents that are being used, which can also affect all monitoring modalities.

The last factor to check, but usually the most frequent reason for loss of MEPs as well as SEPs, is any changes in the anesthesia, such as adding a bolus of anesthetic agent. The addition of neuromuscular blockade will essentially make MEP responses difficult to obtain and also affect the free-running EMG, as no bursts will be seen in case of inadvertent root manipulation. A patient's level of depth of anesthesia should also be carefully checked, e.g. with a BiSpectral Index (BIS) monitor, as readings that are too high or too low can make SEP and MEP responses difficult to obtain. After all this information is quickly obtained and analyzed in correlation to the SEP and MEP changes, the findings are communicated to the surgeon and the anesthesia team and appropriate mitigating steps can be taken in order to avoid impending complications.

## REFERENCES

1. Frank JS, Jones JC, Weigert BJ. The assessment of cervical myelopathy. Spine J. 2006;6(Suppl):S182-9.

2. Dvorak J, Sutter M, Herdmann J. Cervical myelopathy: clinical and neurophysiological evaluation. Eur Spine J. 2003; 12(Suppl 2):S181-7.
3. Daube J, Rubin D. Clinical Neurophysiology, 3rd edition. New York: Oxford; 2009.
4. Merton PA, Morton HB. Stimulation of the cerebral cortex in the intact human subject. Nature. 1980;285:277.
5. Barker AT, Freeston IL, Alinous R, et al. Magnetic stimulation of the human brain. J Physiol. 1985;369:3.
6. Kameyama O, Shibano K, Kawakita H, et al. Transcranial magnetic stimulation of the motor cortex in cervical spondylosis and spinal canal stenosis. Spine. 1985;20: 1004-10.
7. Sutter M, Deletis V, Tamaki T. Current opinions and recommendations on multimodal intraoperative monitoring during spine surgeries. Eur Spine J. 2007;16(Suppl 2):S232-7.
8. Sutter M, Eggspuhler A, Muller A, et al. Multimodal intraoperative monitoring: an overview of proposed methodology based on 1017 cases. Eur Spine J. 2007;16(Suppl 2):S153-61.
9. Bose B, Sestokas AK, Schwartz DM. Neurophysiologic monitoring of spinal cord function during instrumented anterior cervical fusion. Spine J. 2004;4:202-7.
10. Toleikis JR. Intraoperative monitoring using somatosensory evoked potentials. A position statement by the American Society of Neurophysiologic Monitoring. ASNM Website. December 2010.

# Section 2

# Outcomes

Chapter 6

# Natural History of Cervical Spondylotic Myelopathy

*Christopher D Witiw, Michael G Fehlings*

## INTRODUCTION

Cervical spondylotic myelopathy (CSM) is recognized worldwide as the most common cause of spinal cord impairment.[1] This degenerative condition leads to chronic, progressive compressive effects on the cervical spinal cord. Surgical intervention is commonly employed to relieve the compressive forces on the spinal cord in an effort to halt symptomatic progression and potentially reverse some clinical changes. However, an understanding of the natural history of CSM is essential for appropriate implementation of clinical monitoring and treatment planning.

Increasing use of quantitative measures of dysfunction has facilitated objective analysis of the natural history of CSM. Despite this, numerous questions remain regarding disease progression. The natural history is highly variable and difficult to predict on an individual patient basis. The aim of this chapter is to summarize the current understanding of the natural history and risk factors for disease progression in patients who are already exhibiting myelopathy and factors that predict the onset of myelopathic symptoms in patients who are asymptomatic but have evidence of spinal cord compression from cervical spondylosis.

## THE NATURAL HISTORY OF CSM

The natural history of CSM is based upon the symptom progression of patients afflicted with this condition who have not undergone surgical management. Evidence pertaining to the natural history of CSM is derived from prospective and retrospective studies of conservative management. The specifics of this approach may range from no therapy to rest or immobilization or traction therapy. Compliance with these conservative strategies is difficult to verify, and the specific effects of each are generally not well understood. At present, a true study of the natural history of CSM is not available and for various reasons is unlikely to be, so outcomes from these conservative approaches are regarded as providing the best insight into the natural course of the disease.

One of the initial studies of the natural history of CSM was published by Clarke and Robinson in 1956.[2] They described a retrospective review of 120 patients where 26 patients did not have surgical intervention. The temporal progression of myelopathic symptoms in these patients was combined with the progression of the disease prior to surgical intervention in the remaining cohort. Clinical symptomatology was used as the basis of outcome measurement, specifically, motor and sensory symptoms of myelopathy in one or both of the arms and legs. Based upon these purely qualitative measures, they found that new symptoms and signs appeared in 75% of patients; 5% of patients had a rapid onset of symptoms followed by a prolonged quiescent interval, while 20% experienced a slow, steady progression of symptoms. Importantly, of the patients who did not undergo surgery, 50% improved. The information provided by this study was greatly limited by the subjective outcome measures and a paucity of quantitative and objective measures of disease progression, but it provided some of the earliest insights into the highly variable natural history of CSM. Since this early contribution to the body of literature on CSM, objective measures of severity and progression of the myelopathic symptoms have been developed and increasingly utilized. Stronger evidence is now becoming available to help garner a greater appreciation of the clinical course for patients with CSM. The aim of this section of the chapter is to provide an overview of the current understanding of the natural history of CSM in terms of quantitative and semiquantitative measures of neurological and functional outcome from studies of nonoperative management.

## Modified Japanese Orthopedic Association Score

A classic approach to quantifying the neurological assessment of a patient with CSM is the Japanese Orthopedic Association (JOA) score.[3] The JOA has advocated for the use of this scoring system, which quantifies the motor and sensory function of the upper and lower extremities along with bladder function since 1975. The maximum score of 17 signifies normal neurological function. The score is limited, however, by culturally specific criteria, specifically in the upper extremity motor component. The scoring system was translated to English and modified in 1991 in order to include additional components in the lower extremity motor function category and to be more culturally appropriate for North American and European patients.[4] This modified version (the mJOA) has a maximum score of 18, which signifies normal neurological function. The mJOA has largely supplanted the JOA for studies of the natural history of CSM in Western societies (Table 6.1).

Utilizing the mJOA scoring system, Kadaňka et al. conducted a 3-year prospective randomized trial of 66 patients comparing conservative to surgical management of CSM.[5,6] At the 3-year follow-up, the patients were stratified into nonresponders (deterioration of the mJOA score of 1 or more points), responders (no change in the mJOA score or an improvement of 1 point) and very good responders (improvement of the mJOA score of 2 or more points). Classification of patients was as follows: 26.7% of conservatively managed patients were classified as nonresponders, 50% as responders, and 23.3% as very good responders. The mean mJOA score at the outset of the study was 14.6, and the mean mJOA at 3-year follow-up within the conservatively managed group was 14.7, with no significant time-related trend within the group. Furthermore, the results of a 10-year follow-up of the patients from the initial 3-year study have been published.[7] There were 25 patients available for follow-up in the conservatively managed group, and the difference between mean baseline and 10-year follow-up mJOA scores was again not significantly different (Fig. 6.1).

Another prospective study using the JOA as a primary means of neurological assessment was of 60 patients with mild CSM, with JOA scores of 13 or higher who were treated conservatively.[8] The initial mean JOA of this cohort was 14.5 and the mean JOA at the end of the follow-up period was 14.1, with an average follow-up time of 78.9 months. Again, there was no significant difference between the initial and end JOA score. However, 25% of the cases had a deterioration of their clinical status, which was defined as a decline in JOA score to $<13$ with a decrease of at least 2 points.

A retrospective review of 64 conservatively managed patients with CSM, utilizing only the motor extremity component of the JOA score with a mean follow-up period of 6 years, demonstrated improvement in the upper extremity motor score of 1 or more in 55%, no change in 45% and worsening in 0% of those included in the study. Improvement in the lower extremity motor score of 1 or more occurred in 57%, no change was recorded in 39% and worsening was found in 3% of the participants.

**Table 6.1:** Modified Japanese Orthopedic Association score.

| | |
|---|---|
| *I. Motor dysfunction score of the upper extremities* | |
| Inability to move hands | 0 |
| Inability to eat with a spoon but able to move hands | 1 |
| Inability to button shirt but able to eat with a spoon | 2 |
| Able to button shirt with great difficulty | 3 |
| Able to button shirt with slight difficulty | 4 |
| No dysfunction | 5 |
| *II. Motor dysfunction score of the lower extremities* | |
| Complete loss of motor and sensory function | 0 |
| Sensory preservation without ability to move legs | 1 |
| Able to move legs but unable to walk | 2 |
| Able to walk on flat floor with a walking aid | 3 |
| Able to walk up and/or down stairs with a hand rail | 4 |
| Lack of stability but able to walk up and/or down stairs without hand rail | 5 |
| Mild lack of stability but walk unaided with smooth reciprocation | 6 |
| No dysfunction | 7 |
| *III. Sensation* | |
| Complete loss of hand sensation | 0 |
| Severe sensory loss or pain | 1 |
| Mild sensory loss | 2 |
| No sensory loss | 3 |
| *IV. Sphincter dysfunction score* | |
| Inability to micturate voluntarily | 0 |
| Marked difficulty with micturition | 1 |
| Mild to moderate difficulty with micturition | 2 |
| Normal micturition | 3 |
| *Total for normal patient* | 18 |

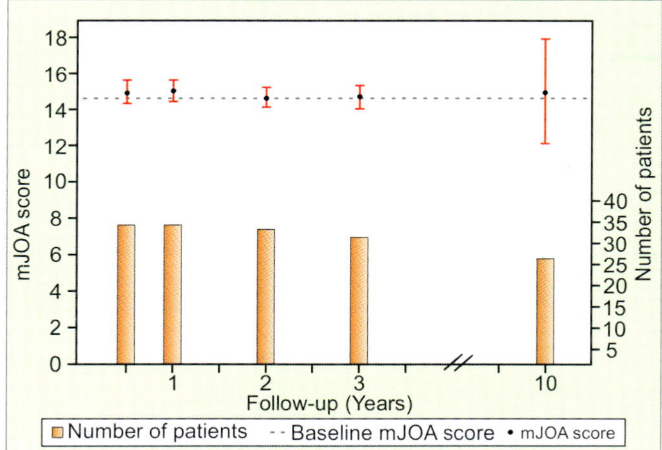


**Fig. 6.1:** Mean modified version of Japanese Orthopedic Association (mJOA) score over a 10-year follow-up of a conservatively managed cervical spondylotic myelopathy patient cohort. No significant time-related trend in mJOA scores was identified over the follow-up period.
*Source*: Figure derived from the data of Kadaňka Z, et al.[5,7]

## Nurick Scale

An alternative to the JOA for quantitative assessment of the symptoms of CSM is the Nurick scale.[9] This six-grade quantitative measure was first described in 1972. It is based upon the severity of a patient's gait impairment, with a score of 0 representing radiculopathic symptoms or signs but no evidence of myelopathy and a score of 1 representing evidence of myelopathy without impairment. Increasing score represents progressive severity of gait dysfunction from myelopathy up to a score of 5, which represents a patient who is chair or bedridden (Table 6.2). Barnes and Saunders[10] utilized this quantitative assessment to retrospectively review a cohort of 45 patients with evidence of myelopathy. They found that 13% of patients had deteriorated, 20% had improved, and 67% were unchanged after a mean follow-up period of 8.2 years.

## Activities of Daily Living

Sampath et al. prospectively evaluated a cohort of 31 patients with conservative management of CSM for 11 months.[11] They used a 4-point scale (none, some, most or all) to assess the extent of participation in their usual work or social activities. The average of the social and work activities gave an overall functional status, with higher scores representing better functional status. After the 11-month follow-up, there was a nonsignificant improvement in overall functional status from 3.26 to 3.68. The

**Table 6.2:** Nurick scale.

| | |
|---|---|
| Signs or symptoms of root involvement but without evidence of spinal cord disease | 0 |
| Signs of spinal cord disease but no difficulty in walking | 1 |
| Slight difficulty in walking that did not prevent full-time employment | 2 |
| Difficulty in walking that prevents full-time employment or the ability to do all housework, but that was not so severe as to require someone else's help to walk | 3 |
| Able to walk only with someone else's help or with the aid of a frame | 4 |
| Chair bound or bedridden | 5 |

investigators also assessed activities of daily living in the study group. They assigned a score of 0–5 to represent how performing activities of daily living worsened the patient's symptoms. These activities comprised lifting heavy weights, standing for >10 minutes, sitting for >10 minutes, sitting in a car and lying down. A score of 0 indicated that none of these activities worsened their symptoms, while 5 represented all of the activities worsening their symptoms. There was a statistically significant increase in scores from 1.84 to 2.47 over the 11-month follow-up period. Kadaňka et al.[7] also reported on changes in activities of daily living scores over the 10-year follow-up period. They found that 56% of patients reported a subjective worsening of their ability to perform activities of daily living between their baseline assessment and 10-year follow-up.

## Timed 10-Meter Walk

As another means of evaluating functional outcome, Kadaňka and colleagues utilized the timed 10-meter walk test to assess a cohort of 25 conservatively treated patients over a 10-year follow-up period.[7] The walk times at baseline and at 10-year follow-up were 7.0 and 7.1 seconds, respectively.

## Summary

It can be seen from these studies using a variety of different quantitative and semiquantitative metrics that the natural history of CSM is such that 20–60% of patients with CSM will experience a neurological deterioration over time (Box 6.1). However, the clinical course is highly variable and the timing and degree of deterioration is difficult to predict for any individual patient with CSM.

**Box 6.1:** Key features of the natural history.

- Our understanding of the natural history of cervical spondylotic myelopathy (CSM) is based upon studies of symptom progression in patients who have had nonsurgical management of their condition. These conservative approaches are numerous and nonstandardized.
- Twenty to sixty percent of patients will experience a neurological deterioration without surgical intervention.
- The clinical course of CSM is highly variable. Some patients experience prolonged periods of clinical quiescence while others have rapid progression of myelopathic symptoms.

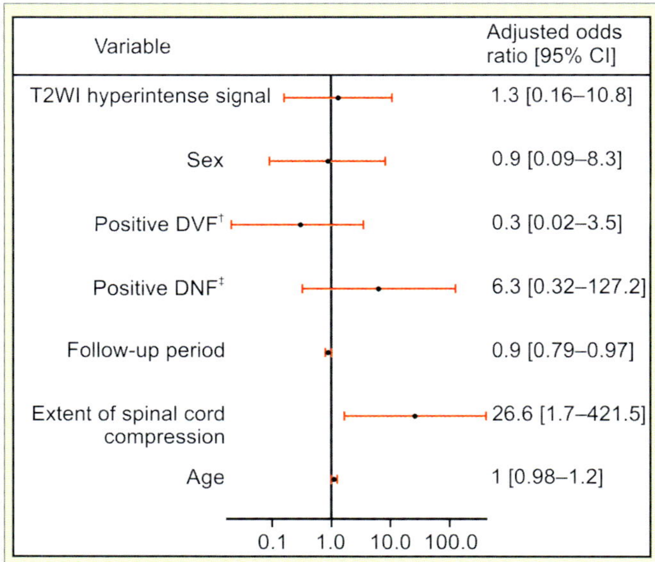


**Fig. 6.2:** Prognostic factors for neurological deterioration in patients with conservatively managed cervical spondylotic myelopathy. Adjusted odds ratios reported by Shimomura T, et al.[12]
†: Developmental factors on plain lateral radiograph (positive = present);
‡: Dynamic factors on plain lateral radiograph (positive = present).
*Source*: Adapted from Karadimas SK, et al.[27]

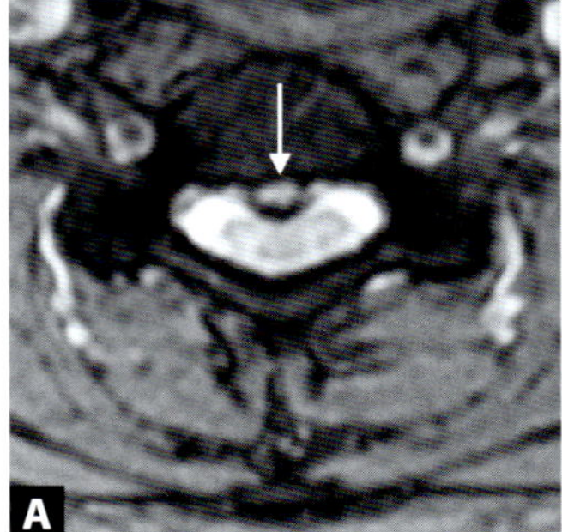


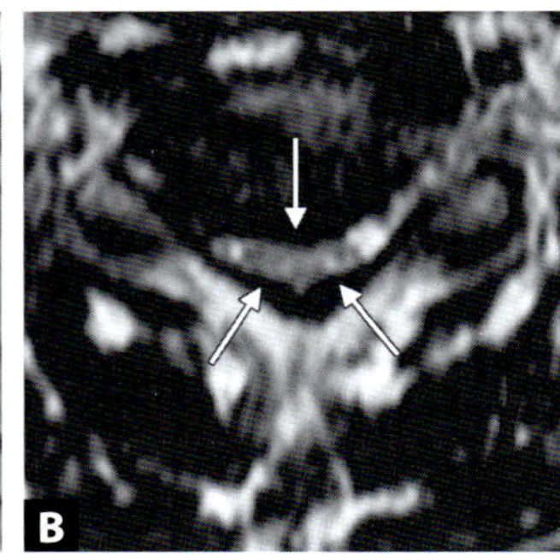


**Figs. 6.3A and B:** T2-weighted magnetic resonance imaging demonstrating the extent of spinal cord compression as defined by Shimomura T, et al.[12] (A) Partial spinal cord compression. White arrow indicates the ventral location of the compressive pathology (B), Circumferential spinal cord compression. Three white arrows indicate the circumferential location of the compressive pathology.

## PROGNOSTIC FACTORS

Despite the capricious natural history of CSM outlined in the previous section, it is essential for clinicians to gain an understanding of the risk factors for progressive neurological deterioration as well as factors that suggest a more favorable clinical course in order to make treatment decisions. The aim of this section of the chapter is to summarize the current understanding of these risk factors that may help guide clinicians in their decision making regarding the timing of clinical follow-up and the threshold for surgical intervention.

### Predictors of Neurological Worsening

Shimomura et al. conducted a prospective study of 56 patients with a mild form of CSM (JOA ≥ 13) to evaluate prognostic factors associated with neurological deterioration (Fig. 6.2).[12] The only prognostic factor that was significantly associated with neurological decline was circumferential spinal cord compression in the maximum compression segment on axial magnetic resonance imaging (MRI). Ten of the 33 patients with circumferential compression deteriorated during follow-up in comparison to 1 of the 23 patients with only partial compression (Odds Ratio: 26.6; 95% confidence interval 1.7–421.5). No significant association was noted between age, gender, follow-up period, developmental, or dynamic canal factors of the cervical spine on plain lateral radiographs or high T2-weighted signal intensity on sagittal MRI (Figs. 6.3A and B).[27]

Yoshimatsu and colleagues[13] evaluated 69 patients with CSM treated nonoperatively over a mean follow-up time of 29 months and found that the only significant predictor of follow-up JOA score was duration of disease. They found that all eight patients in the study who had the symptoms for 5 years or longer experienced worsening during the study period.

### Favorable Predictive Factors

As important as it is to have an awareness of factors that portend neurological deterioration, it is equally important to recognize factors that are predictive of a favorable clinical course when nonsurgical intervention is undertaken.

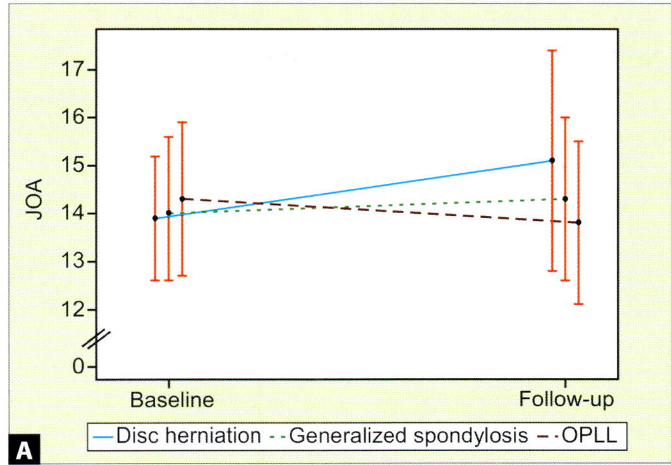


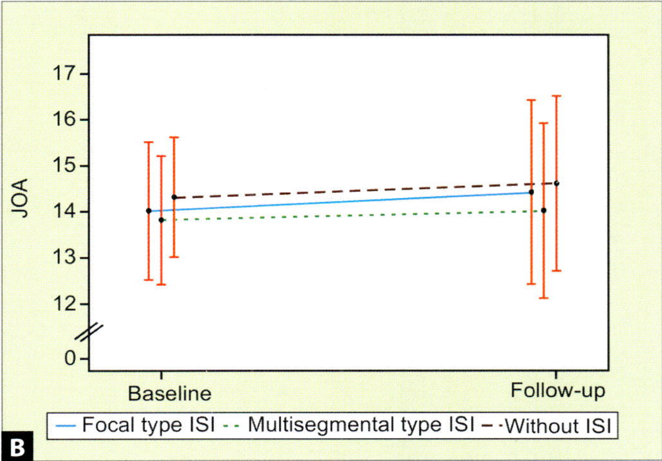


**Figs. 6.4A and B:** (A) The relationship between the nature of the compressive lesion (single level disk herniation, generalized spondylosis or ossification of the posterior longitudinal ligament) and the progression of myelopathic symptoms. No significant difference between the change in Japanese Orthopedic Association (JOA) between the three etiologies. (B) The relationship between the type of T2-weighted image magnetic resonance imaging increased signal intensity (focal, multisegmental, none) and progression of myelopathic symptoms. No significant difference between the change in JOA and the pattern of increased signal intensity. *Source*: Figure derived from the data of Matsumoto M, et al.[17]

A retrospective review of 64 conservatively managed patients revealed that a milder disability, as defined by the motor component of the JOA scale, was associated with a greater likelihood of achieving a motor score of 4 (no disability) with a mean follow-up time of 6 years and 2 months.[14] Additionally, older age, larger transverse area of the spinal cord at the level of compression, and normal values of central motor conduction time to the upper extremities were found to be significant predictors of an improved mJOA score at 3-year follow-up.[6] A higher calculated Pavlov's index was also found to predict improved mJOA score. This index is the ratio of sagittal diameter of the spinal canal to the sagittal diameter of the vertebral body at C5.[15]

## Notable Nonpredictive Factors

Matsumoto et al.[16] conducted a small retrospective review of 17 conservatively managed patients with CSM with follow-up time points at 3 and 6 months and then a final follow-up at a mean of 3.9 years. In this study, the investigators limited the cohort population to patients who had CSM secondary to soft cervical disk herniations (as determined by MRI) while patients with CSM secondary to more generalized spondylosis or ossification of the posterior longitudinal ligament (OPLL) were not included. The baseline JOA in this cohort was 13.6. At 3-month follow-up, the mean JOA had improved to 14.9, then 15.6 at 6-month follow-up, and finally 16.2 at the final assessment. This notable increase in JOA scores from 13.6 to 16.2 and an associated 77% rate of patient satisfaction was suggestive of a more favorable natural history for patients with myelopathy secondary to soft disk herniations rather than more generalized spondylotic processes. However, in contrast to these findings, Matsumoto et al.[17] published another cohort study of 52 patients with mild cervical myelopathy that included generalized spondylosis as well as OPLL in addition to soft disk herniations. In this investigation, they found that there were no statistically significant differences in the JOA score change between baseline and follow-up among the three groups (Fig. 6.4A). Additionally, these authors studied the relationship between increased signal intensity (ISI) on T2-weighted image (T2WI) MRI of the cervical spinal cord and the natural history of CSM. They classified the ISI by pattern and divided the patients into three cohorts. The first group did not have any ISI on their imaging studies, the second group had focal ISI, and the third group had multisegmental ISI. They found no statistically significant change in JOA scores among the three categories of ISI (Fig. 6.4B).

## Summary

Overall, it seems that circumferential spinal cord compression and longer duration of disease are predictive of worsening neurological dysfunction in patients with

**Box 6.2:** Key prognostic features.

- Circumferential cervical spinal cord compression and longer duration of symptoms of myelopathy are predictive of worsening neurological function.
- Milder disability at the time of diagnosis, larger transverse area of the spinal cord at the compressive level, a higher Pavlov's index, and normal central motor conduction time to the upper extremities predict improved neurological function with conservative management.
- Cervical intramedullary T2-weighted image hyperintensity does not appear to predict greater risk of neurological decline with conservative management.

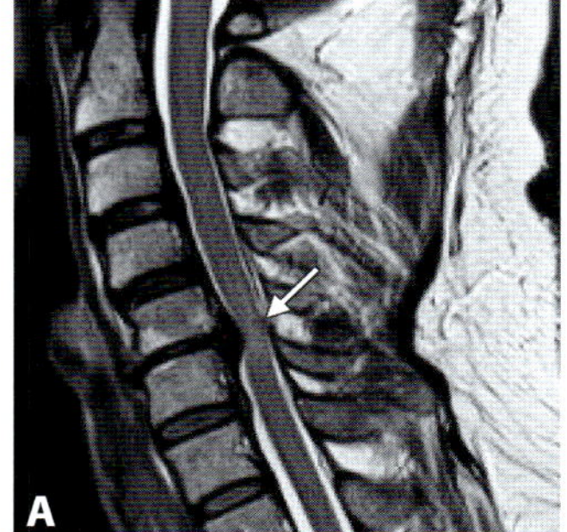

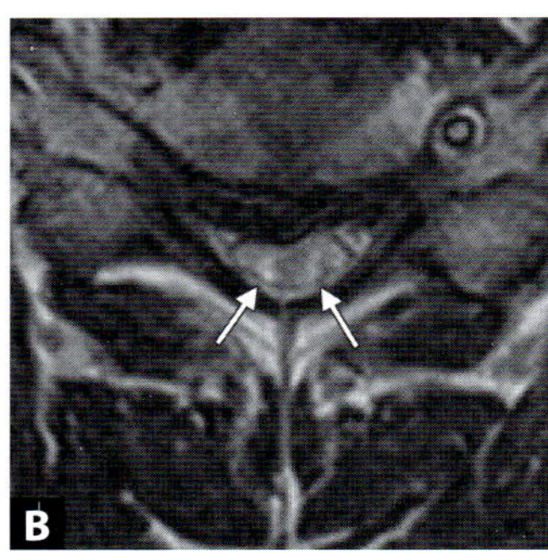


**Figs. 6.5A and B:** T2-weighted magnetic resonance imaging demonstrating signal hyperintensity. (A) Sagittal image with hyperintense intramedullary signal secondary to focal cervical spinal stenosis at C5/6. (B) Axial image at the C5/6 level demonstrating the same hyperintense intramedullary signal.

pre-existing CSM. Milder symptoms, older age, larger transverse area of the spinal cord at the compressive level, higher Pavlov's index, and normal values of central motor conduction time of the upper extremities are suggestive of a more favorable natural history (Box 6.2). Patients with soft cervical disk herniations do not appear to have a significant difference in neurological outcomes in comparison to those with a more generalized spondylotic compressive process, and the presence or absence or pattern of T2WI MRI signal hyperintensity is not predictive of neurological outcome in patients who already have evidence of myelopathy.

## PREDICTORS OF NEUROLOGICAL DYSFUNCTION IN NONMYELOPATHIC PATIENTS

While considerable effort has been invested in the study of the progression of symptoms in patients who initially present with evidence of myelopathy, the majority of patients with degenerative cervical spinal stenosis will never develop myelopathic symptoms. Nine percent of patients >70 years had cervical spinal stenosis on postmortem examination, and 95% of males and 70% of females of the same age range have evidence of cervical spondylosis.[18,19] With the ever-increasing use of radiographic studies, counseling asymptomatic patients with cervical degenerative changes regarding the risk of developing symptoms of myelopathy and its appropriate management is becoming increasingly important for specialists focused on the management of spinal pathology.

Bednařík et al.[20] have addressed this with a prospective study of 199 patients with spondylotic or discogenic compression of the cervical spinal cord without clinical signs or symptoms attributable to cervical spinal cord involvement. The subjects underwent a baseline clinical examination, electrophysiological evaluation, and radiographic imaging, and had prospective follow-up examinations every 6 months for 2 years and every year thereafter. Mean follow-up duration was 44 months. A total of 22.6% of subjects met the primary endpoint of the study, which was detection of clinical signs and symptoms of cervical myelopathy that could be unequivocally attributed to cervical cord dysfunction. Significant risk factors for the development of myelopathy were electromyographic signs of anterior horn cell lesion, prolonged somatosensory-evoked potentials (SEP), prolonged motor-evoked potentials (MEP), MRI with T2WI hyperintensity (Figs. 6.5A and B), and clinically symptomatic radiculopathy. Eight percent of study subjects developed symptomatic myelopathy within 1 year of the time of entry into the study. The significant risk factors for the early (≤12 months) onset of clinical myelopathy were prolonged SEPs, prolonged MEPs, clinically symptomatic radiculopathy and, notably, the absence of MRI with T2WI hyperintensity. Further to this, in a separate investigation of the same cohort of 199 patients, the relationship between trauma and the onset of myelopathic symptoms in patients with asymptomatic cervical spinal compression was studied. No significant association between traumatic episodes and the onset of myelopathy was found.[21]

Fujiyoshi et al.[22] specifically focused an investigation on patients with cervical spinal cord compression from OPLL. They studied an asymptomatic prospective cohort of 27 patients with a spinal canal that measured 12 mm or less on MRI. The baseline JOA score was 17 (normal), and after a mean follow-up period of 59 months none of the subjects developed myelopathy based upon reassessment of the JOA score. In a separate study of

**Box 6.3: Key considerations for patients with asymptomatic degenerative compressive cervical stenosis.**

- Eight percent of these asymptomatic patients will develop myelopathy at 1-year, and 23% at median 44-month follow-up.
- Symptoms of cervical radiculopathy, prolonged somatosensory-evoked potentials or motor-evoked potentials, and electromyelographic signs of anterior horn cell lesions were predictive of the onset of myelopathy within 1 year of initial assessment.
- Patients with cervical intramedullary T2-weighted image hyperintensity are at higher risk for the onset of myelopathy over long-term follow-up.

asymptomatic patients with OPLL, Matsunaga et al.[23] performed a multicenter retrospective cohort study of 156 patients with a mean follow-up time of 10.3 years to determine if there were any radiographic predictors of the onset of myelopathy. They found that 61.5% of the study subjects developed myelopathy and 100% of the patients with cervical spinal canal stenosis of 60% or more developed myelopathic symptoms. However, the authors did not define what they considered to be neurological confirmation of myelopathy and appear not to have used an objective and quantitative means of assessment.

### Summary

Overall, approximately 8% of patients with asymptomatic degenerative compressive cervical canal stenosis will develop clinical myelopathy within 12 months and 23% will have done so at a median follow-up of 44 months (Box 6.3). Prolonged SEPs and MEPs at baseline and clinically symptomatic radiculopathy are significant risk factors for both early onset and later onset of myelopathy; however, the absence of MRI hyperintensity appears to be predictive of early onset of myelopathy while the presence of hyperintensity is predictive of later onset. Specifically, within the population of asymptomatic patients with OPLL, the onset of myelopathy ranges between 0% and 61.5% with a follow-up of 59 months to 10.3 years.[24] However, heterogeneity in the definition of myelopathy makes these results challenging to interpret.

## LIMITATIONS IN NATURAL HISTORY STUDIES

Evidence for the natural history of CSM is derived chiefly from a few small prospective and retrospective studies. These studies use a variety of quantitative and semiquantitative measures of neurological function. However, with the numerous metrics utilized it is difficult to ascertain what is a meaningful clinical deterioration. This is well exemplified by the previously discussed, landmark prospective trial by Kadaňka et al. that demonstrated a nonsignificant change in mJOA scores from baseline to those at the 10-year follow-up time point. Despite this lack of a statistically significant change in scores, over half of the study patients reported a notable worsening in their ability to perform activities of daily living over this time period. Presently, an outcome measure that has been demonstrated as reliable and valid within the CSM population is lacking and the paucity of such a measure has been previously recognized a substantial limitation in the collective literature on the subject of the natural history of CSM.[25]

In addition to the limitations imposed on the natural history literature by the currently available outcome measures, these studies are limited by variable definitions of conservative management or nonoperative care. Nearly all studies with a conservatively managed cohort of CSM patients involve some sort of imposed physical or lifestyle modification as a means of conservative management. For example, the patient population in the retrospective study by Nakamura and colleagues[14] employed a variety of conservative measures for the management of CSM such as Crutchfield's skull traction, cervical bracing, and continuous head halter traction bracing in bed. Other conservative measures include intermittent soft collar immobilization, anti-inflammatory medications, active discouragement of high-risk activities, intermittent bed rest for patients with pain, and avoidance of risky environments.[5] The effects of these conservative measures on the natural course of CSM are variable and not clearly elucidated. Furthermore, it is unclear in the majority of studies how patients were assigned to nonoperative management. In these cases, there is a high potential for selection bias with the possibility of patients with more severe symptoms being preferentially selected for surgical management. It is unlikely that a true natural history study will be published, where no element of modification (be it behavioral or physical) will be employed for the cohort of patients who are undergoing nonsurgical therapy. Large prospective studies with rigorous and defined means of nonoperative management will provide the best evidence and mitigate this limiting factor as we move forward towards a greater understanding of the natural history of CSM. However, it should be noted that as more and more evidence mounts that surgical decompression for the treatment of CSM is associated with significant

**Box 6.4:** Summary of key points.

- The natural history of cervical spondylotic myelopathy (CSM) is highly variable. Twenty to sixty percent of patients will experience a neurological deterioration without operative intervention.
- Circumferential cervical spinal cord compression and longer duration of symptoms of myelopathy are risk factors for neurological worsening in conservatively managed myelopathic patients. Milder disability, larger transverse area at the compression level, a higher Pavlov's index and normal central motor conduction time portend improved neurological function with conservative management.
- Eight percent of asymptomatic patients with degenerative compressive cervical stenosis will become symptomatic by 1-year and 23% at median 44-month follow-up. Radiculopathy and electrophysiological abnormalities are risk factors for short-term symptom onset and cervical intramedullary T2-weighted image hyperintensity is a long-term risk factor.
- Current literature on CSM is insufficient to provide definitive understanding of its natural history and is limited by highly variable means of conservative management and a lack of a quantitative outcome measure that is valid and reliable for detecting meaningful neurological deterioration.

improvements in function and quality-of-life outcomes,[26] the likelihood of a contribution of such a study to the literature becomes less and less.

## CONCLUSION

Despite the significant prevalence and incidence of CSM, the number and quality of clinical studies pertaining to the natural history of this condition have been insufficient to ascertain a definitive understanding of the course of the disease and the risk factors for its symptomatic progression.

The literature currently available relating to the natural history of CSM suggests that about 20–60% of patients with CSM will experience a neurological deterioration over time if they are managed nonoperatively (Box 6.4). The clinical course is variable with some patients experiencing periods of improvement or at least an absence of neurological decline, others enduring a slowly progressive deterioration and still others experiencing a rapid progression of myelopathic symptoms.

Evidence to identify factors that place patients at higher risk for progressive myelopathy is limited. Circumferential spinal cord compression and longer duration of symptoms have been identified as risk factors for neurological decline while milder disability at diagnosis, larger transverse area of the spinal cord at the level of compression, a higher Pavlov's index, and normal values of central motor conduction time are predictive of improvements in mJOA score. The presence or pattern of T2WI MRI signal hyperintensity is not predictive of neurological outcome with nonoperative management in myelopathic patients.

Within the subgroup of patients who have been identified with radiographic evidence of cervical spinal stenosis but who are without clinical symptoms or signs of myelopathy, about 8% will develop these within 12 months. Patients with prolonged SEPs or MEPs or clinical radiculopathy are at greater risk for the development of myelopathy and may be considered for closer clinical follow-up.

Overall, the current studies supplying evidence regarding the natural history of CSM are limited by the influence of varying approaches to conservative management and future studies are likely to be similarly limited. Presently, an outcome measurement tool that is reliable and valid for detecting meaningful clinical deterioration within the CSM patient population is unavailable, but the development of such measure will help to establish consistency in the classification of neurological deterioration in patients with CSM and provide the best opportunity for clinicians to establish a more complete understanding of the natural history of the condition.

## REFERENCES


1. Moore AP, Blumhardt LD. A prospective survey of the causes of non-traumatic spastic paraparesis and tetraparesis in 585 patients. Spinal Cord. 1997;35(6):361-7.
2. Clarke E, Robinson PK. Cervical myelopathy: a complication of cervical spondylosis. Brain. 1956;79(3):483-510.
3. Yonenobu K, Okada K, Fuji T, et al. Causes of neurologic deterioration following surgical treatment of cervical myelopathy. Spine (Phila Pa 1976). 1986;11(8):818-23.
4. Benzel EC, Lancon J, Kesterson L, et al. Cervical laminectomy and dentate ligament section for cervical spondylotic myelopathy. J Spinal Disord. 1991;4(3):286-95.
5. Kadaňka Z, Mareš M, Bednařík J, et al. Approaches to spondylotic cervical myelopathy: conservative versus surgical results in a 3-year follow-up study. Spine (Phila Pa 1976). 2002;27(20):2205-10.

6. Kadaňka Z, Mareš M, Bednařík J, et al. Predictive factors for spondylotic cervical myelopathy treated conservatively or surgically. Eur J Neurol. 2005;12(1):55-63.
7. Kadaňka Z, Bednařík J, Novotný O, et al. Cervical spondylotic myelopathy: conservative versus surgical treatment after 10 years. Eur Spine J. 2011;20(9):1533-8.
8. Sumi M, Miyamoto H, Suzuki T, et al. Prospective cohort study of mild cervical spondylotic myelopathy without surgical treatment. J Neurosurg Spine. 2012;16(1):8-14.
9. Nurick S. The pathogenesis of the spinal cord disorder associated with cervical spondylosis. Brain. 1972;95(1):87-100.
10. Barnes MP, Saunders M. The effect of cervical mobility on the natural history of cervical spondylotic myelopathy. J Neurol Neurosurg Psychiatry. 1984;47(1):17-20.
11. Sampath P, Bendebba M, Davis JD, et al. Outcome of patients treated for cervical myelopathy: a prospective, multicenter study with independent clinical review. Spine (Phila Pa 1976). 2000;25(6):670-6.
12. Shimomura T, Sumi M, Nishida K, et al. Prognostic factors for deterioration of patients with cervical spondylotic myelopathy after nonsurgical treatment. Spine (Phila Pa 1976). 2007;32(22):2474-9.
13. Yoshimatsu H, Nagata K, Goto H, et al. Conservative treatment for cervical spondylotic myelopathy: prediction of treatment effects by multivariate analysis. Spine J. 2001;1(4):269-73.
14. Nakamura K, Kurokawa T, Hoshino Y, et al. Conservative treatment for cervical spondylotic myelopathy: achievement and sustainability of a level of "no disability". J Spinal Disord. 1998;11(2):175-9.
15. Pavlov H, Torg JS, Robie B, et al. Cervical spinal stenosis: determination with vertebral body ratio method. Radiology. 1987;164(3):771-5.
16. Matsumoto M, Chiba K, Ishikawa M, et al. Relationships between outcomes of conservative treatment and magnetic resonance imaging findings in patients with mild cervical myelopathy caused by soft disc herniations. Spine (Phila Pa 1976). 2001;26(14):1592-8.
17. Matsumoto M, Toyama Y, Ishikawa M, et al. Increased signal intensity of the spinal cord on magnetic resonance images in cervical compressive myelopathy: does it predict the outcome of conservative treatment? Spine (Phila Pa 1976). 2000;25(6):677-82.
18. Gore DR, Sepic SB, Gardner GM. Roentgenographic findings of the cervical spine in asymptomatic people. Spine (Phila Pa 1976). 1986;11(6):521-4.
19. Lee MJ, Cassinelli EH, Riew KD. Prevalence of cervical spine stenosis: anatomic study in cadavers. J Bone Joint Surg Am. 2007;89(2):376-80.
20. Bednařík J, Kadaňka Z, Dusek L, et al. Presymptomatic spondylotic cervical myelopathy: an updated predictive model. Eur Spine J. 2008;17(3):421-31.
21. Bednařík J, Sládková D, Kadaňka Z, et al. Are subjects with spondylotic cervical cord encroachment at increased risk of cervical spinal cord injury after minor trauma? J Neurol Neurosurg Psychiatry. 2011;82(7):779-81.
22. Fujiyoshi T, Yamazaki M, Okawa A, et al. Static versus dynamic factors for the development of myelopathy in patients with cervical ossification of the posterior longitudinal ligament. J Clin Neurosci. 2010;17(3):320-4.
23. Matsunaga S, Nakamura K, Seichi A, et al. Radiographic predictors for the development of myelopathy in patients with ossification of the posterior longitudinal ligament: a multicenter cohort study. Spine (Phila Pa 1976). 2008;33(24):2648-50.
24. Wilson JR, Barry S, Fischer DJ, et al. Frequency, timing, and predictors of neurological dysfunction in the nonmyelopathic patient with cervical spinal cord compression, canal stenosis, and/or ossification of the posterior longitudinal ligament. Spine (Phila Pa 1976). 2013;38(22 Suppl 1):S37-54.
25. Kalsi-Ryan S, Singh A, Massicotte EM, et al. Ancillary outcome measures for assessment of individuals with cervical spondylotic myelopathy. Spine (Phila Pa 1976). 2013;38(22 Suppl 1):S111-22.
26. Fehlings MG, Wilson JR, Kopjar B, et al. Efficacy and safety of surgical decompression in patients with cervical spondylotic myelopathy: results of the AO Spine North America prospective multi-center study. J Bone Joint Surg Am. 2013;95(18):1651-8.
27. Karadimas SK, Erwin WM, Ely CG, et al. The pathophysiology and natural history of cervical spondylotic myelopathy. Spine (Phila Pa 1976). 2013;38(22 Suppl 1):S21-36.

Chapter 7

# Influence of Conservative Management on Outcomes

*Jerry Cheriyan, Elizabeth Tanzi, Peter G Passias, Thomas Cheriyan*

## INTRODUCTION

The natural history of cervical spondylotic myelopathy (CSM) and asymptomatic cervical cord compression is highly unpredictable. The proportion of CSM patients who deteriorate within 3–6 years ranges widely from 20% to 62%.[1] Given the highly unpredictable clinical progression of CSM, the optimal management of patients with CSM is controversial, especially in the subset of patients with minimal symptoms and asymptomatic patients with cord compression.[1-3] Cervical spondylotic myelopathy has traditionally been managed surgically as it prevents clinical worsening and improves function, and delay in surgical treatment results in poor outcomes.[4,5] In patients with moderate or severe CSM, surgical treatment is usually recommended. However, in patients with mild, nonprogressive or slowly progressive CSM, the long-term superiority of surgical management over conservative treatment has not been fully established.

## NONOPERATIVE MODALITIES

Nonoperative treatment modalities for CSM patients include rest and cervical immobilization using a soft collar or brace; limitation of high-risk injury activities such as heavy lifting, exercise, and contact sports; and pain management.[3,6,7-9] Patients are also advised to take precautions against whiplash injury, such as adjusting the headrest to the level of the occiput.[7] Cervical traction and manipulation may lead to aggravation of cord compression and should be avoided. Pain management medications in CSM include nonsteroidal anti-inflammatory drugs (NSAIDs), opioid and nonopioid drugs, muscle relaxants, and antidepressants.

Nonsteroidal anti-inflammatory drugs like aspirin and ibuprofen are commonly used in CSM patients to relieve pain as it may reduce swelling and inflammation. However, there is a paucity of clinical evidence supporting their efficacy.[10] Efficacy of NSAIDs might be higher in patients with concomitant acute axial or radicular pain. If axial pain is relieved by NSAIDs in these patients and long-term use is required, regular monitoring of medication side effect is necessary. Cyclooxygenase-2 inhibitors, opioid, or nonopioids may be considered in patients who are at high risk of NSAIDs toxicity.[11]

Acetaminophen may be considered for mild-to-moderate pain due to the favorable efficacy and safety profile of the drug. Opioids may be considered in patients who do not achieve adequate analgesia with NSAIDs and nonopioids. Opioids are advantageous in that they are not associated with end-organ toxicity, provide potent analgesia, and do not have a ceiling dose. However, opioids may have limited benefit in neuropathic pain.[11] Long-term use of opioids carries with it the risk of physical dependence on the drug. The dose of the opioid can be lowered by the concomitant use of a nonopioid.

Muscle relaxants can be used to alleviate pain associated with reactive paraspinal and trapezius muscle spasm. Centrally acting muscle relaxants, including baclophen, cyclobenzaprine, carisoprodol, and tizanidine, result in some sedation and can be beneficial for patients with pain-disrupted sleep.[11] Antidepressants may be of some value in patients with chronic pain. Common side effects of antidepressants include dry mouth, drowsiness, weight gain, sexual dysfunction, urinary retention, and constipation. Tricyclic antidepressants are contraindicated in patients with serious cardiac dysfunction. Anticonvulsants like tiagabine and oxcarbazepine can be considered for neuropathic pain patients; however, these are not approved by the Food and Drug administration for this indication. Although not often used, epidural steroid injections may decrease pain in CSM. It is important to note that there are not sufficient data to support or refute the clinical effectiveness of these pain management modalities in CSM. The side effects of the drugs should be considered when prescribing them for patients (Table 7.1).

## EVIDENCE

A comprehensive review of early longitudinal studies that investigated the progression of CSM with conservative treatment was done by Matz.[12] Lees and Aldren-Turner[13] were among the first to describe the natural history and progression of cervical spondylosis in 1963. In the 44 myelopathy patients, the duration of follow-up ranged from 3 years to 40 years. Among the 28 patients who were treated nonoperatively with cervical immobilization, 61% improved clinically. They also recorded that there were long periods of stability and short periods of exacerbation. Nurick[14] described the outcomes of 91 patients who had CSM. Eighteen (67%) out of the 27 patients underwent conservative treatment with cervical immobilization and rest and maintained good (grade I and II) Nurick scores. Nurick recognized that the severity of disability was established early and the natural history of CSM comprised periods of stability with exacerbation. In the 121 patients with CSM, Clarke and Robinson observed 5% mortality and an average survival of 7 years after diagnosis among these patients.[15] They noted that 75% had stepwise worsening with deterioration, 20% had slow, steady progression, and 5% had initial worsening followed by a stable period.[12,15] Among the 16 patients who underwent conservative therapy with cervical collar, eight showed improvement with none having worsening of symptoms.[3,13] A synopsis of studies as summarized by Matz is given in Table 7.2.[12]

Matsumoto et al.[16] investigated the outcome of conservative treatment in mild CSM patients caused by soft disk herniation confirmed by magnetic resonance imaging (MRI). Mild cervical myelopathy was defined by the Japanese Orthopedic Association (JOA) score of > 10. Out of 27 patients, 17 underwent conservative treatment with cervical bracing and restriction of daily activities for >6 months. There was significant improvement in their mean JOA scores (13.6–16.2). Furthermore, follow-up MRI of these patients demonstrated a spontaneous regression of their disk displacement in 10 patients (59%). Patients who had diffuse-type herniations were more likely to regress spontaneously than focal-type herniations (78% vs. 37%). The remaining 10 patients ultimately underwent decompression surgery due to neurological decline. The mean JOA improved from 14.1 to 16 in this group (Table 7.3).

**Table 7.1:** Common side effects of medication use in management of pain in cervical spondylotic myelopathy.

| *Medication* | *Common side effect* |
|---|---|
| Nonsteroidal anti-inflammatory drugs | Ulcers, gastropathy, renal failure, hypertension, congestive heart failure, cardiovascular events |
| Nonopioid/opioid analgesics | Ulcers, dyspepsia/addiction, impaired cognition |
| Muscle relaxants | Sedation, dry mouth, risk of habituation |
| Antidepressants | Sedation, dry mouth, dizziness, constipation, urinary retention, weight gain, and cardiac conduction changes |
| Anticonvulsants | Dizziness, somnolence, weight gain |
| Epidural corticosteroid injection | Dural puncture, spinal headache, facial flushing, stiff neck, hypertension, chemical arachnoiditis |

*Source*: Adapted from Mazanec D, Reddy A.[11]

**Table 7.2:** Summarization of early observational studies investigating conservative therapy on cervical spondylotic myelopathy.

| *Study* | *Treatment* | *Result summary* |
|---|---|---|
| Lees and Aldren-Turner[13] | Cervical immobilization | 61% improved clinically; observation in 44 CSM patients over 30 years showed long-periods of stability before short-intervals of deterioration |
| Nurick[14] | Cervical immobilization and rest | 18/27 patients remained at good Nurick grades (I and II); age > 60 appeared to be a negative risk factor, especially when compared with surgical decompression ($n$ = 62 good grade patients) |
| Clarke and Robinson[15] | Cervical immobilization and rest | 8 in 16 improved; remainder remained stable |
| Barnes and Saunders | Expectant management | 6 had worsening; 30 unchanged; worsening was associated with greater range of motion and female gender |
| Roberts | Cervical immobilization and rest | 7 improved and 9 did not worsen. Improvement seen in 5 months or not at all. Those who got clinically worse with conservative treatment usually started disabled |

*Source*: Adapted from Matz PG.[12]

**Table 7.3:** Summarization of studies investigating conservative therapy on cervical spondylotic myelopathy with outcome measures.

| *Author* | *Number of patients* | *Outcome measure* | *Therapy* | *Result* |
|---|---|---|---|---|
| Matsumoto et al.[16] | 27 | Japanese Orthopedic Association (JOA) | Cervical immobilization q8h for 3 months and intermittently for 6 months in patients with JOA > 10 (average 13.6) | 17 (59%) improved in JOA grade; 10 patients underwent surgery for worsening neurologic symptoms |
| Matsumoto et al.[6] | 52 | JOA and magnetic resonance imaging (MRI) increased signal intensity | Cervical immobilization q8h for 3 months and intermittently for 6 months in patients with JOA >10 (average 13.6) w/or w/o ISI | Increased signal intensity not related to poor outcome of conservative treatment; JOA remained around 14 over 3 years |
| Nakamura et al.[17] | 64 | JOA | Head halter, cervical immobilization, plaster bed and Crutchfield traction | Improvement in 1 grade in 55% upper extremity and 57% lower extremity |
| Sampath et al.[18] | 62 | Neurologic outcome score, functional status measure, Activities of Daily Living (ADL) scale | Conservative therapy (*n* = 31, included rest, exercise, cervical collar)<br>Surgery (*n* = 31) | Neurologic improvement seen with surgery but not significant compared with conservative. Functional improvement seen with both treatments |
| Yoshimatsu et al.[19] | 69 | Symptoms at first examination compared to final | Rigorous conservative (*n* = 37): continuous cervical traction for 3–4 hours daily for 1–3 months combined with exercise during non-traction hours<br>Nonrigorous conservative (*n* = 32): no defined treatment | Rigorous nonoperative treatment, 38% improved. Only 6% of nonrigorous group showed improvement |
| Bednarik et al.[8] | 49 | Modified JOA and evoked potentials (EP) monitoring | Conservative therapy (*n* = 27, cervical collar, NSAIDs, rest); Surgery (*n* = 22) | No difference in modified JOA scores or aggregate EP potentials at 6 and 24 months |
| Kadanka et al.[21] | 64 | Modified JOA, 10-meter walk times, video evaluate of ADL (self and observer) | Conservative therapy (*n* = 32) included cervical collar, rest, NSAIDs; surgery (*n* = 32) | 10-year follow-up did not show surgery or conservative treatment superior |
| Kadanka et al.[20] | 68 | Modified JOA, 10-meter walk times, video evaluate of ADL (self and observer) | Conservative therapy (*n* = 35) included cervical collar, rest, NSAIDs; Surgery (*n* = 33) | 3-year follow-up did not show surgery or conservative treatment superior |

A second study performed by Matsumoto et al.[6] examined 52 patients with mild cervical myelopathy who underwent nonoperative treatment with a cervical brace. Mild CSM was defined again by a JOA score >10. The patient cohort consisted of 29 patients with spondylosis; 12 had cervical disk herniation and 11 had ossification of the posterior longitudinal ligament. The treatment was similar to a previous study with a cervical collar for >6 months. The average gain in JOA score was 0.4 points +/- 1.9 (range, -5 to +6) with satisfactory outcome in 36 patients (69%). Furthermore, the authors concluded that increased signal intensity noted on MRI was not associated with a poor outcome of nonoperative treatment in patients with mild cervical myelopathy (Table 7.3).

Nakamura et al.[17] reported on 64 patients with CSM treated with nonoperative management. Nonoperative treatment included the following: continuous head halter traction in bed (2 patients), cervical brace (19 patients), plaster bed holding head and trunk (15 patients), and Crutchfield's skull traction (28 patients). Patients were evaluated with the JOA grading system based on lower and upper extremity (0–4 in each category). Their results revealed a rate of "no disability" achieved in 26% in the lower and 27% in the upper extremities. No patients had clinical worsening in the upper extremities and 3% reported clinical worsening in the lower extremities. Furthermore, the improved function was maintained in most patients and some continued to improve during the follow-up period of 3–10 years (Table 7.3).

## OPERATIVE VERSUS CONSERVATIVE MANAGEMENT OF CSM

A summary of published studies that compared outcomes in operative and conservative management is given in Table 7.3.

A prospective, multicenter nonrandomized study by Sampath et al.[18] included 62 patients with cervical myelopathy as their predominant syndrome. Conservative therapy was recommended for 31 (50%) patients, including rest, exercise, and a cervical collar. Forty-three patients (69%) returned for follow-up at a mean of 11 months and completed the Neurologic Outcome Score, Functional Status Measure, and ADL scale. Patients treated with conservative therapy had significant worsening in ability to perform daily activities with worsening of their neurologic symptoms. Functional improvement was noted for both operative and nonoperative groups with significant improvement in social and work categories for surgery compared to the nonoperative group. Despite a greater number of neurologic and non-neurologic sequelae before treatment, surgically treated patients had better outcomes when comparing both groups.

Yoshimatsu et al.[19] investigated symptoms after conservative treatment for CSM for 69 patients. The nonoperative cases were further divided into rigorous versus nonrigorous treatment groups. The rigorous group received continuous cervical traction for 3–4 hours daily for 1–3 months combined with exercise during nontraction hours. Nonrigorous group included 12 patients who refused any nonoperative treatment and the remaining 20 who had no defined treatment. The investigators performed a multivariate analysis, which showed significant correlation between clinical outcome and disease duration with the presence of rigorous conservative treatment. Of those who received rigorous nonoperative treatment, 38% improved. Only 6% of patients who did not undergo rigorous treatment showed improvement. The authors further concluded that only conservative treatment would be effective if performed intensively in selected patients. After conservative treatment, 22 patients continued to have surgical treatment. Approximately 78% of the patients with operative treatment had improved neurologic symptoms. The authors suggested that in treating CSM, due consideration should be given to the patients' disease duration. The authors also suggested intensive conservation treatment to be carried out after sufficient patient education. Surgical treatment is to be considered if there was no change in symptoms or exacerbation of symptoms with conservative treatment.

Bednarik et al.[8] performed a prospective randomized study on 61 patients with 2-year follow-up. Cervical spondylotic myelopathy was confirmed by MRI. The patients were divided into two groups based on the grading of clinical cervical cord involvement. The outcome was measured with a modified JOA and electrophysiological monitoring. The 49 patients with mild and moderate CSM were randomized into groups that underwent either surgical or conservative therapy. Approximately 27 patients underwent nonoperative management, including intermittent cervical immobilization, anti-inflammatory medications, and low-risk activities. The authors concluded that there was no difference in modified JOA scores or electrophysiological potentials between the operative and nonoperative groups at both 6-month and 2-year follow-up.

Kadanka et al.[20] performed a 3-year prospective randomized study of 68 patients randomized into two groups. There were 35 subjects in the nonoperative treatment and 33 patients in the operative treatment groups. Outcome measures were a modified JOA, timed 10-meter walk, and daily activities recorded by video. The video was evaluated by observers blinded to the treatment arm. Patients also performed a subjective assessment at 6, 12, 24, and 36 months. Nonoperative treatment included intermittent immobilization, anti-inflammatory medications, and rest. There was no statistical difference for JOA scores for the operative and nonoperative groups, but there was a difference ($p = 0.034$) in the 10-meter walk. For the nonoperative patients, modified JOA scores improved from 14.6 to 14.7 and 10-meter walk time increased from 7.4 seconds to 7.5 seconds. For the operative patients, modified JOA scores worsened from 14.1 to 13.8 and 10-meter walk times increased from 7.9 seconds to 9.4 seconds. For activities of daily living, the nonoperative group did statistically better at 6 months ($p < 0.05$) and the operative group did statistically better at 6 months regarding self-evaluation ($p < 0.05$). However, by the 3-year follow-up point, there was no statistical difference on average between the nonoperative and operative groups. Kadanka et al.[21] reported the 10-year results of the prospective randomized study rather than 3 years. Comparison of the operative and nonoperative management of mild and moderate forms of CSM did not show a statistical difference at 10-year follow-up. Furthermore, the power analysis shows minimal ability to ascertain which treatment is best for patients with mild and moderate nonprogressive CSM. There was a small number of patients for final evaluation as 17 patients died of natural, unrelated causes during the follow-up.

There were no studies comparing outcomes of conservative treatment based on CSM severity. However, more severe CSM tends to have better outcomes with surgery than conservative treatment, while milder CSM may not benefit as much from surgery.[22] In a comprehensive review and recommendation publication by Rhee et al.,[22] the authors recommended the following:

1. Not routinely prescribing nonoperative treatment as the primary modality in patients with moderate-to-severe myelopathy. (Strength of evidence: Low; Strength of recommendation: Strong).
2. If there is a role for nonoperative treatment as primary treatment modality, it may be in patients with mild CSM. That specific nonoperative treatment would provide benefit over natural history is not clear. Neurologic status should be carefully and vigilantly observed. (Strength of evidence: Low; Strength of recommendation: Weak).
3. In patients with CSM but no ossification of the posterior longitudinal ligament (OPLL), available studies do not address neurologic deterioration secondary to minor trauma. However, in those patients with OPLL, trauma may likely worsen symptoms or initiate symptoms in those previously asymptomatic. (Strength of evidence: Low; Strength of recommendation: Weak).
4. In patients having asymptomatic spondylotic cord compression but no clinical myelopathy, there is no evidence to support or refute neurologic deterioration secondary to minor trauma. (Strength of evidence: Low; Strength of recommendation: Weak).

## CONCLUSION

There is lack of strong evidence regarding the efficacy of conservative treatment of CSM. Conservative treatment cannot be routinely recommended to patients. However, nonoperative treatment might be of some benefit in select patients with mild, nonprogressive or slowly progressive CSM.

## REFERENCES


1. Fehlings MG, Wilson JR, Kopjar B, et al. Efficacy and safety of surgical decompression in patients with cervical spondylotic myelopathy: results of the AOSpine North America prospective multicenter study. J Bone Joint Surg Am. 2013;95:1651-8.
2. Fehlings MG, Arvin B. Surgical management of cervical degenerative disease: the evidence related to indications, impact, and outcome. J Neurosurg Spine. 2009;11:97-100.
3. Kadanka Z, Bednarik J, Vohanka S, et al. Conservative treatment versus surgery in spondylotic cervical myelopathy: a prospective randomised study. Eur Spine J. 2000;9:538-44.
4. Holly LT, Matz PG, Anderson PA, et al. Clinical prognostic indicators of surgical outcome in cervical spondylotic myelopathy. J Neurosurg Spine. 2009;11:112-8.
5. Kong LD, Meng LC, Wang LF, et al. Evaluation of conservative treatment and timing of surgical intervention for mild forms of cervical spondylotic myelopathy. Exp Ther Med. 2013;6:852-6.
6. Matsumoto M, Toyama Y, Ishikawa M, et al. Increased signal intensity of the spinal cord on magnetic resonance images in cervical compressive myelopathy. Does it predict the outcome of conservative treatment? Spine. 2000;25:677-82.
7. Levin K. Cervical spondylotic myelopathy. UpToDate 2013.
8. Bednarik J, Kadanka Z, Vohanka S, et al. The value of somatosensory- and motor-evoked potentials in predicting and monitoring the effect of therapy in spondylotic cervical myelopathy. Prospective randomized study. Spine. 1999;24:1593-8.
9. Adams AE. [Acid-base regulations in cerebrospinal fluid and brain functions]. Hippokrates. 1973;44:323-4.
10. Hirpara KM, Butler JS, Dolan RT, et al. Nonoperative modalities to treat symptomatic cervical spondylosis. Adv Orthop. 2012;2012:294857.
11. Mazanec D, Reddy A. Medical management of cervical spondylosis. Neurosurgery. 2007;60:S43-50.
12. Matz PG. Does nonoperative management play a role in the treatment of cervical spondylotic myelopathy? Spine J. 2006;6:175S-81S.
13. Lees F, Turner JW. Natural history and prognosis of cervical spondylosis. Br Med J. 1963;2:1607-10.
14. Nurick S. The pathogenesis of the spinal cord disorder associated with cervical spondylosis. Brain. 1972;95:87-100.
15. Clarke E, Robinson PK. Cervical myelopathy: a complication of cervical spondylosis. Brain. 1956;79:483-510.
16. Matsumoto M, Chiba K, Ishikawa M, et al. Relationships between outcomes of conservative treatment and magnetic resonance imaging findings in patients with mild cervical myelopathy caused by soft disc herniations. Spine (Phila Pa 1976). 2001;26:1592-8.
17. Nakamura K, Kurokawa T, Hoshino Y, et al. Conservative treatment for cervical spondylotic myelopathy: achievement and sustainability of a level of "no disability". J Spinal Disord. 1998;11:175-9.
18. Sampath P, Bendebba M, Davis JD, et al. Outcome of patients treated for cervical myelopathy. A prospective, multicenter study with independent clinical review. Spine (Phila Pa 1976). 2000;25:670-6.
19. Yoshimatsu H, Nagata K, Goto H, et al. Conservative treatment for cervical spondylotic myelopathy. Prediction of treatment effects by multivariate analysis. Spine J. 2001;1:269-73.
20. Kadanka Z, Mares M, Bednanik J, et al. Approaches to spondylotic cervical myelopathy: conservative versus surgical results in a 3-year follow-up study. Spine (Phila Pa 1976). 2002;27:2205-10; discussion 10-1.
21. Kadanka Z, Bednarik J, Novotny O, et al. Cervical spondylotic myelopathy: conservative versus surgical treatment after 10 years. Eur Spine J. 2011;20:1533-8.
22. Rhee JM, Shamji MF, Erwin WM, et al. Nonoperative management of cervical myelopathy: a systematic review. Spine (Phila Pa 1976). 2013;38:S55-67.

Chapter 8

# Influence of Surgical Intervention on Outcomes

*Hisashi Yoshimoto*

## INTRODUCTION

Recent advances in surgical treatment of cervical myelopathy are conspicuous. Patients suffering from cervical myelopathy can benefit from various sorts of decompression procedures, fusion procedures with/without instrumentation, and even minimally invasive ones.

The history of surgical intervention for cervical myelopathy is very long. Mixter and Osgood[1] reported, for the first time, posterior stabilization using silk threads for unstable traumatic atlantoaxial lesions in 1910. Afterward, many fusion and/or decompression procedures were developed and reported. However, those fumbling procedures had many flaws such as unsatisfactory clinical results, poor bony fusion rates, spinal malalignment, and even serious complications.

As far as decompression procedures are concerned, there was a major breakthrough in the 1970s. To that point the only decompression procedure for cervical myelopathy was laminectomy, which sometimes resulted in cervical kyphosis and instability causing unsatisfactory outcomes. However, Kirita[2] developed a far safer wide laminectomy using a burr; in addition, Oyama and Hattori[3] introduced a Z-shaped laminoplasty preserving the posterior elements of the cervical spine. They improved surgical outcomes of cervical myelopathy considerably. Their rational methods form the basis of today's decompression procedures of the cervical spine.

Regarding fusion procedures, Robinson,[4] Cloward,[5] and Bailey[6] developed sophisticated methods of anterior cervical spine fusion. Those satisfactory clinical results made anterior cervical spine fusion widespread. Southwick and Robinson[7] presented the detailed procedure of the anterior approach to the middle and lower cervical spine. The established anterior surgical approach as well as anterior decompression and fusion procedures themselves also moved cervical reconstructive surgery forward with a leap.

In addition, the long-time and gradual evolution of cervical spine instrumentation should be taken up for discussion. As a primitive spinal instrumentation, wiring procedures were widely utilized to fix the cervical spine posteriorly.[8-12] Luque rectangular rod and wiring has been applied to various pathologies, sites, and extents by many researchers to fix the cervical spine posteriorly.[13,14] The hook-and-rod system[15] and bone cement fixation[16] were also vigorously tried and reported. However, those biomechanical properties were not stable enough, so that they did not necessarily bring patients with cervical spine disorders satisfactory results.

For the last two decades, a plethora of new ideas and challenges provided by many researchers have spectacularly evolved cervical spine instrumentation. The posterior cervical spine systems using lateral mass screws[17-19] and pedicle screws,[20] which are applicable to various pathologies, almost all sites and diverse fusion levels, make it possible to better treat many cervical spine disorders needing fusion. In anterior cervical spine fusion, a plate-and-screw fixation system was first advocated by Orozco and Llovet.[21] It was refined by following anterior plate-screw systems such as the Caspar plate,[22] the cervical spine locking plate,[23] and miscellaneous others. Some have proposed anterior cervical pedicle screw fixation to add more stability to the spinal constructs.[24,25]

Nowadays, some attempts at minimally and/or less invasive surgical procedures for the cervical spine, e.g. skip laminoplasty and microendoscopic decompression, have been made.[26-28] Their final aims are to bring similar neurological improvement with little functional impairment such as reduced range of motion (ROM) of the cervical spine and axial pain owing to surgical approaches.

Thanks to both above-mentioned evolutions of operative techniques, including spinal instrumentation, and exquisite analyses of pathology by advanced diagnostic measures, global surgical outcomes of cervical myelopathy have been greatly improved compared with those at the dawn of cervical spine surgery. However, it is mandatory to evaluate each surgical procedure as to whether it truly contributes to expected clinical outcomes.

In this section, the influence of surgical intervention for cervical myelopathy on outcomes is reviewed in the literature so as to provide readers with an appreciation of the clinical benefits and limitations of surgery for cervical myelopathy. First of all, outcome measures that are appropriate to analyze the influence of surgical intervention for cervical myelopathy on outcome are reviewed. Thereafter, especially in cervical spondylotic myelopathy (CSM), cervical ossification of the posterior longitudinal ligament (OPLL), and rheumatoid arthritis (RA), which are thought to be more prevalent in the clinical situation, surgical outcomes are described with a review of the literature. Relatively rare etiologies such as spinal cord tumor, congenital disorders of the cervical spine, syringomyelia, and miscellaneous others are discussed elsewhere.

## OUTCOME MEASURES

It is very important to accurately and objectively evaluate the surgical outcomes of cervical myelopathy. Utilizing the well-known and widely accepted outcome measures is also recommended to make it easy to compare clinical results among institutes and/or papers.

Kalsi-Ryan et al.[29] comprehensively reviewed outcome measures for cervical myelopathy. Among a number of outcome measures, they divided them into four categories and advocated several for clinical usage as shown below.

### Upper Limb Assessment

1. The shortened version of the Disabilities of the Arm, Shoulder and Hand outcome measure (QuickDASH)[30]
2. The Graded Redefined Assessment of Strength, Sensibility and Prehension (GRASSP)[31]
3. Grip strength.

### Balance

1. Berg Balance Scale.[32]

### Gait

1. 10-meter walk test
2. 30-meter walk test[33]
3. 6-meter walk test.

### Overall Global Status

1. The modified Japanese Orthopaedic Association scale (mJOA)[34,35]
2. Nurick grade[36]
3. The Neck Disability Index (NDI)[37]
4. The Myelopathy Disability Index (MDI)[38]
5. The European Myelopathy Scale[39]
6. Short-Form 36.[40]

**Table 8.1:** Recommendable outcome measures for cervical myelopathy by Kalsi-Ryan et al.[29]

| *Construct* | *Screening* | *Clinical longitudinal* | *Research longitudinal* |
|---|---|---|---|
| Upper limb | GRASSP<br>Grip strength | GRASSP<br>Grip strength<br>QuickDASH | GRASSP<br>Grip strength<br>QuickDASH |
| Balance | | BBS | BBS |
| Gait | 30 MWT | 30 MWT<br>10 MWT<br>6 MWT | 30 MWT<br>10 MWT<br>6 MWT<br>GAITRite analysis |
| Global | NDI<br>mJOA<br>MDI | NDI<br>mJOA<br>MDI | NDI<br>mJOA<br>MDI<br>SF-36 |

(GRASSP: The Graded Redefined Assessment of Strength, Sensibility, and Prehension; Quick DASH: The shortened version of the Disabilities of the Arm, Shoulder, and Hand Outcome Measure; BBS: Berg Balance Scale; 30 MWT: 30 minute walk test; 10 MWT: 10 minute walk test; 6 MWT: 6 minute walk test; NDI: Nurick grade; mJOA: Modified Japanese Orthopaedic Association scale; MDI: Myelopathy Disability Index; SF-36: Short-Form 36.)

After a thorough review of related papers in terms of frequency of use in the literature, validity, reliability, and responsiveness, Kalsi-Ryan concluded that the mJOA, Nurick grade, NDI, MDI, 30-meter walk test were the most suitable for screening and clinical follow-up (Table 8.1). Although there were no studies that evaluated validity, reliability, and responsiveness in patients with cervical myelopathy, they proposed the QuickDASH, GRASSP and grip strength for upper limb assessment, along with the Berg Balance Scale and GAITRite analysis[41] for gait assessment as the supplementary outcome measures of cervical myelopathy.

Recently, the Japanese Orthopaedic Association (JOA) developed a new outcome measure, the Japanese Orthopaedic Association Cervical Myelopathy Evaluation Questionnaire, to comprehensively assess the severity of cervical myelopathy. It is a cervical-myelopathy-specific health-related quality-of-life (QOL) questionnaire that we have never had. It contains 24 questions in five domains such as cervical spine function, upper extremity function, lower extremity function, bladder function, and QOL, along with visual analogue scale scores of various portions of the body.[42,43] These multi-dimensional scales can allow spine surgeons to evaluate the patient status as a whole. Therefore, its increasing use in clinical practices and researches is expected.

In patients with RA, destructive multiple joint lesions make the accurate neurological examination very difficult. To resolve the limitation, Ranawat established a neurological measure to evaluate rheumatoid patients with cervical myelopathy.[44] Casey et al. also developed a functional scoring system, the MDI, for patients with RA.[38] Readers who are going to conduct clinical studies relating to cervical myelopathy are required to be familiar with these outcome measures.

## PREDICTIVE FACTORS OF SURGICAL OUTCOMES

Yoon et al.[45] looked at the predictive factors of laminoplasty for CSM. Their systematic review showed that progressive myelopathy, more severe neurological symptoms and longer duration of symptoms are correlated with poor clinical outcomes. However, increased age did not relate to poor neurological outcomes. Although they reviewed a variety of factors such as spinal alignment and magnetic resonance imaging (MRI) findings, they could not reach any other conclusions to determine the predictive factors affecting the surgical results of laminoplasty for CSM (Figs. 8.1A to F).

Li et al.[46] conducted a systematic review concerning the predictive factors of surgical outcomes in cervical OPLL. They enumerated the traverse area of the spinal cord, spinal cord evoked potentials, the increase of ROM, diabetes, history of trauma, onset of ossification of the ligamentum flavum in the thoracic spine, snake eye appearance in axial plane MRI, and incomplete decompression as predictive factors. However, they could not affirm the correlation with the neurological scores, OPLL type, the preoperative duration of symptoms, focal intra-medullar high signal intensity in T2-weighted images of MRI, progression of OPLL or kyphosis and expansion of the spinal canal because of the differences between each retrieved paper. Finally, they concluded that sex, involved levels, and many imaging measurements did not seem to predict the surgical outcomes.

Yoon et al.[45] and Li et al.[46] pointed out the lack of appropriate statistical analysis in the retrieved papers, that is, stepwise regression analysis and multivariate logistic analysis. They suggested that selection of proper endpoint and statistical analysis by subsequent researchers will facilitate the study to determine predictive factors affecting surgical outcomes (Table 8.2).

## OUTCOMES OF SURGICAL NTERVENTION FOR CSM

### Conservative Versus Surgical Treatment

Most spine surgeons might not doubt the effect of surgical treatment of CSM according to their clinical experiences. However, contrary to our expectation, almost no well-designed prospective studies demonstrated the superiority of surgical treatment to conservative management. Kadanka et al. mentioned in their prospective trial that, in mild and moderate cases of CSM, surgical treatment showed similar outcomes to conservative management.[47,48]

However, in moderate and severe CSM, two cohort studies conducted by Sampath et al.[49] and Yoshimatsu et al.[50] showed that surgical treatments were better than nonsurgical ones. However, those studies involved groups with different baseline symptoms between surgical and nonsurgical groups. Considering that surgical groups showed more severe clinical symptoms, they implied that surgical treatment should have had a larger influence on improvement of symptoms in patients with CSM.

As described above, sophisticated comparisons between conservative and surgical treatment of CSM are scant in the literature. If possible, more prospective studies comparing them are expected to firmly validate the surgical treatment of CSM.

### Anterior Versus Posterior

Lawrence et al. performed a systematic review to compare anterior procedures to posterior ones for multilevel CSM with regard to surgical effectiveness and safety.[51] Although some have favored anterior surgery and others have not, according to their thorough review, they concluded that clinical results of both procedures were similar concerning neurological improvement and rate of complications. They recommended deciding the surgical approach individually from the viewpoint of pathoanatomical variations such as ventral versus dorsal lesion, focal versus diffuse lesion, sagittal profile, and segmental instability. Fehlings et al.[52] supported the conclusions of Lawrence et al. The results of a multicenter study of 264 patients showed no significant differences between anterior and posterior groups with respect to surgical effectiveness and complications.

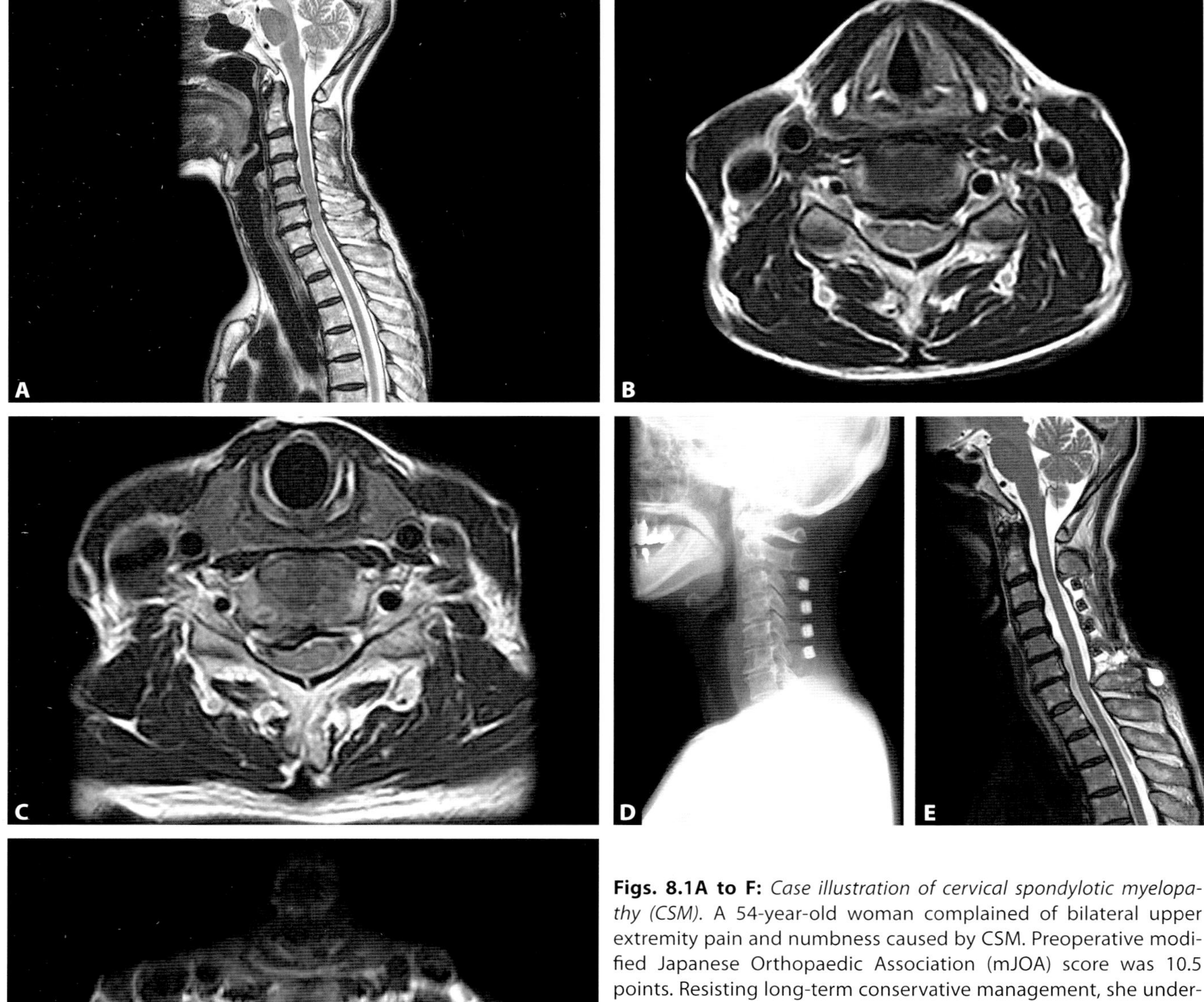

**Figs. 8.1A to F:** *Case illustration of cervical spondylotic myelopathy (CSM).* A 54-year-old woman complained of bilateral upper extremity pain and numbness caused by CSM. Preoperative modified Japanese Orthopaedic Association (mJOA) score was 10.5 points. Resisting long-term conservative management, she underwent C3-C7 double door laminoplasty. Two years after surgery, her mJOA score improved to 15.5 points. The clinical outcome was satisfactory. Note the adequate decompression, posterior shift and recovery of cross-sectional area of the spinal cord in postoperative magnetic resonance imaging (MRI). (A) T2-weighted MRI in the sagittal plane before surgery. (B) T2-weighted MRI in the axial plane at C4/C5 before surgery. (C) T2-weighted MRI in the axial plane at C5/C6 before surgery. (D) Lateral X-ray film after surgery. (E) T2-weighted MRI in the sagittal plane after surgery. (F) T2-weighted MRI in the axial plane at C5/C6 after surgery.

Liu et al. also conducted a systematic review in the same manner.[53] Contrary to the conclusions of Lawrence et al., they concluded that CSM with more than three levels of decompressed lesions should be treated by posterior procedures because of the higher rate of complication in anterior procedures. They stressed that anterior decompression and fusion should be limited to patients with fewer than two levels of involvement.

**Table 8.2:** Predictive factors affecting surgical outcomes of cervical myelopathy.

| | *Factors possibly causing poor outcomes* | *Factors that do not or are unclear to correlate with poor outcomes* |
|---|---|---|
| Yoon et al.[45] (literature review in CSM) | Progressive myelopathy<br>More severe neurological symptoms<br>Longer duration of symptoms | Increased age<br>Diabetes<br>Severity of stenosis<br>More than three levels of decompression<br>Local kyphosis<br>Signal intensity pattern in MRI |
| Li et al.[46] (literature review in OPLL) | Transverse area of the spinal cord<br>SCEPs<br>Increased ROM of the cervical spine<br>History of trauma<br>Concomitant thoracic OLF<br>SEA in MRI<br>Incomplete decompression | Neurological score<br>OPLL type<br>Preoperative duration of symptoms<br>Signal intensity pattern<br>Progression of OPLL<br>Local kyphosis<br>Amount of decompression<br>Sex<br>Involved levels |

(CSM: Cervical spondylotic myelopathy; OPLL: Ossification of the posterior longitudinal ligament; MRI: Magnetic resonance imaging; SCEPs: Spinal cord evoked potentials; ROM: Range of motion; OLF: Ossification of the ligamentum flavum; SEA: Snake eye appearance.)

## Laminectomy Versus Laminoplasty

Laminectomy alone is now uncommonly used to treat CSM because of the highly frequent onset of postlaminectomy kyphosis possibly affecting clinical outcomes, i.e. postoperative axial pain and relapsed myelopathy. Kaptain et al.[54] reported that 21% of patients showed postlaminectomy kyphosis within a 4-year follow-up period. In the literature, the occurrence of postoperative malalignment with or without clinical deterioration ranged from 6% to 30%.[55,56] However, laminectomy with posterior instrumentation and fusion versus laminoplasty seemed to show similar neurological improvement, axial symptoms, and complications according to some systematic reviews.[57,58]

## Influence of Spinal Kyphosis

Smith et al. reported that the severity of CSM was negatively correlated to sagittal alignment of the cervical spine, i.e. C2-C7 sagittal vertical axis.[59] In addition, many reports emphasize that cervical kyphosis reduced outcomes of laminoplasty for CSM.[60,61] However, some researchers mentioned that CSM with local kyphosis did not necessarily show unsatisfactory clinical outcomes of cervical laminoplasty.[62,63] Moreover, Ames and associates stated that correlation between surgical correction of kyphosis for patients with CSM and improvement of health-related QOL scores was not well defined.[64] As a whole, the influence of local kyphosis on surgical outcomes for CSM is still controversial.

## Role of Minimally Invasive and/or Less Invasive Cervical Spine Surgery

Skip laminectomy is one of the alternatives to conventional laminectomy and laminoplasty. Some authors stressed that skip laminectomy showed the same neurological recovery with less impairment of postoperative ROM and axial pain.[26,65] However, a prospective study by Yukawa et al. revealed that skip laminectomy and conventional laminoplasty showed the same neurological recovery, postoperative ROM of the cervical spine and neck pain.[66] Therefore, the clinical superiority of skip laminectomy in terms of postoperative axial symptoms and ROM of the cervical spine is not sufficiently demonstrated.

Some researchers introduced the minimally invasive posterior decompression for CSM and showed excellent clinical results also with regard to postoperative axial symptoms and ROM of the cervical spine. However, owing to short-term clinical results with limited case numbers, the effectiveness of minimally invasive cervical spine decompression is not yet adequately demonstrated.[27,28]

## Selective Versus Wide Decompression

Some clinical challenges were made to lessen the surgical invasiveness for elderly patients with CSM. Kato et al.[67] mentioned that guidance of the somatosensory-evoked potentials to select the responsible site of CSM was very effective when performing posterior decompression for CSM in the elderly. Tsuji and associates[68] selected the decompression levels in consideration of the disappearance of the subarachnoid space in MRI. Their retrospective study comparing selective laminoplasty with conventional C3-7 laminoplasty showed that there was no statistical difference. More studies concerning focal decompression might clarify their effectiveness.

## OUTCOMES FOR SURGICAL INTERVENTION OF CERVICAL OPLL

### Conservative Versus Surgical Treatment

In OPLL with cervical myelopathy, papers comparing conservative and surgical management are lacking. However, in acute spinal cord injury after minor trauma, Gu et al.[69] showed a prospective study comparing laminoplasty with conservative management. Although spontaneous improvement of spinal cord injury often occurred in patients having undergone conservative management, they concluded that laminoplasty showed better clinical results. In addition, Wu et al.[70] conducted a nationwide cohort study comparing conservatively managed cervical OPLL patients and age- and sex-matched people without cervical OPLL. They stated that OPLL patients had 32.16-fold higher risk for acute spinal cord injury. From the viewpoint of the much higher risk of subsequent spinal cord injury, conservative management in symptomatic cervical OPLL patients seems to be limited.

### Anterior Versus Posterior

A systematic review by Xu et al.[71] failed to determine which was superior—anterior or posterior surgery in cervical OPLL—because of the lack of prospective studies, disparity of surgical interventions, heterogeneity of outcome measures, and different qualities of studies. So far, there are no well-designed papers discussing this issue. However, Yamazaki et al.[72], Seichi et al.,[73] Fujiyoshi et al.,[74] and Iwasaki et al.[75] analyzed the limiting factors for indication of laminoplasty for cervical OPLL. They listed cervical kyphosis, hypermobility in the segments of spinal cord compression, thickness of OPLL, and canal occupying ratio as the factors affecting the surgical outcome of laminoplasty for cervical OPLL. Such limiting factors of laminoplasty for cervical OPLL imply that anterior decompression and fusion or posterior decompression with instrumented fusion might be more suitable to achieving better surgical outcomes (Figs. 8.2A to E). Further clinical research is needed.

## OUTCOMES OF SURGICAL INTERVENTION FOR RA

### Conservative Versus Surgical Treatment

Wolfs et al.[76] reported a systematic review concerning outcomes of both surgical and conservative treatment of rheumatoid cervical spine for the first time. They stated that if patients had neurological impairment (Ranawat II, IIIA, IIIB), surgical treatment was better than conservative nonsurgical one. However, in patients without neurological symptoms (Ranawat I), there were no significant differences in surgical outcomes. Some authors insisted that early and prophylactic surgical intervention for patients in Ranawat I and II would remarkably delay exacerbation of QOL and neurological status.[77,78] Some supposed that surgical treatment should improve QOL and mortality of patients in Ranawat IIB,[79-81] whereas others did not.[38] Wolfs et al. stated that they could not decide those issues from the systematic review because of the lack of randomized control studies.[76]

### Decompression, Short Fusion, and Long Fusion

Different patients with RA need different strategies to treat the cervical myelopathy surgically. Therefore, it is not necessarily easy to simply discuss it. However, some of the literature will be reviewed.

Some papers analyzed the clinical results of decompression alone for patients with cervical myelopathy due to RA.[82-84] However, there is no well-designed paper comparing decompression with fusion. Although spinal fusion is usually implemented when operating on patients with cervical myelopathy due to RA, a statistically obvious inferiority of decompression surgery alone could not be affirmed in both atlantoaxial subluxation and subaxial lesion.

In cases of simple atlantoaxial subluxation without advanced stage of RA, C1-C2 posterior fusion through various techniques seems to bring patients mid-term satisfactory results.[85] Even though randomized control trials are lacking in this issue, there seem to be few different opinions in the literature.

An issue of fusion levels is sometimes taken up for discussion. Most papers showed cases having undergone posterior cervical spine fusion within the involved levels. In spite of excellent or good clinical results presented in those papers, there are unresolved problems, such as adjacent segment subluxation possibly causing recurrence of cervical myelopathy.[86] In light of such subsequent exacerbation in shorter life expectancy in patients with RA, some authors proposed occipitothoracic fusion to lessen adjacent segment events in the cervical spine.[80,81]

However, Tanouchi et al.[87] conscientiously reported in their follow-up article that adjacent vertebral fractures occurred in 9 out of 35 patients having undergone occipitothoracic fusion. Diverse discussion continues on this issue. Again, additional well-designed studies are expected to clarify those problems (Figs. 8.3A to H).

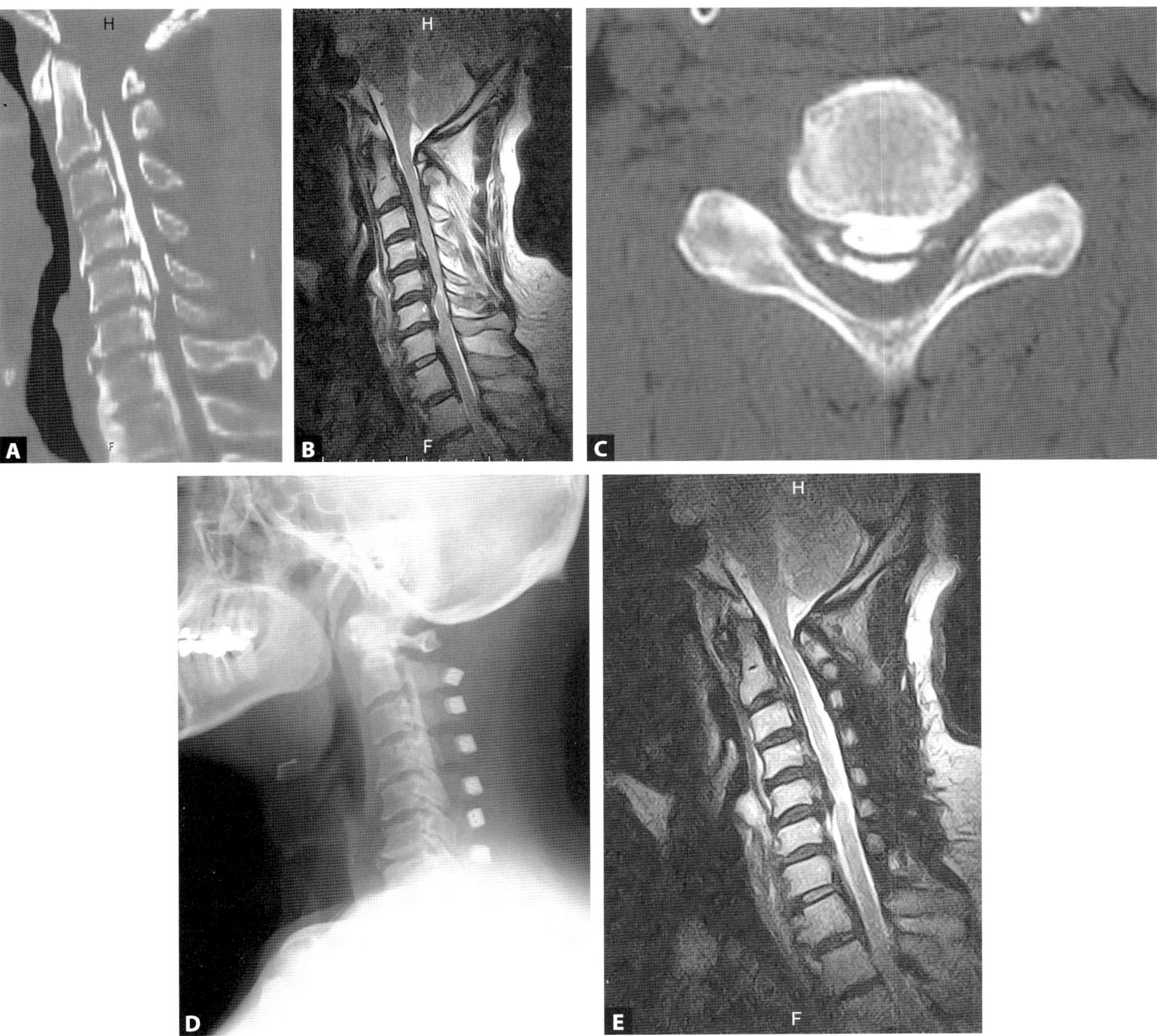


**Figs. 8.2A to E:** *Case illustration of cervical ossification of the posterior longitudinal ligament (OPLL).* A 56-year-old man suffering from deterioration of cervical myelopathy after a mild trauma visited our clinic. Mixed type OPLL from C2 to C6 could be seen. Modified Japanese Orthopaedic Association scale (mJOA) score was 6.5 points. C2-C7 double door laminoplasty was undertaken. At the final survey 4 years after surgery, the mJOA score was 9.5 points. The clinical outcome was not necessarily satisfactory. Huge OPLL, hypermobility at C5/C6 level with the biggest canal occupying rate, and unsatisfactory decompression of the spinal cord were thought to be causes of unsatisfactory neurological recovery. Note the insufficient expansion of subarachnoid space and posterior shift of the spinal cord compared to a cervical spondylotic myelopathy case shown in Figure 8.1. (A) Sagittal reconstruction computed tomography (CT) before surgery. (B) T2-weighted magnetic resonance imaging (MRI) in the sagittal plane before surgery. (C) Plain CT at C5/C6 before surgery. (D) Lateral X-ray film after surgery. (E) T2-weighted MRI after surgery.

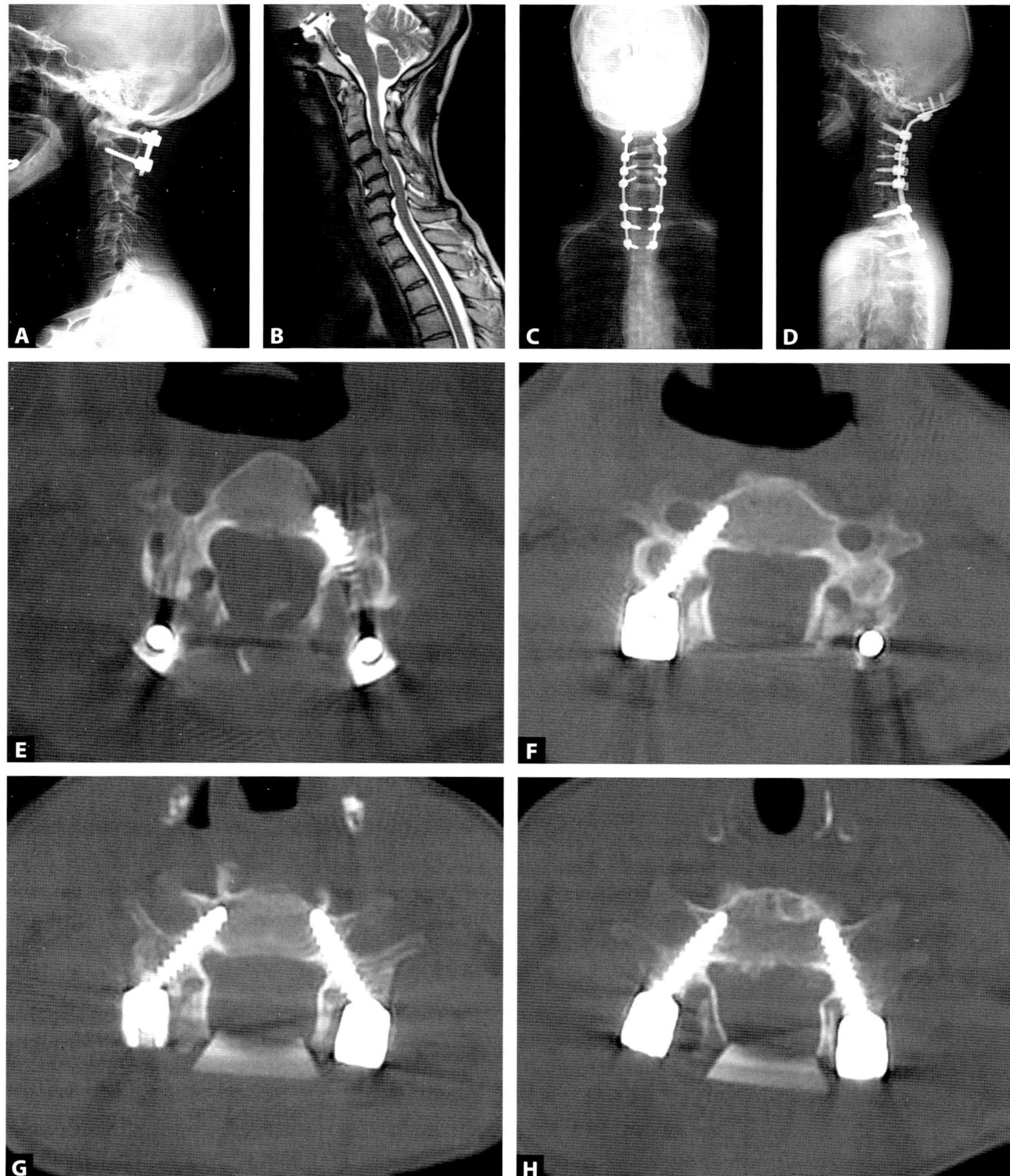


**Figs. 8.3A to H:** *Case illustration of rheumatoid arthritis (RA).* A 53-year-old woman suffered from Ranawat IIIA myelopathy 3 years after C1-C2 posterior fusion for atlantoaxial subluxation due to RA. Although C1-C2 fusion was rigid, marked subaxial subluxation caused obvious spinal cord compression. Just before C1-C2 posterior fusion, the subaxial cervical spine had been free from the obvious involvement of RA. The sites of spinal cord compression were C3/C4 and C5/C6. Because of a rapid spread of subaxial subluxation after the index surgery, decompression with short segmental fusion might result in following adjacent subluxation. Therefore, the author decided to implement occipitothoracic fusion to T3. Two years after the salvage surgery, her symptoms improved to Ranawat I. No additional spine lesions have occurred so far. The clinical outcome was satisfactory. Note all the cervical pedicle screws were in place. (A) Lateral X-ray film before surgery. (B) T2-weighted magnetic resonance imaging before surgery. (C) Anteroposterior X-ray film after surgery. (D) Lateral X-ray film after surgery. (E) Computed tomography (CT) at C3 after surgery. (F) CT at C4 after surgery. (G) CT at C5 after surgery. (H) CT at C6 after surgery.

## REFERENCES


1. Mixter WT, Osgood RB. Traumatic lesions of the atlas and axis. Am J Orthop Surg. 1910;7:348-70.
2. Kirita Y. Posterior decompression for cervical myelopathy due to ossification of the posterior longitudinal ligament [in Japanese]. Surgery (Shujutu). 1976;30:287.
3. Oyama M, Hattori S. A new method of posterior decompression [in Japanese]. Cent Jpn J Orthop Traumat. (Chubuseisaisi). 1973;16:792-94.
4. Robinson RA, Smith GW. Anterolateral cervical disc removal and interbody fusion for cervical disc syndrome. Bull Johns Hopkins Hosp. 1955;96:223-4.
5. Cloward RB. The anterior approach for removal of ruptured cervical disc. J Neurosurg. 1958;23:602-7.
6. Bailey RW. The Cervical Spine. Philadelphia: Lea and Febiger; 1974. pp. 146-56.
7. Southwick WO, Robinson RA. Surgical approaches to the vertebral bodies in the cervical and lumbar lesions. J Bone Joint Surg. 1957;39-A:631-44.
8. Cone W, Turner WG. The treatment of fracture-dislocations of the cervical vertebrae by skeletal traction and fusion. J Bone Joint Surg. 1937;19:584-602.
9. Gallie WE. Features and dislocations of the cervical spine. Am J Surg. 1939;46:495-9.
10. Brooks AL, Jenkins EB. Atlantoaxial arthrodesis by the wedge compression method. J Bone Joint Surg. 1978;60-A:279-84.
11. Rogers WA. Treatment of fracture-dislocation of the cervical spine. J Bone Joint Surg. 1942;24:245-58.
12. Robinson RA, Southwick WO. Surgical approaches to the cervical spine. Instr Course Lect. 1960;17:229-330.
13. Bridwell K. Treatment of markedly displaced hangman's fracture with a Luque rectangle and a posterior fusion in a 71-year-old man. Case report. Spine. 1986;11:49-52.
14. Ransford AO. Craniocervical instability treated by contoured loop fixation. J Bone Joint Surg. 1986;68-B:173-7.
15. Murphy MJ, Daniaux H, Southwick WO. Posterior cervical fusion with rigid internal fixation. Orthop Clin North Am. 1986;17:55-65.
16. Brattstrom H, Granholm L. Atlantoaxial fusion in rheumatoid arthritis: A new method of fixation with wire and bone cement. Acta Orthop Scand. 1976;47:619-28.
17. Roy-Camille R, Saillant G, Mazel C. Internal fixation of the unstable cervical spine by a posterior osteosynthesis with plates and screws. In: Sherk HH, Dunn EJ, Eismont FJ, et al. (Eds). The Cervical Spine, 2nd edition. Philadelphia: JB Lippincott; 1989. pp. 390-403.
18. An HS, Hordin R, Renner K. Anatomic considerations for plate-screw fixation of the cervical spine. Spine. 1991; 16:S548-51.
19. Jeanneret B, Magerl F, Ward EH. Posterior stabilization of the cervical spine with hook plates. Spine. 1991;16:S56-63.
20. Abumi K, Kaneda K. Pedicle screw fixation for nontraumatic lesions of the cervical spine. Spine. 1997;22:1853-63.
21. Orozco Delclos R, Llovet Tapies J. Osteosintesis en las fracturas de raquis cervical. Nota de tecnica. Rev Prtop Traumatol. 1970;14:285-8.
22. Caspar W, Barbier DD, Klara PM. Anterior cervical fusion and Caspar plate stabilization for cervical trauma. Neurosurgery. 1989;25:491-502.
23. Morscher E, Sutter F, Jenny H, et al. Anterior plating of the cervical spine with the hollow screw-plate of titanium. Chirurg. 1986;57:702-7.
24. Aramomi M, Masaki Y, Koshizuka S, et al. Anterior pedicle screw fixation for multilevel cervical corpectomy and spinal fusion. Acta Neurochir (Wien). 2008;150:575-82.
25. Yukawa Y, Kato F, Ito K, et al. Anterior cervical pedicle screw and plate fixation using fluoroscope-assisted pedicle axis view imaging: a preliminary report of a new cervical reconstruction technique. Eur Spine J. 2009;18:911-6.
26. Shiraishi T, Fukuda K, Yato Y, et al. Results of skip laminectomy: minimum 2-year follow-up study compared with open-door laminoplasty. Spine. 2003;28:2667-72.
27. Dahdaleh NS, Wong AP, Smith ZA, et al. Microendoscopic decompression for cervical spondylotic myelopathy. Neurosurg Focus. 2013;35:E8.
28. Minamide A, Yoshida M, Yamada H, et al. Clinical outcomes of microendoscopic decompression surgery for cervical myelopathy. Eur Spine J. 2010;19:487-93.
29. Kalsi-Ryan S, Singh A, Massicotte EM, et al. Ancillary outcome measures for assessment of individuals with cervical spondylotic myelopathy. Spine. 2013;38:S111-22.
30. Beaton DE, Wright JG, Katz JN. Development of the QuickDASH: comparison of three item-reduction approaches. J Bone Joint Surg Am. 2005;87:1038-46.
31. Kalsi-Ryan S, Curt A, Verrier MC, et al. Development of the Graded Redefined Assessment of Strength, Sensibility and Prehension (GRASSP): reviewing measurement specific to the upper limb in tetraplegia. J Neurosurg Spine. 2012;17:65-76.
32. Berg EM, Wood-Dauphinee S, Kesterson L, et al. Measuring balance in the elderly: preliminary development of an instrument. Physiother Can. 1989;41:304-11.
33. Singh A, Crockard HA. Quantitative assessment of cervical spondylotic myelopathy by a simple walking test. Lancet. 1999;354:370-3.
34. Bartels RH, Verbeek AL, Benzel EC, et al. Validation of a translated version of the modified Japanese Orthopaedic Association score to assess outcomes in cervical spondylotic myelopathy: an approach to globalize outcomes assessment tools. Neurosurgery. 2010;66:1013-6.
35. Benzel EC, Lancon J, Kesterson L, et al. Cervical laminectomy and dentate ligament section for cervical spondylotic myelopathy. J Spinal Disord. 1991;4:286-95.
36. Nurick S. The pathogenesis of the spinal cord disorder associated with cervical spondylosis. Brain. 1972;95:87-100.
37. Vernon H, Mior S. The neck disability index: a study of reliability and validity. J Manipulative Physicl Ther. 1991;14:409-15.
38. Casey AT, Crockard HA, Bland JM, et al. Surgery on the rheumatoid cervical spine for the non-ambulant myelopathic patient-too much, too late? Lancet. 1996;347:1004-7.
39. Herdman J, Linzbach M, Krzan M (Eds). The European Myelopathy Score. Berlin: Springer Verlag; 1994.
40. King JT Jr, Roberts MS. Validity and reliability of the Short Form-36 in cervical spondylotic myelopathy. J Neurosurg. 2002;97:180-5.

41. GAITRite Analysis, Homepage; Available at: http://www.gaitrite. com/index.html. Accessed September 13, 2013.
42. Fukui M, Chiba K, Kawakami M, et al. An outcome measure for patients with cervical myelopathy: Japanese Orthopaedic Association Cervical Myelopathy Evaluation Questionnaire (JOACMEQ): Part 1. J Orthop Sci. 2007;12:227-40.
43. Fukui M, Chiba K, Kawakami M, et al. JOA Back Pain Evaluation Questionnaire (JOABPEQ)/JOA Cervical Myelopathy Evaluation Questionnaire (JOACMEQ). The report on the development of revised versions. April 16, 2007. The Subcommittee of the Clinical Outcome Committee of the Japanese Orthopaedic Association on Low Back Pain and Cervical Myelopathy Evaluation. J Orthop Sci. 2009;14:348-65.
44. Ranawat CS, O'Leary P, Pellicci P, et al. Cervical spine fusion in rheumatoid arthritis. J Bone Joint Surg Am. 1979;61: 1003-10.
45. Yoon ST, Raich A, Hashimoto RE, et al. Predictive factors affecting outcome after cervical laminoplasty. Spine. 2013; 38:S232-52.
46. Li H, Jiang LS, Dai LY. A review of prognostic factors for surgical outcome of ossification of the posterior longitudinal ligament of cervical spine. Eur Spine J. 2008;17:1277-88.
47. Kadanka Z, Bednarik J, Novotny O, et al. Cervical spondylotic myelopathy: conservative versus surgical treatment after 10 years. Eur Spine J. 2011;20:1533-8.
48. Kadanka Z, Mares M, Bednanik J, et al. Approaches to spondylotic cervical myelopathy: conservative versus surgical results in a 3-year follow-up study. Spine. 2002;27:2205-10.
49. Sampath P, Bendebba M, Davis JD, et al. Outcome of patients treated for cervical myelopathy. A prospective, multicenter study with independent clinical review. Spine. 2000;25:670-6.
50. Yoshimatsu H, Nagata K, Goto H, et al. Conservative treatment for cervical spondylotic myelopathy. Prediction of treatment effects by multivariate analysis. Spine J. 2001; 1:269-73.
51. Lawrence BD, Jacobs WB, Norvell DC, et al. Anterior versus posterior approach for treatment of cervical spondylotic myelopathy: a systematic review. Spine. 2013;38:S173-82.
52. Fehlings MG, Barry S, Kopjar B, et al. Anterior versus posterior surgical approaches to treat cervical spondylotic myelopathy: outcomes of the prospective multicenter AOSpine North America CSM study in 264 patients. Spine. 2013;38:2247-52.
53. Liu X, Min S, Zhang H, et al. Anterior corpectomy versus posterior laminoplasty for multilevel cervical myelopathy: a systematic review and meta-analysis. Eur Spine J. 2014;23:362-72.
54. Kaptain GJ , Simmons NE , Replogle RE, et al. Incidence and outcome of kyphotic deformity following laminectomy for cervical spondylotic myelopathy. J Neurosurg. 2000;93: 199-204.
55. Hukuda S, Ogata M, Mochizuki T, et al. Laminectomy versus laminoplasty for cervical myelopathy: brief report. J Bone Joint Surg Br. 1988;70:325-6.
56. Herkowitz HN. A comparison of anterior cervical fusion, cervical laminectomy, and cervical laminoplasty for the surgical management of multiple level spondylotic radiculopathy. Spine. 1988;13:774-80.
57. Lao L, Zhong G, Li X, et al. Laminoplasty versus laminectomy for multi-level cervical spondylotic myelopathy: a systematic review of the literature. J Orthop Surg Res. 2013;8:45.
58. Yoon ST, Hashimoto RE, Raich A, et al. Outcomes after laminoplasty compared with laminectomy and fusion in patients with cervical myelopathy: a systematic review. Spine. 2013;38:S183-94.
59. Smith JS, Lafage V, Ryan DJ, et al. Association of myelopathy scores with cervical sagittal balance and normalized spinal cord volume: analysis of 56 preoperative cases from the AOSpine North America Myelopathy study. Spine. 2013;38: S161-70.
60. Suda K, Abumi K, Ito M, et al. Local kyphosis reduces surgical outcomes of expansive open-door laminoplasty for cervical spondylotic myelopathy. Spine. 2003;28:1258-62.
61. Baba H, Maezawa Y, Furusawa N, et al. Flexibility and alignment of the cervical spine after laminoplasty for spondylotic myelopathy. A radiographic study. Int Orthop. 1995;19:116-21.
62. Uchida K, Nakajima H, Sato R, et al. Cervical spondylotic myelopathy associated with kyphosis or sagittal sigmoid alignment: outcome after anterior or posterior decompression. J Neurosurg Spine. 2009;11:521-8.
63. Chiba K, Toyama Y, Watanabe M, et al. Impact of longitudinal distance of the cervical spine on the results of expansive open-door laminoplasty. Spine. 2000;25:2893-8.
64. Ames CP, Blondel B, Scheer JK, et al. Cervical radiographical alignment: comprehensive assessment techniques and potential importance in cervical myelopathy. Spine. 2013; 38:S149-60.
65. Sivaraman A, Bhadra AK, Altaf F, et al. Skip laminectomy and laminoplasty for cervical spondylotic myelopathy: a prospective study of clinical and radiologic outcomes. J Spinal Disord Tech. 2010;23:96-100.
66. Yukawa Y, Kato F, Ito K, et al. Laminoplasty and skip laminectomy for cervical compressive myelopathy: range of motion, postoperative neck pain, and surgical outcomes in a randomized prospective study. Spine. 2007;32:1980-5.
67. Kato Y, Kojima T, Kataoka H, et al. Selective laminoplasty after the preoperative diagnosis of the responsible level using spinal cord evoked potentials in elderly patients with cervical spondylotic myelopathy: a preliminary report. J Spinal Disord Tech. 2009;22:586-92.
68. Tsuji T, Asazuma T, Masuoka K, et al. Retrospective cohort study between selective and standard C3-7 laminoplasty. Minimum 2-year follow-up study. Eur Spine J. 2007;16:2072-7.
69. Gu Y, Chen L, Dong RB, et al. Laminoplasty versus conservative treatment for acute cervical spinal cord injury caused by ossification of the posterior longitudinal ligament after minor trauma. Spine J. 2014;14:344-52.
70. Wu JC, Chen YC, Liu L, et al. Conservatively treated ossification of the posterior longitudinal ligament increases the risk of spinal cord injury: a nationwide cohort study. J Neurotrauma. 2012;29:462-8.
71. Xu J, Zhang K, Ma X, et al. Systematic review of cohort studies comparing surgical treatment for multilevel ossification of posterior longitudinal ligament: anterior vs posterior approach. Orthopedics. 2011;33:e397-402.

72. Yamazaki A, Homma T, Uchiyama S, et al. Morphologic limitations of posterior decompression by midsagittal splitting method for myelopathy caused by ossification of the posterior longitudinal ligament in the cervical spine. Spine. 1999;24:32-4.
73. Seichi A, Chikuda H, Kimura A, et al. Intraoperative ultrasonographic evaluation of posterior decompression via laminoplasty in patients with cervical ossification of the posterior longitudinal ligament: correlation with 2-year follow-up results. J Neurosurg Spine. 2010;13:47-51.
74. Fujiyoshi T, Yamazaki M, Kawabe J, et al. A new concept for making decisions regarding the surgical approach for cervical ossification of the posterior longitudinal ligament: the K-line. Spine. 2008;33:E990-3.
75. Iwasaki M, Okuda S, Miyauchi A, et al. Surgical strategy for cervical myelopathy due to ossification of the posterior longitudinal ligament: part 1. Clinical results and limitations of laminoplasty. Spine. 2007;32:647-53.
76. Wolfs JF, Kloppenburg M, Fehlings MG, et al. Neurologic outcome of surgical and conservative treatment of rheumatoid cervical spine subluxation: a systematic review. Arthritis Rheum. 2009;61:1743-52.
77. Ronkainen A, Niskanen M, Auvinen A, et al. Cervical spine surgery in patients with rheumatoid arthritis: long-term mortality and its determinants. J Rheumatol. 2006;33:517-22.
78 Schmitt-Sody M, Kirchhoff C, Buhmann S, et al. Timing of cervical spine stabilization and outcome in patients with rheumatoid arthritis. Int Orthop. 2008;32:511-6.
79. Nannapaneni R, Behari S, Todd NV. Surgical outcome in rheumatoid Ranawat class IIIB myelopathy. Neurosurgery. 2005;56:706-15.
80. Matsuyama Y, Kawakami N, Yoshihara H, et al. Long-term results of occipitothoracic fusion surgery in RA patients with destruction of the cervical spine. J Spinal Disord Tech. 2005;18:S101-6.
81. Tanouchi T, Shimizu T, Fueki K, et al. Neurological improvement and prognosis after occipitothoracic fusion in patients with mutilating-type rheumatoid arthritis. Eur Spine J. 2012; 21:2506-11.
82. Suda Y, Saitou M, Shioda M, et al. Cervical laminoplasty for subaxial lesion in rheumatoid arthritis. J Spinal Disord Tech. 2004;17:94-101.
83. Ogawa H, Hosoe H, Hori H, et al. Postoperative cervical kyphosis after atlantoaxial fixation and cervical expansive laminoplasty at one time. J Spinal Disord Tech. 2006;19:607-11.
84. Mukai Y, Hosono N, Sakaura H, et al. Laminoplasty for cervical myelopathy caused by subaxial lesions in rheumatoid arthritis. J Neurosurg. 2004;100:7-12.
85. Nagaria J, Kelleher MO, McEvoy L, et al. C1-C2 transarticular screw fixation for atlantoaxial instability due to rheumatoid arthritis: a seven-year analysis of outcome. Spine. 2009;34:2880-85.
86. Matsunaga S, Sakou T, Onishi T, et al. Prognosis of patients with upper cervical lesions caused by rheumatoid arthritis: comparison of occipitocervical fusion between c1 laminectomy and nonsurgical management. Spine. 2003;28: 1581-7.
87. Tanouchi T, Shimizu T, Fueki K, et al. Adjacent-level failures after occipito-thoracic fusion for rheumatoid cervical disorders. Eur Spine J. 2014;23:635-40.

# Section 3

# Distinct Diagnostic Etiologies

Chapter 9

# Cervical Amyotrophy

*Venu M Nemani, Han Jo Kim*

## INTRODUCTION

Cervical spondylosis is very common, affecting the majority of people over the age of 65 years. Most people are asymptomatic with regard to neurological sequelae; however, some go on to develop symptoms and signs of either spinal cord compression (myelopathy) or nerve root compression (radiculopathy). In rare cases, however, cervical spondylosis causes severe upper extremity muscle atrophy without significant sensory symptoms. Keegan first described this pathology in a report in 1965, and described it as "dissociated motor loss in the upper extremities with cervical spondylosis." In his series, his patients complained of difficulty in raising their upper extremities due to severe muscle atrophy of their deltoid, biceps, and supinator muscles, with minimal sensory deficit and no long tract signs.[1] Crandall and Batzdorf estimated that <7% of patients with cervical spondylotic myelopathy present with minimal sensory loss, and they described this as a "motor system type of myelopathy."[2] Sobue first described this as cervical spondylotic amyotrophy (CSA), defined by dissociated motor loss with no, or minimal, sensory disturbance, and radicular pain in the upper extremities (although usually this is transient). Objective signs of lower extremity hyper-reflexia were also acceptable according to their definition.[3,4]

The precise pathophysiology of this disorder remains incompletely understood, leaving some uncertainty when counseling patients on the natural history as well as discussing the treatment options. In this chapter, we discuss the current literature on CSA including diagnosis and workup, as well as the current knowledge of both nonsurgical and surgical treatment options.

## CLINICAL PRESENTATION

Cervical spondylotic amyotrophy remains a relatively rare clinical entity, with its description being limited to several case series and no reports on its incidence in the population. Most literature has come from Japan with few reports from North America. The age of the onset of neurological symptoms is typically between 30 and 60 years, with men more frequently affected than women.

Cervical spondylotic amyotrophy is always associated with weakness and severe atrophy and wasting of the upper limb musculature without sensory involvement. It can present as a proximal-type, distal-type, or diffuse type with clinical symptoms depending on the precise pattern of muscle involvement. Patients with proximal-type wasting typically have weakness of the muscles around the scapula, deltoid, and biceps, and complain of difficulty with shoulder abduction and external rotation (positive arm-drop sign). Patients with distal-type CSA present with atrophy of the triceps, forearm musculature, and hand intrinsics and complain of difficulty extending the wrist and first finger (positive wrist-drop sign). There are also patients who have a diffuse type with more widespread myotomal involvement of the upper extremity. Also, a patient with CSA was described recently with dropped head syndrome from atrophic posterior neck and shoulder girdle muscles.[5]

## PATHOPHYSIOLOGY

Two different anatomic lesions have been proposed to be responsible for CSA: the ventral nerve root versus anterior horn motor neurons. Keegan's initial report on CSA described impingement on the ventral motor root from the uncovertebral joint.[1] However, subsequent studies using magnetic resonance imaging (MRI)[6] and delayed enhanced computed tomography (CT) scanning[7] suggested that impingement on the anterior horn was the cause of CSA. Due to the close anatomical relationship of these two structures, it is more than likely that both are involved to varying degrees in different patients, and subsequent studies have demonstrated this. Fujiwara et al.

examined 32 patients with unilateral CSA and found that 88% had impingement on the anterior horn, 66% had impingement on the ventral nerve root, and 53% had impingement on both.[8] Interestingly, their surgical outcomes were inferior in those patients with impingement on both structures compared to those with isolated impingement on the ventral motor root. Shinomiya et al. also showed radiologic and electrophysiologic evidence of both ventral motor root and anterior horn compression in CSA.[9]

Other studies have suggested that the location of the pathology may be different in proximal- versus distal-type CSA. Fujiwara et al. showed in their series that no patients with distal-type CSA had impingement only against the ventral nerve root; rather, these patients all had either isolated impingement against the anterior horn or combined pathology at both the anterior horn and ventral nerve root.[8] Another study used both MRI and recorded epidural spinal cord responses in patients with distal-type CSA and also found evidence of widespread selective gray matter lesions with no or less involvement of the cervical nerve roots.[10]

Finally, the pathophysiology causing the neurological injury itself remains unclear. While there is evidence for direct compression from spondylosis, others have proposed vascular insufficiency to the anterior horn cell at the paramedian compression as the underlying etiology.[11] The anterior horn is located in a watershed zone, in the terminal territory of the sulcal arteries, and is known to be vulnerable to the effects of diminished circulation.[12] Given the multilevel involvement often seen on MRI in the territory of the anterior spinal artery in patients with CSA, Zhang et al. investigated whether anterior spinal artery occlusion could be responsible for the "snake eyes" appearance of the cord on MRI in patients with CSA or cervical spondylotic myelopathy. Using CT angiogram, they found no definitive evidence for complete anterior spinal artery occlusion causing CSA in their series.[13] This, however, does not rule out a secondary dynamic compression of the anterior spinal artery or other vessels as a result of mechanical impingement from disk-osteophyte complexes that could result in ischemia of the anterior horn. More evidence is needed to ultimately define the true root of pathology in patients with CSA.

## PHYSICAL EXAMINATION

In addition to a standard physical examination of the cervical spine, the examination in patients with suspected CSA should particularly focus on inspection of the entire upper extremity and shoulder girdle for wasting and atrophy, and on manual muscle testing (MMT) of both upper and lower extremities and maneuvers to detect signs of myelopathy. Patients with CSA should have no, or very minimal, sensory deficits, and the examiner should confirm this by carefully testing light touch and two-point discrimination. The posterior column pathways should also be spared, so proprioception and vibration sense should be intact. Finally, a careful cranial nerve examination should be performed to rule out bulbar muscle involvement and the possibility of a motor neuron disorder. Specifically, the examiner should check for tongue atrophy or fasciculations, dysarthria, or dysphagia. These signs, in addition to diffuse muscle atrophy and weakness of neck flexor muscles, are all characteristic for amyotrophic lateral sclerosis (ALS) rather than CSA.

## IMAGING AND ELECTRODIAGNOSTIC STUDIES

As with all disorders affecting the cervical spine, radiographic evaluation should begin with plain X-rays of the cervical spine that can demonstrate cervical spondylosis. It is important to rule out instability with flexion/extension views, and oblique views may show osteophyte formation at the uncovertebral joints that may be responsible for compression of exiting ventral nerve roots. Computed tomography scanning will show the bony pathology in more detail; however, the mainstay of imaging is MRI, which can reveal impingement on the cord or nerve roots by either bone or disk, as well as any intramedullary signal change in the spinal cord. In addition to areas of focal impingement, the dimensions of the spinal canal also should be noted as canal stenosis over many levels may dictate the surgical approach necessary for adequate decompression (laminoplasty with foraminotomy vs. anterior cervical discectomy and fusion).

Kameyama et al. used MRI to demonstrate intrinsic cord pathology in three patients with CSA.[6] In this study, MRI examination showed linear high-signal intensity lesions within the compressed spinal cord, extending to more than one segment on sagittal images. Additionally, axial images showed the so-called "snake-eyes" appearance, referring to small symmetric intramedullary high-signal-intensity areas corresponding to the anterior horns (Figs. 9.1A to F). Lesions extending over multiple levels are key as single-level lesions are unlikely to cause significant

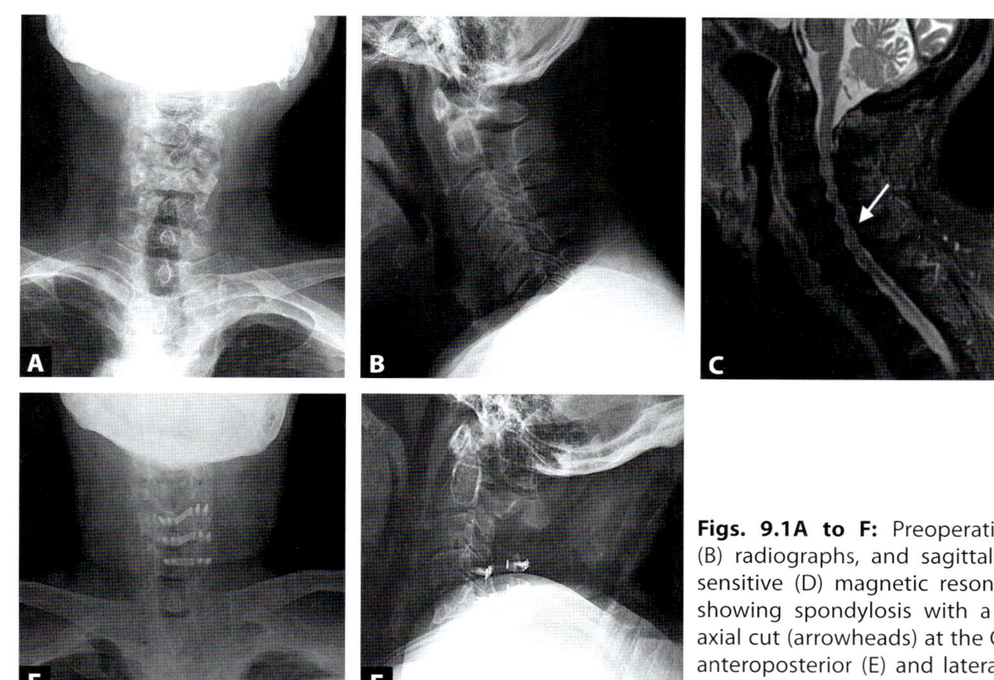


**Figs. 9.1A to F:** Preoperative anteroposterior (A) and lateral (B) radiographs, and sagittal fat-suppressed (C) and axial fluid-sensitive (D) magnetic resonance imaging of the cervical spine showing spondylosis with a typical "snake eyes" lesion on the axial cut (arrowheads) at the C5-6 level (arrow in C). Postoperative anteroposterior (E) and lateral (F) radiographs after a C2 and C7 partial laminectomy, C3 laminectomy, and C4-6 laminoplasty.

muscular atrophy due to innervation from multiple spinal levels, although these MRI changes are not found (or are below the limit of detection) in all patients with CSA.[14]

In one of the larger series on patients with CSA, Uchida et al. found that patients with distal-type CSA more commonly had high-signal-intensity MRI changes compared to patients with proximal-type CSA (66.7% vs. 35.7%, respectively, $p < 0.01$). Further, they also found that central compressive lesions were more likely to demonstrate T2 high-intensity cord signal change than paramedial or foraminal lesions (85.0% vs. 22.7% vs. 11.1%, $p < 0.05$), which is consistent anatomically with the central location of the spinal cord and anterior horn cells, versus the more lateral location of the ventral nerve root.[15] However, it remains unclear how evidence of T2 high-intensity cord signal change relates to the biological activity of the spinal cord and the anterior horn.

When there is no detectable signal change on MRI, the diagnosis of CSA is based on history, physical examination, and the electrodiagnostic studies, which are a key part of the diagnostic workup for CSA. Electromyography (EMG) shows denervation potentials and a decrease in the number of motor unit potentials in the affected muscles. Importantly, thoracic paraspinal muscles and lower limb muscles should not be affected in these patients, which can be clearly demonstrated by EMG.[16] Imajo et al. have measured compound muscle action potentials (CMAPs) from the deltoid and biceps brachii in patients with proximal-type CSA, and have used these measurements to predict the outcomes of both conservative[17] and surgical[16] management. As of yet, no one has reported on using CMAPs to define the severity of disease or to predict outcome after conservative or surgical treatment in distal-type CSA, which typically has a worse prognosis than proximal-type CSA.[8,15,18]

## DIFFERENTIAL DIAGNOSIS

The signs and symptoms of CSA can easily be confused with those of other diseases.[19] Making the diagnostic distinction between CSA and another disorder is critical before deciding to proceed with conservative, and especially surgical, intervention for CSA. Most notably, the motor neuron diseases, the most common of which is ALS, can be difficult to distinguish from CSA. Adding to the diagnostic dilemma is that both diseases preferentially affect middle-aged and elderly individuals, and that cervical spondylosis and ALS can be present in the same individual.

In the early stages, making a definitive diagnosis and distinguishing between the two entities can be difficult. Physical examination can be used to determine whether there is posterior column involvement (diminished vibratory sense or proprioception) that would rule out a pure motor neuron disease. Also, EMG analysis can be particularly helpful in this scenario, as changes are diffused in patients with ALS but should only be found in the affected atrophic muscles in patients with CSA. Above all else, patients in whom the diagnosis is unclear should be examined repeatedly over a period of time to observe for progression or changes in clinical symptoms until the diagnosis is certain. Cervical spondylotic amyotrophy follows a self-limited course with motor weakness that does not progress beyond a few myotomes, and with symptoms that usually stabilize for years after an initial progressive course. This is in contrast to ALS, which may begin focally but eventually progresses to involve the entire body and bulbar musculature and is progressive.

Cervical spondylotic amyotrophy should also be distinguished from Hirayama's disease (also known as monomelic amyotrophy or juvenile muscular atrophy of the distal extremity), which is similarly characterized by the insidious onset of asymmetric upper extremity weakness and muscular atrophy, usually without sensory changes.[20] The pathologic lesion also is in the anterior horn of the spinal cord, mostly commonly at C7 and T1.[21] Magnetic resonance imaging in the neutral position can show subtle cord atrophy, but the pathological hallmark of Hirayama's disease is anterior displacement of the cord with dynamic compression of the lower cervical cord, with epidural venous plexus engorgement.[21,22]

Finally, disorders affecting the brachial plexus or peripheral nerves that cause weakness and/or atrophy should be ruled out, such as brachial plexopathy from trauma, Parsonage-Turner syndrome, posterior interosseous nerve palsy, Cubital-Tunnel syndrome, or carpal tunnel syndrome. Even comparatively benign problems such as rotator cuff tears can cause atrophy and mimic proximal-type CSA. Given that treatment for these other diseases differs drastically from the treatment for CSA, it is critical to have a firm diagnosis before proceeding with targeted treatment.

## CONSERVATIVE TREATMENT

Unfortunately, there is no consensus on the optimal management of CSA. There have been several reports by Japanese surgeons on the outcomes of conservative treatment for CSA. Nagata et al. described 120 patients who were treated with a combination of cervical traction, neck immobilization using a collar, physical therapy, and administration of vitamin B12 or E.[23] They concluded that they were able to achieve recovery of shoulder function in 58% of their patients. Importantly, however, their study was limited only to those patients with proximal-type CSA.

More recently, Imajo et al. used CMAPs from the deltoid and biceps brachii muscles and correlated their findings with their MRI findings in 21 patients who underwent conservative therapy for proximal-type CSA.[17] Unfortunately, the specifics of their conservative treatment regimen were not included, other than that "most patients received medication, including vitamin B12." At an average of 30 months' follow-up, they found that 8 patients completely recovered their strength and 13 patients had incomplete recovery. They also concluded that patients with CMAP amplitude in the affected limb that was at least 50% that of the normal limb were able to fully recover muscle function with conservative treatment.

Another recent study reported on 90 patients (55 proximal-type, 24 distal-type) who underwent conservative treatment for CSA with 2–3 weeks of cervical traction. At discharge, they found good or excellent results in 46.7% (42 patients). At mean follow-up of 5 years, 51 patients avoided surgery, of whom 66.7% (34 patients) had good or excellent results.[24] The authors examined these patients further and found that patient age <50 years, symptom duration <6 months, single-level stenosis (vs. multiple levels), and foraminal stenosis (vs. central stenosis) were all predictive of success with conservative treatment.

## OPERATIVE TREATMENT

The indications for operative treatment of CSA have not yet been well defined. Inui et al. attempted nonoperative treatment first using traction, and then offered surgery to those patients who failed conservative treatment.[24] Another group recommended surgery on initial presentation if patients had very severe muscle atrophy or if their symptoms were longstanding, based on risk factors that they identified to be associated with a poor outcome from surgical treatment.[18] Currently, there is not enough information on the natural history of untreated CSA and long-term outcomes of those undergoing conservative treatment to define strict indications for operative treatment.

Several different procedures have been used in patients with CSA, including anterior cervical decompression and fusion (ACDF), laminoplasty, and posterior foraminotomy (often combined with laminoplasty). The argument for ACDF is that the offending lesions are almost always anterior; however, as described earlier, the spinal level responsible for the symptoms is not always clear from the imaging. In these situations, some argue that a posterior decompression of the spinal canal at all levels with selective foraminotomies at levels with foraminal stenosis is the best procedure. Unfortunately, the heterogeneity of patients in previously reported series makes a determination of the optimal procedure impossible. In patients in whom there are clearly only one or two affected levels with ventral lesions and sufficient space available for the cord, ACDF or anterior cervical corpectomy and fusion (ACCF) is likely the best procedure. When three or more levels are affected, there is a narrow spinal canal, and the patient has maintained cervical lordosis and the absence of neck pain, then laminoplasty with foraminotomy is probably a better option. Ultimately, surgeons must look carefully at all of the available information from the history, physical examination, and diagnostic studies to identify the offending lesion(s) and formulate an appropriate surgical strategy.

There have been several studies examining the outcomes of surgical treatment of CSA.[8,10,15,16,18,24-27] Fujiwara et al. performed laminoplasty in 32 patients with CSA (22 also had foraminotomy) and reported improvement in muscle power in 78% of patients, although, interestingly, 92% of proximal-type patients showed improvement versus only 38% of distal-type patients.[8] Uchida et al. reported on 51 patients who underwent surgical decompression (39 ACDF, 12 laminoplasty + foraminotomies). They found that proximal-type CSA patients with a long preoperative period and central rather than foraminal stenosis had worse outcomes.[15] In the largest series reported to date, Inui et al. treated 90 patients with CSA, with a protocol beginning with cervical traction for 2–3 weeks, and then indicated for surgery those patients who failed conservative management. In their series, 34 patients underwent an operation: 22 patients had a laminoplasty and selective foraminotomy, 5 patients had laminoplasty alone, and 7 had ACDF.[24] They found that 82% had postoperative improvement in their neurologic symptoms, but they were unable to determine the specific factors that were associated with a good outcome.

More recent studies have attempted to identify the factors associated with a poor outcome after surgical treatment of CSA. Imajo et al. used CMAPs from the deltoid and biceps brachii and central motor conduction time in a series of patients with proximal-type CSA, and found that patients with a good to excellent surgical outcome had CMAP amplitudes of at least 30% compared to the contralateral side.[16] Another group retrospectively reviewed 59 patients who underwent a variety of procedures, and found that symptom duration [odds ratio (OR) = 1.263], preoperative MMT grade (OR = 0.169), and distal-type CSA (OR = 9.223) were all associated with an increased risk of a poor surgical outcome.[18]

Several other studies have shown worse outcomes after surgical treatment of distal-type CSA compared to proximal-type CSA,[8,15] although at least one showed no difference.[24] In one of the larger series looking specifically at patients with distal-type CSA, Tauchi et al. reviewed 17 patients treated with surgery (11 laminoplasty, 1 laminoplasty + foraminotomy, 3 ACDF, 2 laminectomy + posterior spinal fusion). They had excellent results in 41% (7 patients), but in the subgroup of patients with preoperative MMT grade $< 3$, excellent recovery was only achieved in 30%.[25] Possible reasons for the inferior outcomes in distal-type CSA include impingement against the anterior horn (in distal-type CSA), which cannot regenerate like the ventral nerve root, and also the longer distance to the atrophied hand muscles (in distal-type CSA) compared to the deltoid and biceps (in proximal-type CSA). Further evidence, preferably prospective, is needed to better determine the factors that influence the outcome after surgery for CSA.

In patients who have had a poor outcome despite surgical decompression, there are unfortunately few options. However, Kumar et al. recently reported on eight patients with proximal-type CSA who underwent transfer of the trapezius, pectoralis major, latissimus dorsi, and Steindler's procedure to restore shoulder and elbow function.[28] With this salvage procedure, they reported that at 3 to 6 months' follow-up all patients had obtained satisfactory functional recovery and had improvement of 28 points in the Japanese version of the disabilities of the arm, shoulder and hand score. However, it is unclear whether this improvement would persist at long-term follow-up given the potentially progressive nature of the weakness in patients with CSA.

## CONCLUSION

Cervical spondylotic amyotrophy is a difficult to treat disorder characterized by upper extremity muscle atrophy and weakness without sensory deficit or myelopathy. More research is needed to better define the pathophysiology, as this may improve our ability to provide targeted nonsurgical and surgical treatments. Currently, there is no evidence favoring ACDF versus posterior decompression using laminoplasty with selective foraminotomy in the treatment of CSA. For one- or two-level ventral lesions without canal stenosis, ACDF will likely be effective. For lesions >2 levels with concomitant canal stenosis, laminoplasty with selective foraminotomy will provide effective decompression.

## REFERENCES

1. Keegan JJ. The cause of dissociated motor loss in the upper extremity with cervical spondylosis. J Neurosurg. 1965; 23(5):528-36.
2. Crandall PH, Batzdorf U. Cervical spondylotic myelopathy. J Neurosurg. 1966; 25(1):57-66.
3. Sobue I, Kato H, Yanagi T. Clinical characteristics and classification of cervical spondylotic myelopathy. Rinsho Seikeigeka. 1975;10:999-1006.
4. Yanagi T, Kato H, Sobue I. Clinical characteristics of cervical spondylotic amyotrophy. Rinsho Shinkeigaku. 1976; 16:520-8.
5. Ahdab R, Creange A, Benaderette S, et al. Cervical spondylotic amyotrophy presenting as dropped head syndrome. Clin Neurol Neurosurg. 2009;111(10):874-6.
6. Kameyama T, Ando T, Yanagi T, et al. Cervical spondylotic amyotrophy. Magnetic resonance imaging demonstration of intrinsic cord pathology. Spine (Phila Pa 1976). 1998; 23(4):448-52.
7. Fujiwara K. Cervical spondylotic amyotrophy with intramedullary cavity formation. Spine (Phila Pa 1976). 2001; 26(10):E220-2.
8. Fujiwara Y, Tanaka N, Fujimoto Y, et al. Surgical outcome of posterior decompression for cervical spondylosis with unilateral upper extremity amyotrophy. Spine (Phila Pa 1976). 2006;31(20):E728-32.
9. Shinomiya K, Komori H, Matsuoka T, et al. Neuroradiologic and electrophysiologic assessment of cervical spondylotic amyotrophy. Spine (Phila Pa 1976). 1994;19(1):21-5.
10. Kaneko K, Taguchi T, Toyoda K, et al. Distal-type cervical spondylotic amyotrophy: assessment of pathophysiology from radiological findings on magnetic resonance imaging and epidurally recorded spinal cord responses. Spine (Phila Pa 1976). 2004;29(9):E185-8.
11. Ito T, Tsuji H, Tamaki T, et al. The clinical consideration of the dissociated motor loss syndrome (Keegan) in diseases of the cervical spine. Nippon Seikeigeka Gakkai Zasshi. 1980;54:135-51.
12. Gilles FH, Nag D. Vulnerability of human spinal cord in transient cardiac arrest. Neurology. 1971;21(8):833-9.
13. Zhang Z, Wang H. Is the "snake-eye" MRI sign correlated to anterior spinal artery occlusion on CT angiography in cervical spondylotic myelopathy and amyotrophy? Eur Spine J. 2014;23(7):1541-7.
14. Iizuka Y, Iizuka H, Mieda T, et al. Prognostic factors for cervical spondylotic amyotrophy: are signs of spinal cord involvement associated with the neurological prognosis? Spinal Cord. 2014;52(5):364-7.
15. Uchida K, Nakajima H, Yayama T, et al. Anterior and posterior decompressive surgery for progressive amyotrophy associated with cervical spondylosis: a retrospective study of 51 patients. J Neurosurg Spine. 2009;11(3):330-7.
16. Imajo Y, Kato Y, Kanchiku T, et al. Prediction of surgical outcome for proximal-type cervical spondylotic amyotrophy novel mode of assessment using compound action potentials of deltoid and biceps brachii and central motor conduction time. Spine (Phila Pa 1976). 2012;37(23):E1444-9.
17. Imajo Y, Kato Y, Kanchiku T, et al. Pathology and prognosis of proximal-type cervical spondylotic amyotrophy: new assessment using compound muscle action potentials of deltoid and biceps brachii muscles. Spine (Phila Pa 1976). 2011;36(7):E476-81.
18. Tauchi R, Imagama S, Inoh H, et al. Risk factors for a poor outcome following surgical treatment of cervical spondylotic amyotrophy: a multicenter study. Eur Spine J. 2013;22(1):156-61.
19. Kim HJ, Tetreault LA, Massicotte EM, et al. Differential diagnosis for cervical spondylotic myelopathy: literature review. Spine (Phila Pa 1976). 2013;38(22 Suppl 1):S78-88.
20. Tashiro K, Kikuchi S, Itoyama Y, et al. Nationwide survey of juvenile muscular atrophy of distal upper extremity (Hirayama disease) in Japan. Amyotroph Lateral Scler. 2006;7:38-45.
21. Chen CJ, Chen CM, Wu CL, et al. Hirayama disease: MR diagnosis. AJNR Am J Neuroradiol. 1998;19(2):365-8.
22. Pinho J, Machado C, Oliveira TG, et al. Dynamic myelopathy in Hirayama disease. Spine J. 2014;14(11):2789-90.
23. Nagata K, Ohashi T, Ishibasi K, et al. Effectiveness of conservative treatment for Keegan type upper extremity dysfunction. Seikei Saigai Geka. 1996;39:131-7.
24. Inui Y, Miyamoto H, Sumi M, et al. Clinical outcomes and predictive factors relating to prognosis of conservative and surgical treatments for cervical spondylotic amyotrophy. Spine (Phila Pa 1976). 2011;36(10):794-9.
25. Tauchi R, Imagama S, Inoh H, et al. Characteristics and surgical results of the distal type of cervical spondylotic amyotrophy. J Neurosurg Spine. 2014:1-6.
26. Takebayashi T, Yoshimoto M, Ida K, et al. Minimum invasive posterior decompression for cervical spondylotic amyotrophy. J Orthop Sci. 2013;18(2):205-7.
27. Zhang JT, Yang da L, Shen Y, et al. Anterior decompression in the management of unilateral cervical spondylotic amyotrophy. Orthopedics. 2012;35(12):e1792-7.
28. Kumar KK, Doi K, Hattori Y, et al. Reconstruction of shoulder and elbow function using multiple muscle transfers for cervical spondylotic amyotrophy. Spine (Phila Pa 1976). 2014;39(21):E1269-75.

Chapter 10

# Rheumatologic Disorders of the Cervical Spine

*Afshin E Razi, Lana Nirenstein, Yong Kim*

## RHEUMATOID ARTHRITIS

Rheumatoid arthritis (RA) is a chronic inflammatory autoimmune disorder that typically affects many organs, including the small joints of the hands and feet. Rheumatoid arthritis is the most common source of inflammatory disease of cervical spine. Classically, it is the upper cervical spine that is most affected. The three hallmark disorders of the cervical spine most appreciated are atlantoaxial subluxation (AAS), vertical settling, and subaxial subluxation.

Rheumatoid arthritis is relatively common, affecting 0.5–1.5% of the US population. Women are twice as likely as men to develop RA. Although the etiology of RA still remains unsolved, it is highly likely that it is a multifactorial disease with a strong genetic basis. It is thought that the disease is triggered by exposure of an immunogenetically susceptible host to an arthritogenic microbial antigen. The rheumatoid factor is the immunoglobulins (IgM) that are produced by the body against autologous IgG. An inflammatory response cascade is then initiated, resulting in a proliferative and erosive synovitis that progresses to destruction of articular cartilage and pannus formation. Rheumatoid arthritis has drastic systemic effects. It reduces life expectancy, and patients afflicted with this disease report becoming disabled within a decade of the disease onset. However, the natural course is varied and unpredictable, and may either be chronic and progressive or characterized by intermittent bouts of flares and remission. Aggressive medical therapy prior to cartilage destruction may prevent or delay joint damage. Therefore, the timely start of pharmacotherapy such as newer immunological mediators can slow progression of the disease.

Rheumatoid arthritis leads to pannus formation and chronic synovial inflammation, resulting in joint destruction or severe incompetence of the osseous structures, ligaments, and tendons. The cervical spine is the second most affected site after the metatarsophalangeal joints. Garrod first reported involvement of the cervical spine in 36% of patients with RA in 1890.[1] Kornblum et al. acknowledged the link between RA and cervical spine instability in 1952.[2] In the cervical spine, the disease is manifested as subluxation, instability, and spinal cord compression. Patients may complain of pain, instability, and neurologic deficits. Rawlins et al. estimated that between 17% and 86% of RA patients have cervical spine involvement, depending on the patient population and diagnostic criteria. In addition, the cervical spine disease is chronologically associated with RA, often seen within 2 years of the onset of RA with a prevalence of 12%.[3] Atlantoaxial instability with myelopathy arises in 2.5% of patients with RA with disease after about 14 years.[4] Three patterns of instability in the rheumatoid spine have been described: AAS, atlantoaxial impaction or cranial settling, and subaxial subluxation. Each may be present in isolation or may exist in combination with the other forms of instability. Riise et al. documented a mean observation time from the diagnosis of RA to AAS of 3.9 years.[5] Pellicci et al. reported that 43% of their patients presented with radiographic evidence of rheumatoid disease of the cervical spine at the start of study.[6] Atlantoaxial subluxation was seen in 61%, AAS combined with subaxial subluxation in 20%, and subaxial subluxation in 11%. On the follow-up study, it was evident that cervical subluxation occurred more in patients with erosions of the hands and feet. Several studies have shown that the severity of cervical spine involvement correlates with male gender, high seropositivity, rheumatoid nodules, vasculitis, high-dose steroid therapy, and severity of peripheral joint disease.[7-10]

The ultimate danger is spinal cord or brain stem compression and subsequent paralysis or death. Sunahara et al. reported on 21 patients with RA and myelopathy secondary to AAS who refused surgery.[11] There was no improvement, and 76% of them had evidence of deterioration in follow-up. Furthermore, all became bedridden within 3 years after the onset of myelopathy and the cumulative probability of survival was 0% in 7 years following the onset of myelopathy. Another study reported that RA patients with AAS had an eight times higher mortality rate than those without AAS.[5] Hence, it is imperative to identify patients with a high chance of neurologic deterioration and to intervene surgically to prevent catastrophic, permanent neurologic compromise.

Boden et al. followed 73 RA patients with cervical spine disease over an average of 7.1 years. Of these, 58% became paralyzed. The majority of patients who were treated nonoperatively deteriorated neurologically, and all died within 4 years. Of those who were treated operatively, 71% had neurologic improvement with initial neurologic class directly correlating to postoperative neurologic outcome.[12]

## PATHOPHYSIOLOGY

There are 22 separate synovial joints in the cervical spine, including the atlanto-occipital, atlantoaxial, and facet (apophyseal) joints. Each is a potential target of RA. The atlanto-occipital and atlantoaxial joints do not have any intervertebral disks or uncovertebral joint of Luschka. The C1-C2 facet joints are also orientated in an axial direction. There are several important ligaments that help with the stability of the atlantoaxial segment. The primary restraint is the transverse ligament. There is synovium noted between the transverse ligament and the odontoid. The secondary stabilizer is the alar ligament located between the odontoid process and the occiput. Another stabilizer is the apical ligaments, which provide support for the occiput-atlantoaxial articulation. Complete resection of the transverse ligament causes 4–5 mm of anterior C1-C2 subluxation as long as the secondary stabilizers are intact. It is only after the secondary stabilizers are damaged that there is >10 mm of subluxation.

Several inflammatory factors mediate the cascade of pathologic processes of RA disease. These include several growth factors, cytokines, and metalloproteinases. These factors are involved in activation and proliferation of synoviocytes and result in destruction of articular cartilage, tendons, ligaments, and subchondral bone. As the synovitis advances, there is bone erosion and ligamentous laxity, causing mechanical instability of the cervical spine. The most common presentations of cervical spine disease include AAS (65%), cranial settling (20%), subaxial subluxation (15%), or a combination.

### Atlantoaxial Subluxation

The synovial joints are damaged by pannus formation, which is a fibrous inflammatory tissue observed in RA. Pannus formation and synovitis can degrade the mechanical integrity and strength of the transverse, alar and apical ligaments. Over time, the compromised ligaments can become overly stretched or even rupture from the repetitive strain and the weight of the head. The most common place for the transverse ligament to rupture is at the site of synovial bursa, which separates it from the posterior face of the odontoid process. Chronic inflammation leads to decalcification of nearby bone, allowing the ligament to avulse off the insertion site of the atlas.

Subluxation can also be caused by erosion of the odontoid process, another classic feature of RA. There are three locations where this erosion may take place: anteriorly at the synovial joint with the anterior arch of the atlas, posteriorly at the synovial joint with the transverse ligament, and superiorly at the insertion of the apical ligament. Asymmetric erosion guides the way to several different radiographic patterns of instability, including anterior (most common), posterior (7%), or lateral subluxation with rotatory component (20%).

Atlantoaxial subluxation is identified in nearly half of all RA patients. In the majority of cases, the atlas translates anteriorly on the axis. This can be recognized on a cervical spine lateral radiograph as an increased anterior atlantodental interval (AADI) and decreased posterior atlantodental interval (PADI).

Unfortunately, AAS is progressive. As the atlas moves away from the axis, the space available for the cord (SAC) decreases. Initially, the deformity may be dynamic, only becoming apparent on flexion views and reducible in its early stages. The SAC decreases as the anterior atlantodental interval increases and the posterior atlantodental interval (PADI) decreases. As the disease progresses, pannus may become interposed between the atlas and the dens, blocking reduction and transforming a dynamic deformity into a fixed one. The pannus behind the odontoid may decrease the PADI, resulting in reduction of the SAC. Subluxation can eventually cause cord compression and neurologic compromise due to myelopathy.

### Cranial Settling

This phenomenon is also known as basilar invagination, rostral migration of the dens, atlantoaxial impaction, translocation of the dens, vertical settling, or superior migration of the dens. In brief, it results from diseased atlanto-occipital and atlantoaxial joints. Disease involvement softens the articulations and can lead to collapse of the lateral masses, resulting in cephalad translation of the odontoid process and ultimately cranial settling. The prevalence is estimated to be between 5% and 32%, and appears after AAS. Compared with the other instability patterns, cranial settling seems to be the most ominous and carries the highest risk of myelopathy.

Impingement of the first cervical nerves leads to occipitocervical pain, while ventral pressure on the medulla oblongata can compromise and injure cranial nerves or cause sudden death by harming the respiratory center. The vascular supply is also at risk. The anterior spinal artery and vertebral artery can be compressed, leading to immediate neurologic deficits, transient ischemic attacks, or vertebrobasilar insufficiency. As atlantoaxial impaction progresses, the dens is driven further into the foramen magnum and AAS may decrease, a phenomenon known as "pseudostabilization".[13] This phenomenon indicates worsening of the disease, which can be interpreted as improvement of the anatomic subluxation.

### Subaxial Subluxation

Facet joints are destabilized when RA weakens their facet capsules and interspinous ligaments. Destabilization leads to anterior subaxial subluxation. This is followed by osteophyte formation, ankylosis, bone collapse, and kyphosis. A typical "staircase" deformity is seen when there is multilevel involvement with an associated kyphosis. Although moderate to severe degenerate disk disease is observed in this population of patients, it is not due to synovitis. This instability pattern occurs last in the trilogy described and affects nearly a quarter of patients living with RA.

Subaxial subluxation can also be appreciated following upper cervical fusion in RA patients, most frequently observed at the C2-C3 and C3-C4 levels. The subluxation may not be readily visible on lateral radiographs, but it can be elicited on flexion and extension radiographs.

## CLINICAL PRESENTATION

Although most patients with rheumatoid involvement of the cervical spine are asymptomatic, most will develop neck pain. Patients usually describe the discomfort as a deep pain radiating into the occipital, retro-orbital, or temporal areas. When pain is referred to the face or ears, it is often the result of irritation of the C2 nerve, the nucleus of the spinal trigeminal tract, or the greater auricular nerve. When patients complain primarily of subocciput pain, it is due to involvement of the lesser occipital nerve (C1); when the pain is located at the occipital region, it is usually due to the greater occipital nerve (C2). The incidence of occipital headache is higher in patients with cranial settling. There are also uncommon symptoms such as vertigo, visual disturbances, tinnitus, loss of equilibrium, diplopia, and dysphagia due to vertebrobasilar insufficiency or spinal cord compression at the cervicomedullary junction. Patients with cranial settling also have a higher incidence of myelopathy, brain stem dysfunction, and cranial nerve involvement.

Patients may also report experiencing their head fall forward during neck flexion. A clunk may be experienced during extension, which represents spontaneous reduction of a subaxial subluxation. This phenomenon has been termed the Sharp-Purser test. Therefore, obtaining a thorough history is crucial.

Unlike radiographic changes, neurologic deficits tend to occur later in the course of RA, affecting patients who are late middle aged. Objective neurologic deficits are harder to elicit, due to multiple joint involvement with decreased painful range of motion, neuropathy, and muscle wasting. Signs of myelopathy should be aggressively monitored, such as gait changes, clumsiness in performing fine motor tasks, or bowel and bladder dysfunction. Other classic physical exam findings include hyperreflexia, upgoing toes (also known as a Babinski sign), a positive Hoffman's sign, and Lhermitte's sign. Serial physical examination is recommended, including subtle findings such as loss of proprioception and spasticity.

Several classification systems have been developed to assess cervical spine disease in patients with RA. Most of these classifications are limited due to many limitations secondary to associated disabilities such as deformities, arthritic changes, and neuropathy. Some reported classification systems include the American Rheumatological Association, the Steinbrocker, and the Ranawat classification. The Ranawat classification is frequently used to group RA patients with cervical spine disease according to their physical findings. This system is helpful in establishing a baseline neurologic function, planning surgery, and predicting postoperative outcome and neurologic recovery. Class I includes patients with neck pain but no neurologic deficits. Class II includes patients with subjective complaints, such as weakness and dysesthesia. Class

III describes patients with objective weakness and long tract signs. Class III is further divided into two groups: Class IIIA patients are ambulatory and class IIIB are not.[14]

## RADIOGRAPHIC EVALUATION

Screening radiographs are not accepted as the standard of care, and the importance of preoperative screening for cervical disease in RA patients continues to be debated. However, radiographs are recommended in some groups of high-risk patients who will be receiving endotracheal intubation. Suggested films include lateral, anteroposterior, open mouth, lateral flexion, and extension views. Plain radiographs are often difficult to assess due to bony overlap, osteopenia, and odontoid erosions. Riew et al. evaluated radiographs of patients with rheumatoid disease of cervical spine.[15] The most simply recognized markers were the hard palate, definitely visible on 93% of X-rays, and the atlas, definitely seen in 88% of cases. The tip of the dens was the least clearly distinguishable marker. Therefore, attention should be given to identify several markers on the lateral view. These include the clivus, hard palate, opisthion (the dorsal border of the foramen magnum), basion (the ventral border of the foramen magnum), atlas, pedicle of axis, and tip of the dens.

The AADI is measured from the posterior aspect of the ring of the atlas to the anterior aspect of the dens. The normal value is <3 mm.[16] The AADI is commonly used to assess patient with RA, and surgical modalities have been recommended based on this measurement. Many studies have suggested a threshold of 8–10 mm for surgical intervention.[17-19] However, other studies have indicated that AADI is not a consistent measurement.[20,21] As indicated previously, the odontoid process migrates cranially as the disease progresses, giving a false indication of improved AADI.[13,22] Furthermore, this measurement is limited due to variations in the diameter of the atlas and pannus posterior to the dens. The PADI is measured from the posterior aspect of the dens to the anterior border of the posterior ring of the atlas. Boden et al. showed that 60% of patients with AAS and neurologic compromise had an AADI <9 mm in contrast to 96% of patients with AAS and Ranawat III who had PADI of ≤13 mm.[12] Those with a Ranawat II had a mean PADI of 13 mm and Ranawat I had 15 mm. This study showed that a PADI of ≤14 mm had a 97% sensitivity and 52% specificity compared to an AADI of >8 mm with a 59% sensitivity and 58% specificity in recognizing those with paralysis.

Atlantoaxial impaction or cranial settling can be diagnosed through a variety of radiographic measurements. One measurement frequently used is McGregor's line. It is seen on a lateral radiograph as the line between the hard palate and the opisthion. Protrusion of the dens beyond this landmark by >4.5 mm confirms atlantoaxial impaction. However, odontoid erosion can mask the impaction. Other measurements include McRae's line and Chamberlain's line. The Ranawat method was created to gauge the collapse at the atlantoaxial articulation. It is the vertical distance between the lines drawn across the transverse axis of the atlas and the C2 pedicle. Values of <15 mm in men and <13 mm in women are suggestive of settling. The Redlund-Johnell value represents the occiput to C2 changes. Clark et al. illustrated another technique by dividing the odontoid process into three stations.[19] Typically, the cranial third of the dens is at the level or next to the ring of the atlas (station I). In station II, the middle third of dens is at the level of the ring, and in station III the inferior third of the dens is at the level of the ring, indicating severe cranial settling.

Riew et al. showed that a combination of Clark's stations, the Ranawat index, and the Redlund-Johnell value had sensitivity of 94% and a negative predictive value of 91%, much higher compared to one single measurement. They also suggested that if any of these values are positive for cranial settling, another neurodiagnostic test (computed tomography [CT] or magnetic resonance imaging [MRI]) should be performed.[15]

Radiographic analysis of a cervical spine with subaxial subluxation demands attention to the sagittal plane as well posterior column changes, such as facet joint erosions and widening. Boden et al. showed that subluxation with a SAC (measured similar to PADI) of ≤14 mm correlates with risk of neurologic compromise and less favorable postoperative neurologic recovery. In 1995, Yonezawa et al. described subaxial subluxation as >2 mm or 20% listhesis of vertebral body diameter corresponding to progression of myelopathy.[23]

Additional imaging modalities include MRI, which provides the greatest detail of the cervical spine, providing information on the spinal cord compression or pathology, soft tissue lesions, and epidural tissues such as periodontoid pannus. It is the best study to evaluate spinal cord compression. Therefore, this test should be done on any patient with any abnormal neurologic or radiographic finding. The cervicomedullary angle (CMA) is the angle obtained from the line along the anterior cervical spine and the line drawn along the long-axis of the medulla. This value is normally between 135° and 175°. In the presence of progressive craniocervical disease, the brain stem develops an apex anterior deformity. As the CMA falls below 135°, there is an increased correlation with cervicomedullary compression or myelopathy.[24,25] Furthermore, dynamic MRI has also been investigated. Reijnierse et al. showed that canal stenosis on the flexion can influence spinal cord compression at this junction if there is some encroachment on neutral MRI.[26]

Computed tomography scans are also commonly used to delineate a detailed bony anatomy, especially for perioperative planning such as evaluation of vertebral artery anomaly. This diagnostic tool has also been shown to correlate more with neurologic deficits than AADI measurement. Computed tomography myelography is needed in those who have contraindications to MRI.[27]

## TREATMENT OPTIONS

With knowledge of the natural history of RA and predictors of paralysis and neurologic recovery, decisions can be made regarding surgical intervention. It is now well-established that 50% of patients with atlantoaxial instability by AADI are asymptomatic, patients with more severe neurologic dysfunction have a poorer prognosis, and there is a 10% chance of sudden death in RA. The goals of management for patients with rheumatoid cervical spine disease are to recognize atlantoaxial instability, prevent the development of irreversible neurologic dysfunction, and prevent sudden death caused by unrecognized neural compression.[21]

### Nonoperative Management

Patients with RA of the cervical spine benefit from early medical intervention and regular follow-up that includes cervical spine radiographs. Research has demonstrated that early use of combination disease-modifying antirheumatic drug (DMARD) therapy can prevent or delay the onset of AAS.

Soft cervical collars represent a valid treatment option for patients with mild occipitocervical pain and may also be appropriate for use in elderly or ill patients who are poor surgical candidates. However, they do not restrict cervical motion and do not slow or alter the course of the disease. The combination of multiple modalities such as patient education, physical therapy, symptomatic treatment, and DMARDs can achieve and sustain pain relief in many patients. Physical therapy revolves around isometric strengthening of neck muscles and postural training. However, neurologic function has been observed to decline in patients with spinal cord myelopathy treated with soft collar. Santavirta et al. showed that 1 out of 34 patients with rheumatoid cervical spine had improvement in pain when treated nonoperatively, but all had neurologic deterioration.[28] Marks et al. reported on patients with RA and cervical myelopathy, most of whom were treated nonoperatively and died in short-term follow-up.[29] Four patients underwent surgical treatment, three of whom had excellent outcomes.

### Pharmaceutical

The role of pharmaceutical agents in preventing cervical pathology is controversial. Winfield et al. reported a 10% incidence of AAS in RA patients treated with gold or penicillamine after a 2-year follow-up. Paimela et al. found that the incidence of AAS was 9% and cranial settling was 4%; RA patients were treated with DMARDs for a minimum of 2 years. Neva et al. performed a prospective randomized study following RA patients for 2 years, treated with either a single DMARD or a combination DMARD. After 2 years, there were no patients with AAS or cranial settling in the combination group. However, in the single DMARD group, there was an incidence of 6.6% AAS and 2.2% cranial settling. The early results of systemic drug therapy appear promising, but pharmacological treatment of this disease still requires more investigation with longer follow-up.[30-32]

### Surgical Management

Two goals are recognized in the surgical management of rheumatoid disease of the cervical spine. The spine must be stabilized via a solid fusion and the neural elements must be decompressed. Appropriate surgical candidates are patients with intractable pain, neurologic deterioration, or evidence of instability. Neurologic deterioration includes weakness, gait disturbance, and loss of fine motor coordination. Boden et al. recommend surgery, even in the absence of neurologic compromise, if any of the following radiographic risk factors is present: AAS with a PADI ≤14 mm, atlantoaxial impaction evidenced by odontoid migration >5 mm rostral to McGregor's line, or subaxial subluxation canal diameter ≤14 mm.[21]

Therefore, it is important to recognize radiographic predictors for paralysis in RA patients in order to intervene surgically in a timely fashion. These findings include a PADI that is < 14 mm, subaxial canal diameter of < 14 mm, subaxial anterior subluxation (>2 mm) and axial shortening, or evidence of cranial settling. Furthermore, MRI findings of either a CMA of < 135°, a spinal cord diameter of <6 mm in flexion or less, or a SAC of < 13 mm, have also been associated with a poor prognosis for paralysis.

Surgical outcomes of patient with RA have improved over the past decade, largely due to earlier diagnosis of myelopathy and more efficient referral patterns. However, there are both radiographic markers and clinical factors that have been shown to be associated with a poor neurologic recovery despite surgical intervention. Those with more severe preoperative neurologic dysfunction have inferior postoperative neurologic improvement. For example, patients with a higher Ranawat class have a worsening prognosis for neurologic recovery. As another example, patients with class III have a worse prognosis compared to class II and more so when comparing class IIIb to IIIa.[12,33-35] Casey et al. also showed that patients with Ranawat IIIB had worse outcomes in postoperative complication rate, length of hospital stay, functional outcome, and survival.[36]

Furthermore, the location of pathology can also affect the prognosis. Cranial settling combined with AAS has been shown to have a worse prognosis than isolated AAS or subaxial subluxation. Other studies have shown the importance of preoperative radiographic markers. Patients with isolated AAS and a PADI of >14 mm have a better chance of recovery compared to those with a PADI of <10 mm, who have a poor prognosis. Those with AAS and cranial settling tend to have a better neurologic outcome if the PADI is at least 13 mm. Similarly, patients with subaxial subluxation and postoperative canal diameter of <14 mm have less favorable neurologic recovery. Magnetic resonance imaging studies showed that those with a spinal cord area of ≥ 44 mm had good neurologic recovery. Moreover, several elements have not been associated with neurologic recovery, including age, gender, duration of disease or neurologic compromise before surgery, and AADI.[34]

## General Surgical Considerations

Patients with RA tend to have poor nutritional status, poor skin, poor healing profile, and osteopenic bone. This may originate from chronic steroid use and/or chronic systemic disease. The nutritional status should be assessed preoperatively and appropriate treatment should be undertaken.

One of the most critical aspects of surgery is the perioperative airway management. Wattenmaker et al. found that 14% of RA patients undergoing surgery had upper-airway obstruction after extubation from a nonfiberoptic intubation compared to 1% in fiberoptic-intubated patients.[37] Awake fiberoptic intubation is preferably fiberoptic guided if the spinal cord is compressed and the spine is unstable. Wattenmaker et al. have recommended continuing intubation postoperatively for a minimum of 12 hours, more so for patients undergoing transoral surgery.

### *Atlantoaxial Subluxation*

A posterior atlantoaxial fusion is recommended if the subluxation is reducible. However, if the subluxation is irreducible, the cause of compression must be investigated. If the compression is posterior, a laminectomy is performed. If an anterior compression is bony, a single-stage transoral decompression and posterior stabilization should be considered. If the anterior compression is due to periodontal pannus, anterior transoral decompression should be considered. Grob et al. noted that 19 of 22 patients had significant pannus desorption on a follow-up MRI, after a solid upper cervical fusion without anterior decompression. If the patient continues to have a neurologic deficit postoperatively after stand-alone C1-C2 fusion, a follow-up MRI is recommended. If the diagnostic test demonstrates that the pannus has not resolved, a second-stage anterior transoral resection procedure is then recommended. Most common postoperative complications are cerebrospinal fluid leakage and meningitis. Other complications include bleeding, postoperative tongue swelling, wound dehiscence, postoperative instability, and neurologic worsening.[38,39]

A variety of posterior fusion techniques are possible when treating AAS. Traditionally, posterior C1-C2 fusions are done using sublaminar or interspinous wiring. These techniques include Gallie, modified Gallie, and Brooks wiring. The sublaminar wires and cables carry a potential risk of cord injury and hardware breakage as well as cutting out through the soft bone. Magerl's transarticular screw technique provides a more rigid internal fixation. It is mandatory to obtain a CT scan to assess the pedicular anatomy and its relation to the vertebral artery. This technique carries a high risk of vertebral artery and cord injury.[40,41] Moskovich and Crockard described a technique using Halifax interlaminar clamps with interposed bone graft.[42] In 2001, Jürgen Harms described a novel C1-C2 posterior instrumentation technique using the C1 lateral mass and the C2 pedicle by using polyaxial screws and rods. There have been several modifications to this technique.[43,44]

### *Cranial Settling*

Early surgery following the diagnosis of atlantoaxial impaction is recommended due to the high-risk of neurologic compromise seen in this pattern of instability. Neurologic evidence or cord compression visualized on MRI are powerful reasons to proceed to operative management. Preoperative use of halo traction is recommended to reduce the atlantoaxial impaction and reduce the need for foramen magnum decompression or odontoid resection. An occipitocervical fusion is carried out using wires or screws attaching to the occiput caudal to the superior nuchal line and connected to a construct with subaxial fixation. If preoperative traction is unsuccessful in reducing the impaction, a transoral odontoid resection or C1 laminectomy may be considered.

### *Subaxial Subluxation*

Surgical candidates include patients who present with neurologic deficit and asymptomatic patients with a subaxial canal diameter <14 mm. Subaxial subluxation can also occur after upper cervical fusion. One study showed that the rate of subaxial subluxation was 36% 2.6 years after a Occ-C2 fusion but 5.5% about 9 years after C1-C2 fusion.[45]

Reducible subluxations can be fused posteriorly or anteriorly. Irreducible subluxations must be treated with an anterior decompression and fusion. Posterior fusions should be considered following a laminectomy. The extent of fusion is not obvious and should be deliberated carefully secondary to the progressing nature of RA. When subaxial and AAS occur together, the fusion construct should be extended to the lowest diseased level. This serves to decrease the risk of the junctional degeneration.

### *Surgical Outcome*

The mortality rate, reoperation rate, and neurologic improvement appear to be similar across types of procedures. Overall postoperative mortality rate has been reported between 10% and 11%. Reoperation rate is about 3–10%, and overall neurologic recovery between 38% and 72%, with a worse prognosis in the case of severe disease, worse in Ranawat class IIIB. Fusion rates also vary for different procedures, from 50% to 100%.[19,34,35,46-48]

## DIFFUSE IDIOPATHIC SKELETAL HYPEROSTOSIS

Diffuse idiopathic skeletal hyperostosis (DISH) is a musculoskeletal condition that is characterized by spinal stiffness and back pain. This relatively common disorder is a systemic bone-generating disease with primary spinal clinical and radiographic features. It is a disease that usually targets patients >50 years of age and a real male predominance has been observed. An autopsy series published in 1987 reported that 28% of subjects with an average age of 65 years had evidence of DISH.[49] However, some authors have argued that the disease actually starts much sooner, between 20 and 40 years of age, but requires time to mature and become clinically and radiographically significant.[50]

The effort to identify the genetic etiology of DISH has been largely unsuccessful. Although the bone formation observed in DISH is similar to several seronegative spondyloarthropathies, no connection to HLA-B27 has been forged.

Diffuse idiopathic skeletal hyperostosis is identified on X-rays by the presence of flowing ossification along the anterolateral margins of at least four contiguous vertebrae without the presence of spondyloarthropathy or degenerative spondylosis. Interestingly, bony changes are identified on the right side of the thoracic spine.

Patients typically suffer from chronic mild pain in the mid to low back with accompanying stiffness. Some patients may also suffer from extra spinal tendonopathies, particularly Achilles tendonitis. Nevertheless, many patients maintain a relatively benign clinical course and remain asymptomatic throughout the course of their disease.

Cervical spine involvement is less common than that of the thoracic and lumbar spine. The primary complaints may be pain and stiffness. Radiographic evidence of disease is more common in the lower cervical spine. Frequently, there is hyperostosis and loss of elasticity of the anterior paravertebral tissues, particularly the anterior longitudinal ligament. Ligamentum flavum overgrowth, unchecked calcification of the posterior longitudinal ligament and mild straightening of the cervical spine may occur, leading to cervical spine stenosis and myelopathy. Syndesmophytes are identified symmetrically along the anterior anterolateral vertebral bodies.

Occasionally, cervical spine disease may exert an impact on nearby soft tissue structures, especially when large osseous syndesmophytes are present. Dysphagia, hoarseness, and obstructive sleep apnea have all been identified as potential sequelae of DISH.

Surgical management of DISH is rarely recommended, in part because the disease is less painful than other rheumatologic diseases of the cervical spine. This is thought to be the result of an ankylosis that prevents painful motion. Surgery is indicated if myelopathy, painful deformity, or impingement develops. Resection of syndesmophytes is palliative if the bony outgrowths are impinging on anterior structures. In the setting of cervical stenosis with concurrent myelopathy, laminoplasty can be carried out if there is preserved lordosis. Otherwise, anterior decompression and fixation may be performed.

Patients with DISH are at an increased risk from fracture and instability from relatively minor trauma. There is usually a delay in diagnosis, and a high incidence of immediate and delayed neurologic compromise has been noticed. Due to the ankylosis of adjacent vertebral segments proximal and distal to the fracture, fracture segments can become unstable from the increased lever arms.

In the cervical spine, the canal diameter, alignment and mobility of motion segments must be carefully analyzed to rule out trauma. Hyperextension mechanisms are not uncommon. Fractures of the odontoid process and AAS have been identified, but are not classic injury patterns.

## PSORIATIC ARTHRITIS

Psoriatic arthritis (PsA) is an inflammatory arthritis of the axial and appendicular joints that is diagnosed in 6–48% of individuals afflicted with psoriasis. Patients usually develop the disease in their fourth decade of life, and both sexes are affected equally.

Investigations studying the genetic basis of PsA have pointed toward inciting environmental factors such as trauma and infection. A robust inflammatory cascade occurs in both the skin and synovium. A common link between the two tissues may lie in their biomechanics. The dermal epidermal interface and tendon bone junctions are engineered to resist shear stress at high-stress areas. In individuals with psoriasis and PsA, both of these regions are laden with clonally expanded T4 and T8 lymphocytes.[51] In addition, psoriatic synovium contains a high expression of matric metalloproteinase, adhesion molecules, and vascular markers.

The severity of the arthritis is not correlated to the extent of skin involvement. Radiographic features include ankylosis, erosions, and fluffy periostitis. The disease usually follows a moderate course, but nearly half of afflicted patients will develop arthritis severe enough to destroy joint architecture.

Approximately 14% of patients affected by PsA demonstrate axial skeleton involvement, either spinal or sacroiliac (SI). These patients may develop sacroiliitis, syndesmophytes, paravertebral ossification, and discovertebral pathology. The pattern of the inflammatory arthritis changes in the cervical spine is also characterized by ankylosis, syndesmophytes, and ligamentous ossification. Salvarani et al. described the changes of the cervical spine in 57 patients with PsA.[52] Two patterns of cervical disease were appreciated. The first group demonstrated erosive changes and/or subluxating changes similar to RA. The second group had changes like those visualized in ankylosing spondylitis (AS). Many patients complain of neck pain and stiffness. In a study of 160 Finnish patients, Laiho and Kauppi were able to identify the incidence of the clinically relevant radiographic features of diseased cervical spines. The authors identified cervical disease in 18% of patients. The most common pathology seen was apophyseal joint ankylosis. The next most frequent radiographic feature identified was anterior AAS, followed by atlantoaxial impactions.[53]

## ANKYLOSING SPONDYLITIS

Ankylosing spondylitis is a chronic and progressive seronegative inflammatory arthritis of unknown etiology whose primary target is the axial skeleton, particularly the SI joints. The SI joints are involved early in the disease, followed by the spread of disease into the paravertebral zygapophyseal joints and intervertebral disk spaces.

Ankylosing spondylitis affects young adults, usually between their third and fourth decades in life, with a predilection for males. The incidence has been estimated to be 1 to 2 cases per 1,000. The disorder has also been shown to have a strong genetic basis and is linked to HLA-B27.

Much of the pathology manifests as an enthesopathy, which leads the way for fibrosis and calcifications at tendon insertion sites and eventual ankylosis. This pathological fusion alters the sagittal balance and frequently causes a hyperkyphotic deformity.

The cervical spine becomes rigid late in the disease. A hyperkyphotic deformity or flexion deformity at the cervicothoracic junction can subsequently develop.

Cervical spine problems are thought to be more prevalent in women. Range of motion becomes restricted in the sagittal plane. Chin-brow angle, occiput-to-wall distance and gaze angle are all measurement techniques used to evaluate the deformity of the cervical spine. Most patients remain neurologically intact with normal deep tendon reflexes. However, there is a risk of developing a progressive cauda equina syndrome late in the disease.[54]

Patients with cervical spine involvement are also at risk for developing AAS, cervical spine fractures, and cervical spine stenosis. Management is largely nonoperative and supportive, consisting of nonsteroidal anti-inflammatory drugs and collars.

Unlike RA in which pannus leads to bony erosion, the spine in AS becomes ankylosed as the disease ascends from the SI joints. Overt calcification of the longitudinal ligaments creates the pathognomonic "bamboo spine" deformity associated with this disease. The rigid spine is forced to act like one long bone and predisposes patients to spinal fractures. Therefore, it not is surprising that patients with AS are up to four times more likely to sustain spinal fractures. There is a high incidence of associated neurologic damage, which can result from a number of causes, such as dislocation displacement, epidural hematomas, or impingement by the ossified ligamentum flavum.[55,56] It is estimated that the risk of spinal cord injury in patients with AS is 11 times greater than that of an individual without the disorder.

Most acute fractures are the result of low-energy mechanisms, such as a fall from standing. The majority occurs in the cervical spine, usually at C5-C6 or C6-C7. This area is vulnerable to injury because of the obliquity of its facet joints and its location between an immobile thoracic spine and mobile head. Three quarters of the injuries result from hyperextension mechanisms, and it has been postulated that an increased kyphotic alignment makes the spine more vulnerable to a hyperextension injury. Fracture lines can extend through intervertebral disks as well as the body, due to the inelasticity of the diseased disk and calcified surrounding annulus.

## REFERENCES


1. Wasserman BR, Moskovich R, Razi AE. Rheumatoid arthritis of the cervical spine—clinical considerations. Bull NYU Hosp Jt Dis. 2011;69(2):136-48.
2. Kornblum D, Clayton ML, Nash HH. Nontraumatic cervical dislocations in rheumatoid spondylitis. J Am Med Assoc. 1952;149(5):431-5.
3. Paimela L, Laasonen L, Kankaanpää E, et al. Progression of cervical spine changes in patients with early rheumatoid arthritis. J Rheumatol. 1997;24(7):1280-4.
4. Moskovich R, Shott S, Zhang ZH. Does the cervical canal to body ratio predict spinal stenosis? Bull Hosp Jt Dis. 1996; 55(2):61-71.
5. Riise T, Jacobsen BK, Gran JT. High mortality in patients with rheumatoid arthritis and atlantoaxial subluxation. J Rheumatol. 2001;28(11):2425-9.
6. Pellicci PM, Ranawat CS, Tsairis P, et al. A prospective study of the progression of rheumatoid arthritis of the cervical spine. J Bone Joint Surg Am. 1981;63(3):342-50.
7. Lipson SJ. Cervical myelopathy and posterior atlantoaxial subluxation in patients with rheumatoid arthritis. J Bone Joint Surg Am. 1985;67(4):593-7.
8. Zeidman SM, Ducker TB. Rheumatoid arthritis. Neuroanatomy, compression, and grading of deficits. Spine (Phila Pa 1976). 1994;19(20):2259-66.
9. Kauppi M, Konttinen YT, Honkanen V, et, al. A multivariate analysis of risk factors for anterior atlantoaxial subluxation and an evaluation of the effect of glucocorticoid treatment on the upper rheumatoid cervical spine. Clin Rheumatol. 1991;10(4):413-8.
10. Meijers KA, Cats A, Kremer HP, et al. Cervical myelopathy in rheumatoid arthritis. Clin Exp Rheumatol. 1984;2(3): 239-45.
11. Sunahara N, Matsunaga S, Mori T, et al. Clinical course of conservatively managed rheumatoid arthritis patients with myelopathy. Spine (Phila Pa 1976). 1997; 22(22):2603-7; discussion 2608.
12. Boden SD, Dodge LD, Bohlman HH, et al. Rheumatoid arthritis of the cervical spine. A long-term analysis with predictors of paralysis and recovery. J Bone Joint Surg Am. 1993;75(9):1282-97.
13. Casey AT, Crockard HA, Geddes JF, et al. Vertical translocation: the enigma of the disappearing atlantodens interval in patients with myelopathy and rheumatoid arthritis. Part I. Clinical, radiological, and neuropathological features. J Neurosurg. 1997;87(6):856-62.
14. Ranawat CS, O'Leary P, Pellicci P, et al. Cervical spine fusion in rheumatoid arthritis. J Bone Joint Surg Am. 1979;61(7): 1003-10.
15. Riew KD, Hilibrand AS, Palumbo MA, et al. Diagnosing basilar invagination in the rheumatoid patient. The reliability of radiographic criteria. J Bone Joint Surg Am. 2001;83-A(2):194-200.
16. Fielding JW, Cochran G van B, Lawsing JF, et al. Tears of the transverse ligament of the atlas. A clinical and biomechanical study. J Bone Joint Surg Am. 1974;56(8):1683-91.
17. Weissman BN, Aliabadi P, Weinfeld MS, et al. Prognostic features of atlantoaxial subluxation in rheumatoid arthritis patients. Radiology. 1982;144(4):745-51.
18. Rana NA. Natural history of atlantoaxial subluxation in rheumatoid arthritis. Spine (Phila Pa 1976). 1989;14(10): 1054-6.
19. Clark CR, Goetz DD, Menezes AH. Arthrodesis of the cervical spine in rheumatoid arthritis. J Bone Joint Surg Am. 1989;71(3):381-92.

20. Collins DN, Barnes CL, FitzRandolph RL. Cervical spine instability in rheumatoid patients having total hip or knee arthroplasty. Clin Orthop Relat Res. 1991;(272):127-35.
21. Boden SD. Rheumatoid arthritis of the cervical spine. Surgical decision making based on predictors of paralysis and recovery. Spine (Phila Pa 1976). 1994;19(20):2275-80.
22. Casey AT, Crockard HA, Stevens J. Vertical translocation. Part II. Outcomes after surgical treatment of rheumatoid cervical myelopathy. J Neurosurg. 1997;87(6):863-9.
23. Yonezawa T, Tsuji H, Matsui H, et al. Subaxial lesions in rheumatoid arthritis. Radiographic factors suggestive of lower cervical myelopathy. Spine (Phila Pa 1976). 1995;20 (2):208-15.
24. Breedveld FC, Algra PR, Vielvoye CJ, et al. Magnetic resonance imaging in the evaluation of patients with rheumatoid arthritis and subluxations of the cervical spine. Arthritis Rheum. 1987;30(6):624-9.
25. Bell GR, Stearns KL. Flexion-extension MRI of the upper rheumatoid cervical spine. Orthopedics. 1991;14(9):969-73; discussion 973-4.
26. Reijnierse M, Breedveld FC, Kroon HM, et al. Are magnetic resonance flexion views useful in evaluating the cervical spine of patients with rheumatoid arthritis? Skeletal Radiol. 2000;29(2):85-9.
27. Raskin RJ, Schnapf DJ, Wolf CR, et al. Computerized tomography in evaluation of atlantoaxial subluxation in rheumatoid arthritis. J Rheumatol. 1983;10(1):33-41.
28. Santavirta S, Kankaanpää U, Sandelin J, et al. Evaluation of patients with rheumatoid cervical spine. Scand J Rheumatol. 1987;16(1):9-16.
29. Marks JS, Sharp J. Rheumatoid cervical myelopathy. Q J Med. 1981;50(199):307-19.
30. Winfield J, Young A, Williams P, et al. Prospective study of the radiological changes in hands, feet, and cervical spine in adult rheumatoid disease. Ann Rheum Dis. 1983;42(6):613-8.
31. Paimela L, Laasonen L, Kankaanpää E, et al. Progression of cervical spine changes in patients with early rheumatoid arthritis. J Rheumatol. 1997;24(7):1280-4.
32. Neva MH, Kauppi MJ, Kautiainen H, et al. Combination drug therapy retards the development of rheumatoid atlantoaxial subluxations. Arthritis Rheum. 2000;43(11):2397-401.
33. Casey AT, Crockard HA, Bland JM, et al. Predictors of outcome in the quadriparetic nonambulatory myelopathic patient with rheumatoid arthritis: a prospective study of 55 surgically treated Ranawat class IIIb patients. J Neurosurg. 1996;85(4):574-81.
34. Zoma A, Sturrock RD, Fisher WD, et al. Surgical stabilisation of the rheumatoid cervical spine. A review of indications and results. J Bone Joint Surg Br. 1987;69(1):8-12.
35. Peppelman WC, Kraus DR, Donaldson WF, et al. Cervical spine surgery in rheumatoid arthritis: improvement of neurologic deficit after cervical spine fusion. Spine (Phila Pa 1976). 1993;18(16):2375-9.
36. Casey AT, Crockard HA, Bland JM, et al. Surgery on the rheumatoid cervical spine for the nonambulant myelopathic patient-too much, too late? Lancet. 1996;347(9007):1004-7.
37. Wattenmaker I, Concepcion M, Hibberd P, et al. Upper-airway obstruction and perioperative management of the airway in patients managed with posterior operations on the cervical spine for rheumatoid arthritis. J Bone Joint Surg Am. 1994;76(3):360-5.
38. Grob D, Würsch R, Grauer W, et al. Atlantoaxial fusion and retrodental pannus in rheumatoid arthritis. Spine (Phila Pa 1976). 1997;22(14):1580-3; discussion 1584.
39. Zygmunt S, Säveland H, Brattström H, et al. Reduction of rheumatoid periodontoid pannus following posterior occipitocervical fusion visualised by magnetic resonance imaging. Br J Neurosurg. 1988;2(3):315-20.
40. Grob D, Jeanneret B, Aebi M, et al. Atlantoaxial fusion with transarticular screw fixation. J Bone Joint Surg Br. 1991; 73(6):972-6.
41. Wang C, Yan M, Zhou H, et al. Atlantoaxial transarticular screw fixation with morselized autograft and without additional internal fixation: technical description and report of 57 cases. Spine (Phila Pa 1976). 2007;32(6):643-6.
42. Moskovich R, Crockard HA. Atlantoaxial arthrodesis using interlaminar clamps. An improved technique. Spine (Phila Pa 1976). 1992;17(3):261-7.
43. Aryan HE, Newman CB, Nottmeier EW, et al. Stabilization of the atlantoaxial complex via C-1 lateral mass and C-2 pedicle screw fixation in a multicenter clinical experience in 102 patients: modification of the Harms and Goel techniques. J Neurosurg Spine. 2008;8(3):222-9.
44. Jacobson ME, Khan SN, An HS. C1-C2 posterior fixation: indications, technique, and results. Orthop Clin North Am. 2012;43(1):11-8, vii.
45. Kraus DR, Peppelman WC, Agarwal AK, et al. Incidence of subaxial subluxation in patients with generalized rheumatoid arthritis who have had previous occipital cervical fusions. Spine (Phila Pa 1976). 1991;16(10 Suppl):S486-9.
46. Santavirta S, Konttinen YT, Laasonen E, et al. Ten-year results of operations for rheumatoid cervical spine disorders. J Bone Joint Surg Br. 1991;73(1):116-20.
47. Krieg JC, Clark CR, Goetz DD. Cervical spine arthrodesis in rheumatoid arthritis: a long-term follow-up. Yale J Biol Med. 1993;66(3):257-62.
48. Moskovich R, Crockard HA, Shott S, et al. Occipitocervical stabilization for myelopathy in patients with rheumatoid arthritis. Implications of not bone-grafting. J Bone Joint Surg Am. 2000;82(3):349-65.
49. Boachie-Adjei O, Bullough PG. Incidence of ankylosing hyperostosis of the spine (Forestier's disease) at autopsy. Spine (Phila Pa 1976). 1987;12(8):739-43.
50. Resnick D, Shapiro RF, Wiesner KB, et al. Diffuse idiopathic skeletal hyperostosis (DISH) [ankylosing hyperostosis of Forestier and Rotes-Querol]. Semin Arthritis Rheum. 1978;7(3):153-87.
51. Loffredo S, Ayala F, Marone G, et al. Immunopathogenesis of psoriasis and pharmacological perspectives. J Rheumatol Suppl. 2009;83:9-11.
52. Salvarani C, Macchioni P, Cremonesi T, et al. The cervical spine in patients with psoriatic arthritis: a clinical, radiological and immunogenetic study. Ann Rheum Dis. 1992;51 (1):73-7.
53. Laiho K, Kauppi M. The cervical spine in patients with psoriatic arthritis. Ann Rheum Dis. 2002;61(7):650-2.
54. Kubiak EN, Moskovich R, Errico TJ, et al. Orthopaedic management of ankylosing spondylitis. J Am Acad Orthop Surg. 2005;13(4):267-78.
55. Westerveld LA, Verlaan JJ, Oner FC. Spinal fractures in patients with ankylosing spinal disorders: a systematic review of the literature on treatment, neurological status and complications. Eur Spine J. 2009;18(2):145-56.
56. Mundwiler ML, Siddique K, Dym JM, et al. Complications of the spine in ankylosing spondylitis with a focus on deformity correction. Neurosurg Focus. 2008;24(1):E6.

Chapter 11

# Ossification of the Posterior Longitudinal Ligament

*Nikhil A Sahasrabudhe, Russell G Strom, Michael L Smith*

## INTRODUCTION

Ossification of the posterior longitudinal ligament (OPLL) is a pathologic condition that primarily affects the cervical and thoracic spine. Ligament overgrowth and ossification may lead to axial pain, myelopathy, or radiculopathy. Ossification of the posterior longitudinal ligament is more common in East Asians, with a prevalence of 4.3% in Japan, 3.6% in Korea, and 2.8% in Taiwan. A prevalence of 0.12% has been reported in North American Caucasians, but this may be an underestimate as the condition is not as well defined and studied as it is in Asia.[1] In North America, OPLL is thought to be sporadic, but epidemiologic studies from Japan have shown familial associations, common gene mutations, and higher prevalence with specific metabolic disorders. Ossification of the posterior longitudinal ligament typically presents in patient 50 years of age and older, predominantly affecting males with a ratio of 2:1.[2]

## PATHOPHYSIOLOGY AND ETIOLOGY

The posterior longitudinal ligament (PLL) runs along the posterior aspect of the vertebral bodies and marks the anterior border of the spinal canal. Normal PLL consists mainly of collagen and elastin. In OPLL, the normal architecture is disrupted with heterotopic ossification. The process begins with PLL hypertrophy, with ventral and dorsal layers forming. The ossified dorsal layer consists of endochondral bone with immature marrow. The deep layer consists of fibrocartilaginous tissue that acts as a center of bone formation. As the ventral layer proliferates and thickens, new bone formation occurs at the ossifying front between the ventral and dorsal layers.[3] The ossified ligamentous overgrowth causes spinal canal stenosis, with the potential for myelopathy or radiculopathy.

Multiple genes have been implicated in the pathogenesis of OPLL.

*Col11A2*: Polymorphisms in the gene encoding collagen α2 (XI), *COL11A2*, have been associated with OPLL. Collagen XI assembles with Collagen II to form a major part of the ligament structure. Specific polymorphisms are thought to cause alternative splicing, which can be either protective against or permissive of the heterotopic ossification seen in OPLL.[4]

*Col6A1*: Similarly, specific polymorphisms with the gene for collagen 6α1, located on chromosome 21, have been shown to be associated with OPLL. Collagen VI is a protein found in the extracellular matrix, and its overproduction could potentially provide a matrix in which osteoblasts can proliferate.[5]

*TGFβ*: Data for gene polymorphisms for *TGFβ* have been inconsistent. However, one study of in vitro cultured cell lines showed that administration of *TGFβ* halted OPLL cell proliferation.[6,7]

*BMP2*: Polymorphism analysis of *BMP2* has shown certain polymorphisms associated with the onset and extent of OPLL, and other polymorphisms to be associated with the extent of OPLL. Administration of *BMP2* to cultured OPLL cell lines has been shown to stimulate osteoblastic differentiation.[8]

*NPPS*: Nucleotide pyrophosphatase was originally characterized in a mouse model of OPLL and subsequently in human cell lines. Its normal function is the production of inorganic pyrophosphate, a known inhibitor of calcification. Certain polymorphisms have been associated with both the presence and severity of OPLL.[9,10]

Multiple other gene polymorphisms and proteins have been implicated in the pathogenesis of OPLL, but it is unclear how OPLL arises from these. The pathogenesis of OPLL is likely multifactorial, a combination of genetic predispositions and environmental triggers.

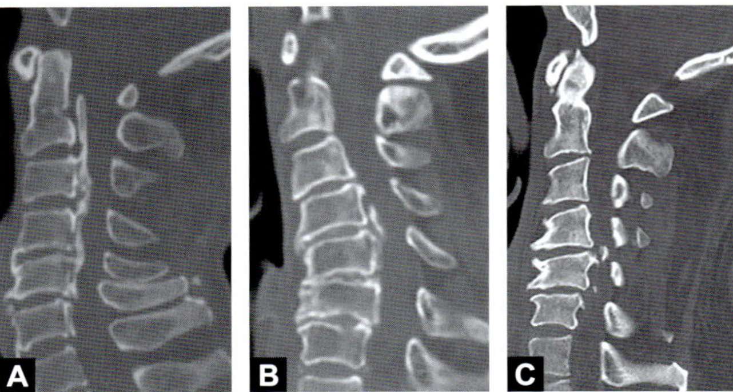


**Figs. 11.1A to C:** (A) Continuous ossification of the posterior longitudinal ligament (OPLL) with a single ossified mass spanning vertebral bodies and intervening disk spaces. (B) Segmental OPLL with ossified masses primarily dorsal to vertebral bodies and skipping the disk spaces. (C) Focal OPLL with the ossified mass dorsal to the disk space only. A fourth subtype is "mixed," which has a combination of continuous and segmental.

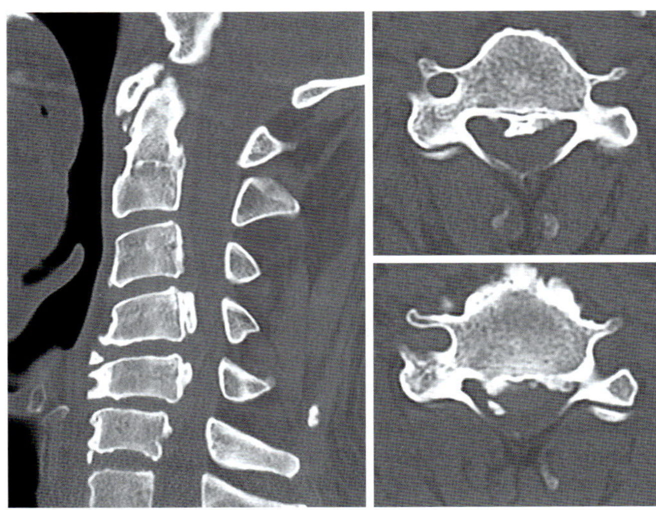

**Fig. 11.2:** Preoperative sagittal and axial computed tomography showing segmental ossification of the posterior longitudinal ligament with ossification behind the bodies of C4 and C5 with sparing of the posterior longitudinal ligament overlying the C4-5 disk space. Noted the separate focus of calcification posteriorly on the right, suggesting some dural involvement.

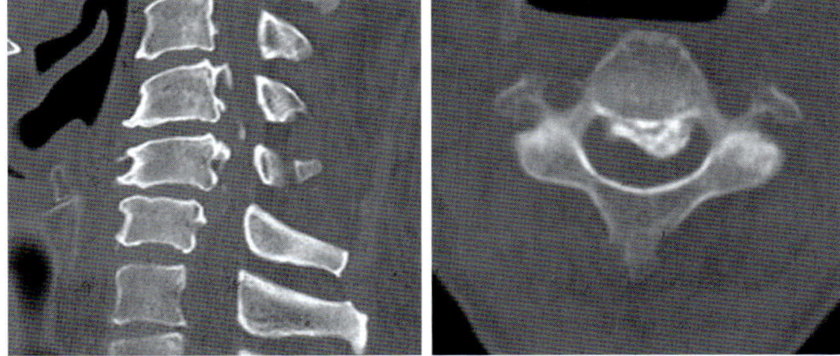

**Fig. 11.3:** The sagittal image to the left shows a focal calcification dorsal to the ossified posterior longitudinal ligament with a hypodense area in between (double-layer sign). The axial image on the right shows eccentric calcification leadings to a "C" shape, forcing the dura to curve over (single-layer sign).

## CLINICAL AND RADIOGRAPHIC EVALUATION

Ossification of the posterior longitudinal ligament can present with symptoms of cervical or thoracic myelopathy, radiculopathy, or axial pain. Early symptoms are typically paresthesias in the hands, followed by discomfort. In patients with a long segment of OPLL, a major complaint may be neck stiffness. Myelopathy slowly progresses with loss of dexterity and gait imbalance. Occasionally, patients experience an acute exacerbation of myelopathy after even minor cervical trauma (central cord syndrome). The risk of neurologic deterioration after trauma correlates with the extent of canal stenosis and the amount of cervical mobility.[11] The ossified ligament contributes to "static" compression, and cervical mobility contributes to "dynamic" compression.[12]

Ossification of the posterior longitudinal ligament can be seen on plain radiographs, computed tomography (CT), and magnetic resonance imaging (MRI). In each modality, OPLL is diagnosed as an ossified mass posterior to the vertebral body causing stenosis of the spinal canal. Lateral radiographs can be useful in determining the extent of canal narrowing. A normal cervical canal measures approximately 17 mm in the anterior-posterior (A-P) dimension.[13] Multiple studies have correlated the extent of A-P stenosis with the presence of myelopathy. According to Sasaki et al., patients with 40% canal stenosis are at risk of myelopathy.[14] In another study, all 45 patients with 60% stenosis had signs of myelopathy.[15]

Although OPLL can be diagnosed and followed with lateral radiographs, CT is more sensitive for detection. Computed tomography can better define the subtype of OPLL (Figs. 11.1A to C) and reveal laterality of compression (Fig. 11.2). Computed tomography can also help determine dural penetrance. Dural penetrance is the extension of the ossification into the intradural space. The double-layer and single-layer signs may suggest this (Fig. 11.3). The double-layer sign consists of a hypodense layer between the posterior aspect of the vertebral body, representing the dura, and an intradural linear calcification. It is best appreciated in the sagittal plane. The single-layer sign describes a central ossified mass with partial lateralization causing the dura to fold over. This is seen in the

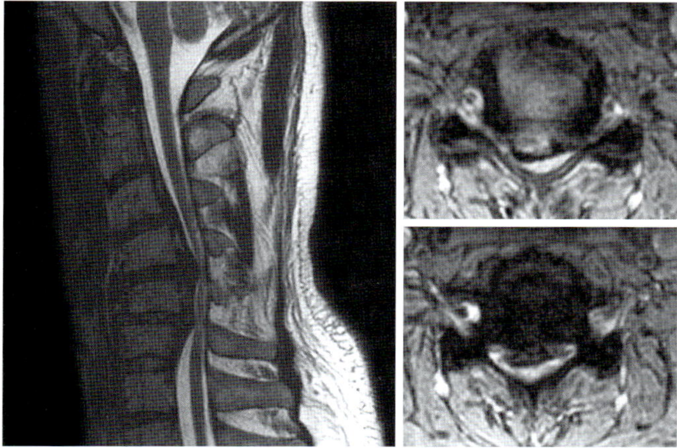

**Fig. 11.4:** T2-sagittal and axial imaging showing severe canal stenosis and compression of cervical cord at C4-5 and C5-6. The T2 signal abnormality and volume loss suggest cord atrophy.

axial plane. Dural penetrance correlates with a higher incidence of cerebrospinal fluid (CSF) leak and can be useful in operative planning.[16]

Magnetic resonance imaging is the most sensitive for evaluating cord compression and intrinsic cord changes such as edema or myelomalacia (Fig. 11.4).[17] Ossification of the posterior longitudinal ligament lesions is hypointense and may mimic more common spondylosis changes such as disk-osteophyte complexes. Therefore, OPLL must be kept in the differential and CT imaging obtained to confirm the appropriate diagnosis.

## TREATMENT OF OSSIFICATION OF POSTERIOR LONGITUDINAL LIGAMENT

### Conservative Treatment

Conservative treatment of OPLL consists of pain management with medications such as nonsteroidal anti-inflammatory drugs. Conservative management should be offered to individuals who have radiographic evidence of OPLL without signs or symptoms of myelopathy. Age >70 or multiple comorbidities that make a patient a poor operative candidate should be taken into consideration as well. In general, there is no role for bracing or epidural steroid injections.[17]

### Surgical Treatment

Ossification of the posterior longitudinal ligament may be treated with posterior, anterior, or combined posterior-anterior approaches.

#### *Posterior Approaches*

Posterior options include laminectomy, laminectomy with fusion, and laminoplasty. All rely on indirect decompression by allowing the cervical cord to fall away from the ventral compression. For this reason, posterior approaches are contraindicated in the setting of a fixed kyphotic deformity.

Laminectomy alone can be considered in patients who have normal cervical alignment and do not require multilevel or wide decompression. A narrow laminectomy preserving the facets helps maintain stability postoperatively. In a long-term follow-up of 44 patients who underwent laminectomy for OPLL, 1- and 5-year neurologic improvement-over-baseline rates were 44.2% and 42.9%, respectively. At 10 years, the rate dropped to 32.8%. Risk factors for poor outcomes include age >70, preoperative severe myelopathy, and history of trauma. Forty-seven percent of these patients developed kyphotic deformity.[18]

Because of the risk of post-laminectomy kyphosis and neurologic deterioration, cervical laminectomy is often coupled with posterior instrumented fusion. Stabilization can be achieved with pedicle screws, lateral mass screws, or wiring techniques. Posterior fusion is utilized in the setting of instability or when adequate decompression risks instability.

Laminoplasty allows for posterior decompression, maintenance of stability, and preservation of motion. A 3-year study of 20 patients who underwent laminoplasty showed a mean 42% increase in A-P canal diameter with a preservation of normal range of motion in 83%.[19] There is, however, a concern for deterioration in the long term. Similar to laminectomy, poor prognostic indicators are age, extent of preoperative myelopathy, and trauma.[19]

#### *Anterior Approaches*

Anterior approaches for OPLL include anterior cervical discectomy and fusion (ACDF), single or multilevel corpectomy, or a hybrid construct with corpectomy and ACDF. These allow direct decompression via resection of the OPLL mass. Combined A-P approaches are sometimes needed, as in the case of multilevel corpectomy (Fig. 11.5). A posterior approach allows additional decompression if needed. In cases of two or more level corpectomy, where subsidence and failed fusion are of concern, supplemental posterior arthrodesis and fixation can maximize the chance for successful healing in anatomic alignment.

There is evidence that anterior approaches are associated with superior neurologic outcomes compared to

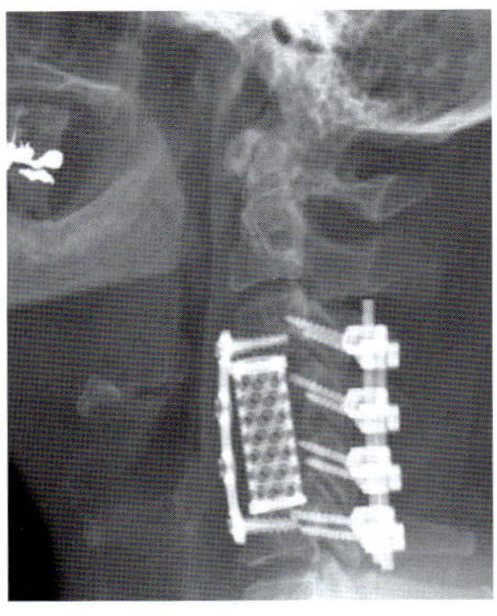
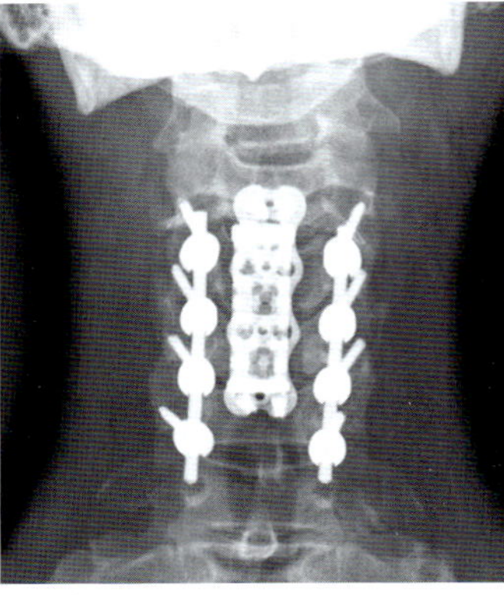

**Fig. 11.5:** Postoperative imaging for the patient in Figure 11.3. Anterior decompression and restoration of alignment are accomplished with a two-level corpectomy and stabilization with titanium mesh cage and anterior plate. The construct is supplemented with posterior fusion and lateral mass fixation.

posterior approaches. In multiple series comparing posterior and anterior approaches, patients undergoing anterior decompressions had overall better outcomes.[13,20] In a study of 75 patients, those receiving anterior decompression had a mean improvement in the neurosurgical cervical spine scale (NCSS) of 78%, compared to 46.1% in patients with posterior decompression. At later follow-up, posterior patients had a decrease in the NCSS; however, anterior patients had a marginal increase. [21] Posterior decompression has also been associated with a higher incidence of progression of OPLL when compared to conservatively managed patients.[22]

Anterior decompression may offer better neurologic outcomes but can be technically more challenging. Compared to posterior approaches, there is an increased risk of CSF leak because the OPLL mass adheres to the ventral dura. The incidence of CSF leak ranges from 4.3% to 32% in the literature.[23] In a retrospective analysis of 126 OPLL cases, patients with dural ossification had a 63.6% incidence of CSF leak.[24] Primary suture repair of anterior dura is difficult; lacerations may increase the size of the defect. More commonly, onlay repairs with gelatin foam or fascial graft and a sealant such as fibrin glue are used. Postoperatively, the patient may require bed rest with head elevation, application of pressure dressings, serial wound aspirations, or CSF diversion temporarily with a lumbar drain or permanently with a shunt.

## CONCLUSION

Ossification of the posterior longitudinal ligament should be considered in the workup for cervical myelopathy. Computed tomography is essential in its accurate diagnosis when there is concern for OPLL on MRI or X-ray. Current surgical treatment paradigms offer improved outcomes for patients with symptomatic OPLL, with the data suggesting that anterior approaches provide superior outcomes, tempered by surgical challenge. At this time there are no known effective preventive measures or reliable methods for identifying at-risk patients.

## REFERENCES


1. Inamasu J, Guiot BH, Sachs DC. Ossification of the posterior longitudinal ligament: an update on its biology, epidemiology, and natural history. Neurosurgery. 2006;58(6):1027-39; discussion 1039.
2. Sasaki E, Ono A, Yokoyama T, et al. Prevalence and symptom of ossification of posterior longitudinal ligaments in the Japanese general population. J Orthop Sci. 2014;19(3):405-11.
3. Tsuyama N. Ossification of the posterior longitudinal ligament of the spine. Clin Orthop Relat Res. 1984(184):71-84.
4. Maeda S, Ishidou Y, Koga H, et al. Functional impact of human collagen alpha2(XI) gene polymorphism in pathogenesis of ossification of the posterior longitudinal ligament of the spine. J Bone Miner Res. 2001;16(5):948-57.
5. Kong Q, Ma X, Li F, et al. COL6A1 polymorphisms associated with ossification of the ligamentum flavum and ossification of the posterior longitudinal ligament. Spine (Phila Pa 1976). 2007;32(25):2834-8.
6. Kawaguchi Y, Furushima K, Sugimori K, et al. Association between polymorphism of the transforming growth factor-beta1 gene with the radiologic characteristic and ossification of the posterior longitudinal ligament. Spine (Phila Pa 1976). 2003;28(13):1424-6.
7. Inaba K, Matsunaga S, Ishidou Y, et al. Effect of transforming growth factor-beta on fibroblasts in ossification of the posterior longitudinal ligament. In Vivo. 1996;10(4):445-9.
8. Kon T, Yamazaki M, Tagawa M, et al. Bone morphogenetic protein-2 stimulates differentiation of cultured spinal ligament cells from patients with ossification of the posterior longitudinal ligament. Calcif Tissue Int. 1997;60(3):291-6.
9. Nakamura I, Ikegawa S, Okawa A, et al. Association of the human NPPS gene with ossification of the posterior longitudinal ligament of the spine (OPLL). Hum Genet. 1999;104(6):492-7.
10. Koshizuka Y, Kawaguchi H, Ogata N, et al. Nucleotide pyrophosphatase gene polymorphism associated with ossification of the posterior longitudinal ligament of the spine. J Bone Miner Res. 2002;17(1):138-44.
11. Matsunaga S, Sakou T, Hayashi K, et al. Trauma-induced myelopathy in patients with ossification of the posterior longitudinal ligament. J Neurosurg. 2002;97(2 Suppl):172-5.
12. Yoshii T, Yamada T, Hirai T, et al. Dynamic changes in spinal cord compression by cervical ossification of the posterior longitudinal ligament evaluated by kinematic computed tomography myelography. Spine (Phila Pa 1976). 2014;39(2):113-9.

13. Epstein N. Diagnosis and surgical management of cervical ossification of the posterior longitudinal ligament. Spine J. 2002;2(6):436-49.
14. Sasaki E, Ono A, Yokoyama T, et al. Prevalence and symptom of ossification of posterior longitudinal ligaments in the Japanese general population. J Orthop Sci. 2014;19(3):405-11.
15. Matsunaga S, Nakamura K, Seichi A, et al. Radiographic predictors for the development of myelopathy in patients with ossification of the posterior longitudinal ligament: a multicenter cohort study. Spine (Phila Pa 1976). 2008; 33(24):2648-50.
16. Epstein NE. Identification of ossification of the posterior longitudinal ligament extending through the dura on preoperative computed tomographic examinations of the cervical spine. Spine (Phila Pa 1976). 2001;26(2):182-6.
17. Epstein NE. Laminectomy for cervical myelopathy. Spinal Cord. 2003;41(6):317-27.
18. Kato Y, Iwasaki M, Fuji T, et al. Long-term follow-up results of laminectomy for cervical myelopathy caused by ossification of the posterior longitudinal ligament. J Neurosurg. 1998;89(2):217-23.
19. Morimoto T, Matsuyama T, Hirabayashi H, et al. Expansive laminoplasty for multilevel cervical OPLL. J Spinal Disord. 1997;10(4):296-8.
20. Yonenobu K, Hosono N, Iwasaki M, et al. Neurologic complications of surgery for cervical compression myelopathy. Spine (Phila Pa 1976). 1991;16(11):1277-82.
21. Kawano H, Handa Y, Ishii H, et al. Surgical treatment for ossification of the posterior longitudinal ligament of the cervical spine. J Spinal Disord. 1995;8 (2):145-50.
22. Takatsu T, Ishida Y, Suzuki K, et al. Radiological study of cervical ossification of the posterior longitudinal ligament. J Spinal Disord. 1999;12(3):271-3.
23. Mazur M, Jost GF, Schmidt MH, et al. Management of cerebrospinal fluid leaks after anterior decompression for ossification of the posterior longitudinal ligament: a review of the literature. Neurosurg Focus. 2011;30(3):E13.
24. Fengbin Y, Xinyuan L, Xiaowei L, et al. Management and outcomes of cerebrospinal fluid leak associated with anterior decompression for cervical ossification of the posterior longitudinal ligament with or without dural ossification. J Spinal Disord Tech. 2013. [Epub ahead of print].

# Chapter 12

# Os Odontoideum

*Peter G Passias, Cyrus M Jalai*

## INTRODUCTION

Although much surrounding the current understanding of os odontoideum, an abnormality of the cervical spine, remains equivocal, the strict definition remains uniform across the literature: os odontoideum is a rare condition marked by hypoplasia of the odontoid process coupled with an independent ossicle representing the odontoid that is discontinuous from C2 and above the superior facets of the axis.[1,2] It also displays with smooth circumferential cortical margins, and although rare, it is the most common disorder of odontoid processes. Although the definition of the condition retains a historical basis, there remains much debate regarding the etiology and surrounding factors. The term "os odontoideum" was first coined by Giacomini in 1886, and since then the processes leading to the development of the disorder have been extensively debated in the literature.[3] Indeed, the pathogenesis of the condition is believed to be either congenital in nature, or, perhaps more commonly accepted, the result of remote trauma. Supporters of the congenital etiology view the presentation of os odontoideum as the result of the failed fusion between the odontoid and axis vertebrae during embryonic development.[4] Those who advocate for an acquired or traumatic etiology state that the ossicle originates from a fracture or injury to the odontoid, followed by ligament contraction and suppression of blood supply.[5]

Regardless of the etiology, affected patients may develop neurological symptoms consistent with craniovertebral junction (CVJ) instability.[4] The subsequent management of os odontoideum, whether it is conservative or surgical, should aim to achieve simultaneous neural decompression and stabilization of the CVJ. The variety of techniques for the management of the condition are familiar to most surgeons, yet retain ranges of applicability, effectiveness, and safety. Thus, a thorough understanding of the potential developmental origins of os odontoideum, coupled with effective radiographic determination of the disorder, is crucial to make a recommendation.

Os odontoideum, manifested as atlantoaxial instability, also has a documented influence on the onset of cervical myelopathy.[6,7] This chapter aims, therefore, to provide an outline of the various etiologies, both congenital and acquired, that have been proposed for os odontoideum, as well as the most updated surgical techniques, clinical outcomes, and potential pathological complications associated with os odontoideum.

## DEFINITION AND PATHOGENESIS

Os odontoideum is a rare anomaly of the second cervical vertebrae in which the odontoid process is separated from the body of the axis by a small transverse gap.[8] The ossicle is independent from the hypoplastic dens, is of variable size, and has smooth osseous margins. Distinct anatomical types of os odontoideum—orthotopic and dystopic—are considered.[9] Orthotopic os odontoideum is characterized by the presence of the ossicle in the position of the normal odontoic; the ossicle is considered dystopic if is presents near the occiput in the area of the foramen magnum.[9] Despite the concrete understanding of the anatomical presentation of os odontoideum, debate persists concerning its pathogenesis. Evidence for both congenital and post-traumatic origins is copious, with various levels of radiographic and clinical support on both sides.

### The Congenital Theory

During embryological development, the caudal and cephalic portions of C1 and C2, respectively, fuse to eventually form the odontoid process. The cartilaginous odontoid process and the body of the axis fuse into one mass by the 8th week of fetal development.[10] Numerous ossification centers start to appear over the course of intrauterine maturation, at the odontoid and at the proatlas.[10] Ossification of the proatlas usually begins at 2–5 years postnatal and ultimately fuses permanently with the odontoid around 10–13 years.[11] Failures of fusion of the protatlas in humans can present in the form of ossiculum terminale persistens of Bergman's, in which the tip of the odontoid process fails to ossify with the odontoid base. The ossiculum terminale represents the third ossification of the odontoid process and arises from the centrum of the proatlas. Failure of fusion of the ossiculum terminale is considered similar to the phenomenon of os odontoideum, also thought to result from fusion failure between the sclerotomes proatlas and C1.[1]

Currently, proponents for a congenital cause of os odontoideum have proposed a number of independent mechanisms accounting for the etiology of the disorder. Firstly, fusion failure between ossification centers during embryonic development can account for the independent ossicle observed in pathological patients.[12] With regard to fusion failure, it is hypothesized that either the secondary ossification center fails to fuse with the body of the odontoid process, or that the odontoid body fails to fuse with the body of the axis.[12] Embryologically, the proatlas is formed from the fourth occipital sclerotome, which consequently develops into the lateral atlantal masses, the superior aspect of the posterior atlas ring, and the apex of the dens. The first cervical sclerotome develops into the anterior arch of the atlas, the interior aspect of the posterior arch of the atlas, and the dens. The second cervical sclerotome turns into the body of the axis. Typically, the dens are separated from the axis body by a cartilaginous band and the neural central synchondrosis, and the failure of any of the fusions is believed to form an os odontoideum.[12,13] The second theory is associated with incomplete migration of the dens from the centrum of the atlas to the centrum of the axis, with subsequent failure of fusion.[14] Third, proponents for the congenital etiology of os odontoideum point to radiograph evidence displaying interdigitations between the anterior arch and the dens as indication of lack of segmentation during embryonic development.[15] Further support for the congenital etiology of os odontoideum derives from the presence of an ossiculum terminale persistens—a small radiodense ossicle at the tip of the dens.[1,16] These two conditions resemble one another in that both may be considered as consequences of fusion failure between C1 and the sclerotomes proatlas.

### *Down Syndrome*

Down syndrome (trisomy 21) is the most common chromosomal abnormality occurring during development. Irregular metabolism of mucopolysaccharides and deficient growth hormone levels in Down syndrome patients can lead to osseous malformation during development.[1] Effectively, ligamentous laxity associated with the condition is believed to account for the major pathological symptoms: hip dysplasia, patellar instability, and cervical instability.[17] Indeed, deformities in the upper cervical spine have been noted since the work of Tishler and Martel in 1965, and the reported incidence of atlantoaxial instability among this population is 10–20%.[18] Reports also indicate that 10–30% of Down syndrome patients also display wider atlantodens interval (ADI) than traditionally noted, often 4–5 mm, due to hyperlaxity atlantoaxial and occiput-C1 levels.[19-21] Isolated cases of instability at the occiput-C1 junction have been identified radiographically in adult and children with Down syndrome. Os odontoideum is a well-described cause for this observed instability and stenosis.[17]

### *Morquio Syndrome*

Morquio syndrome, known also as mucopolysaccharidosis type IV, is a genetic tissue disorder due to the absence or reduced activity of lysosomal hydrolase resulting in the accumulation of mucopolysaccharides in the ligamentous system.[22] Clinically, the disorder is manifested with joint hypermobility and disproportionate dwarfing dysplasia. Typically, spinal cord compression in the thoracolumbar region and abnormal development at the CVJ present in children with the syndrome. This latter area, specifically at the C1-C2 level, is more severe due to the localized soft tissue. In Morquio syndrome, the odontoic process is detached from its basal portion, and the atlas is generally narrowed and thickened.[22] Further, atlantoaxial instability is largely universal in individuals with this condition.

### *Klippel-Feil Syndrome*

Certain os odontoideum lesions appear to be congenital in nature due to associations with another major congenital malformation, Klippel-Feil. This syndrome features congenital fusion of any two cervical vertebrae. Sherk and Dawoud observed a case of hypermobility at C1-C2 associated with an os odontoideum coupled with a Klippel-Feil anomaly below C2, suggesting a connection between the two conditions.[23] In an additional case report, Morgan et al. observed a Klippel-Feil type II fusion of C2-C3 accompanied by an os odontoideum in a young boy.[24] Further cervical X-rays of the boy's father and grandmother revealed comparable os odontoideum and Klippel-Feil fusions of C2 and C3, indicating an autosomal dominant pattern of condition inheritance.[24]

### *Larsen Syndrome*

Larsen syndrome is a rare genetic connective tissue disorder, caused by mutations of the filamin B gene on chromosome 3p14.3.[25] It is a cytoskeletal protein permitting communication between the cytoskeleton and cell membrane, mediating the anatomically correct growth of the skeletal features. Mutations in the filament B gene had been associated with various osteochondrodysplasias, potentially manifesting in multiple joint dislocations, distinct facial anomalies, heart defects, and, importantly, abnormalities of the cervical spine.[17,25] Patients with Larsen syndrome are equally at risk for cervical kyphosis, instability, and anterior subluxation, which have been reported to predispose individuals to development of traumatic os odontoideum.[26,27] Given the risks associated with the disorder, immediate imaging of the cervical spine to look for the onset of such abnormalities is recommended after diagnosis.[17]

### *Pseudoachondroplasia*

Pseudoachondroplasia (PSACH) is a rare autosomal dominant osteochondrodysplasia due to mutations in the gene encoding the cartilage oligomeric matrix protein. It presents clinically with rhizomelic dwarfism, limb and vertebral deformity, joint laxity, and premature osteoarthritis. Pseudoachondroplasia patients are known to have higher rates of os odontoideum and hypoplasia of the dens, and cervical instability in these subjects is estimated to be around 10–20%.[28] Shetty et al. have also described upper cervical instability at C1 and C2 in PSACH patients and corresponding os odontoideum.[29] Furthermore, atlantoaxial instability secondary to os odontoideum can cause severe clinical complications, notably cervical myelopathy; researchers who have observed myelopathy onset in PSACH patients correlate it with os odontoideum and increased degrees of instability.[2,29]

### *Achondroplasia*

Achondroplasia, an autosomal dominant disorder, is the most common form of skeletal dysplasia. It is characterized by abnormal endochondral bone formation, manifested physically in micromelic short stature and a unique facial appearance.[30] A major concern in individuals with achondroplasia is spinal canal stenosis in adults, which can progress into upper cervical instability with associated neurological complications.[31] Yukata et al. present a case in which an os odontoideum was diagnosed in an achondroplastic child, hypothesizing that a link between a mutation in the FGFR-3 gene, which regulates skeletal growth, and the failed fusion of the odontoid process could be supportive of the congenital theory for the disorders.[32]

## The Acquired/Traumatic Theory

While the evidence surrounding the congenital theory emphasizes the presence of various ossification centers, proponents of the acquired theory highlight the nonunion between the dens and the body of C2 as being unrelated to any known centers. Os odontoideum would, then, be improbable as a consequence of a developmental irregularity. Indeed, os odontoideum functionally resembles a C2 fracture at the base of the dens producing a weakened C1-C2 complex and associated instability.[1] Moreover, it has been hypothesized that excessive movement at the time of ossification of the dens base would be required for the production of an os odontoideum, further nullifying a congenital origin for the disorder.[33]

Prevailing evidence of a post-traumatic etiology to the disorder stems from Fielding et al. who posit that a C2 fracture at the base of the dens leading to C1-C2 complex instability, contraction of alar ligaments, and injury to vascular supply contribute to the formation of an isolated ossicle, the os odontoideum.[9,12] Their argument is based on the observation that the ossicle is most frequently located at the base of the dens along the lines of biomechanical stress, and not near the synchondrosis, where a congenital incomplete fusion would be likely to occur.[12] Another key component of the acquired theory of os odontoideum is the enlargement of the anterior tubercle of the atlas.

Further support for acquired os odontoideum following acute injury has been provided in a number of cases, which identify normally developed odontoid processes via radiographic inspection prior to trauma and subsequent vascular injury to the dens and odontoid bone resorption.[9,34,35] For instance, Clemens et al. reported a case in which a 31-year-old man complained of neck and lumbar pain without neurological abnormalities following a fall. Dynamic plain X-rays revealed an os odontoideum and gross atlantoaxial instability.[36] A more contemporaneous case supporting the acquired theory comes from Wang and Wang, who observed computed tomography (CT) confirmation of a formation of an os odontoideum 6 years after an initial injury, the radiographs for which displayed no osseous injury and an intact odontoid initially.[4] The subject presented with normal neck motion following the trauma, yet reported severely restricted motion 6 years afterward.[4] The authors hypothesized that injury to the epiphysis between the two postnatal odontoid ossification centers caused a union failure, producing the os odontoideum.[4]

There have also been attempts by authors to attribute impaired vascular supply to acquired cases of os odontoideum. Factors including avascular necrosis following trauma, interrupted blood supply to the proximal part of the odontoid resulting in osseous absorption, and C1 anterior arch hypertrophy have all been proposed explanations for post-traumatic os odontoideum.[37-39]

## CLINICAL PRESENTATION: HISTORY AND PHYSICAL EXAMINATION

Despite the persistent debate surrounding the etiology of os odontoideum, sequestration in one of the two camps has little influence on the clinical presentation, diagnosis, and subsequent management of the condition; more important is the awareness of the presentation of the disorder, as well as the potential risks associated with atlantoaxial instability and best treatment approach.

Clinical symptoms will appear if atlantal displacement exceeds the limit of reserve space at the atlantoaxial articulation. Os odontoideum has a range of clinical manifestations, encompassing occipital neuralgia, vertebrobasilar ischemia, and cervical myelopathy.[36] The report from Klimo et al. identifies the major presenting clinical symptoms of os odontoideum. In their study of 78 pediatric and adult patients with the condition, neck pain was the most common symptom (64%), accompanied often by headaches.[5] It has been further reported that pain in some cases, occipital or cervical, is the only clear symptom.[8] Additional clinical presentations of os odontoideum include lower cranial nerve dysfunctions, bower and bladder dysfunction, motor weakness, hypersensitivity and hyperalgesia at upper and lower limps with variable onset. Sleep apnea syndrome has also been identified as a possible consequence of CVJ instability associated with an os odontoideum.[40]

Neurological symptoms are not necessarily associated with os odontoideum, but have still been identified. Since the space in the atlantoaxial articulation is present in childhood, many patients will not complain of neurological deficit even when the instability is present.[1] Neurological symptoms present due to bulbospinal compression at rest and during motion. Impingement of the bulbospinal junction on the os odontoideum may also be responsible for sensory motor deficits consistent with myelopathy.[1] Neurological signs and symptoms include transient myelopathy, tetraplegia, paresis, and central cord syndrome.[8]

Cervical myelopathy is also a well-recognized clinical outcome downstream of an initial diagnosis of os odontoideum. Dens or transverse atlantal ligament hypertrophy superimposed on a hypoplastic posterior arch can predispose an individual to developing cervical myelopathy.[41,42] Trauma in the form of occipital injury has also been implicated in cases of cervical myelopathy due to dens hypertrophy.[42]

Many patients with os odontoideum are asymptomatic, and thus experience a delayed diagnosis.[43] In such cases, discovery of the ossicle is often an incidental finding on radiographs. Asymptomatic patients are usually neurologically intact and may exhibit a degree of atlantoaxial instability.[8]

### Diagnosis

Os odontoideum can present with a wide range of clinical symptoms and signs, and therefore, researchers have identified three predominant groups of patients with the condition: (1) those with occipitocervical pain alone, (2) those presenting with myelopathy as well, and (3) those with intracranial symptoms or signs suggestive of posterior circulatory ischemia.[36,44] Asymptomatic patients do occur, and have discovered their condition incidentally; Klimo et al. reported that 15% of the cases in their series were asymptomatic.[7]

A rare radiographic diagnosis, os odontoideum has nevertheless been characterized bivalently based on the position of the dens tip: orthotopic, in which an ossicle moves with the anterior arch of C1, or dystopic, which defines an ossicle that is functionally fused to the basion.[9] Most commonly, the dystopic os odontoideum may sublux anterior to C1's arch.[9] When examining for os odontoideum, a detailed history and physical and neurological exam should be completed on all patients complaining of neck pain to detect indicators of cervical instability and subtle myelopathies.[45] Initial imaging should follow, including cervical radiographs consisting of an open-mouth odontoid view, a lateral cervical view, and flexion/extension views.[43] Further radiographic confirmation in the form of magnetic resonance imaging is then recommended. Incidental discovery of os odontoideum is not unusual, and it is often not considered as a possible condition until imaging is obtained. The presence of the disorder is suggested primarily after plain cervical spine X-rays, which have been deemed sufficient for diagnosis.[46] Tomography and CT also have documented use to define the osseous anatomy of os odontoideum. High-resolution multiplanar CT scan is necessary to provide the detailed anatomy of the fragment as well as any additional cervical or cerebral abnormalities. Plain dynamic flexion/extension X-rays are used to assess the degree of abnormal motion between C1 and C2, a further confirmatory tool for the diagnosis of the condition. These images often display anterior instability, defined as >3 mm of C1-C2 motion, with subluxation of the os odontoideum in relation to C2.[47] There is, however, a lack of literature describing the sensitivity or specificity of imaging studies for the diagnosis of os odontoideum. Beyond studies reporting patients undergoing static plain cervical spine X-rays, CTs, and MRIs, there is no mention of additional imaging needed for os odontoideum diagnosis.

## Management

Given the rarity of the condition, proper management of os odontoideum remains uncertain. Further, the gap of knowledge regarding the long-term natural history of the disorder complicates the proscription of a certain recommendation. Patients with an incidental diagnosis of os odontoideum either with or without C1-C2 instability who have neither symptoms nor neurological signs can be managed with consistent clinical and radiographical surveillance.[48] Alternatively, surgical intervention is advocated for radiographically unstable os odontoideum, regardless of the presence or absence of symptoms.

### *Conservative Approach*

The universal goal of the various management strategies for os odontoideum has been the stabilization of the observed instability at the C1-C2 vertebral level. Patients without neurological symptoms and instability at C1-C2 on flexion/extension images can be managed nonoperatively without clinical consequence. Sabat et al. report the case of a 17-year-old patient with CVJ-tuberculosis associated with an os odontoideum, wherein conservative treatment in the form of cervical traction followed by a halo-vest resulted in uneventful recovery.[49] In an analysis of 37 cases in which 20 patients were treated conservatively for os odontoideum while the rest underwent occipitocervical or atlantoaxial fusion, after 8 years of follow-up it was found that there were no differences among patients' outcomes between the two treatments, leading to the recommendation that patients with local and transient symptoms (pain in the neck and head, torticollis) should receive nonoperative treatment.[50] These modalities often include cervical traction, physical therapy, occasional collar use, and anti-inflammatory medications.

### *Surgical Approach*

Most investigators of os odontoideum prefer surgical management in the form of stabilization and fusion of potential C1-C2 instability associated with the disorder, the primary concern being the increased risk for future spinal cord injury. In recent years, increased understanding of spinal biomechanics has provided a more profound understanding of approaches to the CVJ. These developments translate into increased utilization of spinal fusions and implementation of instrumentation for the management of the disorder. The main issue, then, is not whether surgical intervention is required, but when. For instance, Arvin et al. recommended that patients, save for adolescents with the potential for growth and increased deformity, with os odontoideum associated with neurological deficit and radiographic evidence of instability accept surgery.[8]

Several main surgical options exist for the treatment of os odontoideum: anterior resection of the os fragment, posterior atlantoaxial fusion, posterior atlantoaxial wiring and fusion, posterior occipitocervical wiring and fusion, posterior Magerl screw fixation and fusion, and Harms' technique of C1-C2 fusion.[1] Wiring techniques, although rather antiquated, remain effective for pediatric patients. The posterior approach is advocated for the management of reducible C1-C2 dislocation, which is more commonly associated with os odontoideum pathology.[1]

Introduced in 1979, the Magerl technique provides atlantoaxial fixation by means of C1-C2 transarticular screw fixation. An advantage of this approach is the immediate obliteration of rotational movement at the atlantoaxial joint, yet the technical difficult of this surgical form prevents its widespread use.[51] However, studies reporting successful implementation of the Magerl technique observe less postoperative pain due to biomechanical stability compared traditional atlantoaxial arthrodesis techniques.[51,52]

The less invasive technique is Harms', which has become the most prominent form for stabilization in adult populations contemporaneously.[53] The technique involves bilateral insertion of minipolyaxial screws in the lateral head of C1 and through the pars interarticularis into the pedicle of C2.[54] This is a technically innovative procedure, although it is not as susceptible to anatomical variations as Magerl's is, with follow-up data indicating solid fusion in patients.[54]

Anterior surgical approaches for managing os odontoideum also exist. The transoral-transpalatopharyngeal approach can be used for ventral decompression of irreducible os odontoideum.[55] This approach involves an incision in the pharyngeal wall over the C1 tubercle, followed by a soft palate incision from the posterior margin of the palatal bone to the superior margin of the uvula.[1] After the detachment of the longuscolli muscles, the decompression can be carried out with the cervical vertebrae exposed.

In an effort to limit the complications associated with the transoral approach, such as pharyngeal wound dehiscence and infection, endoscopic-assisted transoral approach has been implemented. This transnasal technique permits access to the ventral part of C1 and C2, and is delineated by the nasopalatine line, which connects the most inferior point on the nasal bone to the most posterior point on the hard palate in the midsagittal plane.[1] Preoperative planning for this approach is especially important. The patient's head is placed in the neutral position in terms of the CVJ. An access hole is initially introduced in the posterior portion of the nasal septum that permits bilateral access to the nasopharynx. Then, the sphenoid sinus is opened to enlarge the working area such that the ventral arch of C1 is exposed and readily accessed.[56]

A third anterior approach used to gain access to the ventral aspect of the CVJ is the higher anterior cervical retropharyngeal approach. This approach facilitates ventral decompression with anterior cervical fusion without the need for subsequent posterior fixation.[1] In this technique, an incision is made inferior to the mandible, exposing the platysma muscle, which is cut so as to expose the submandibular gland. The digastric muscles beneath are retracted, along with the hypoglossal nerve and pharyngeal muscles, so as to expose the anterior portion of the C1 and C2 vertebrae.[57] Fixation of the atlantoaxial joint with C1-C2 intrafacetal fusion and transarticular screw insertion is then possible.

## CONCLUSION

Os odontoideum is a rare condition of the upper cervical spine and is defined by its contentious pathogenesis and poorly understood natural history. Consequently, it is difficult for consulting physicians to make informed recommendations to their patients. Further complicating the matter is the variable clinical presentation of patients with os odontoideum, potentially accompanied by associated downstream conditions, such as atlantoaxial instability or cervical myelopathy. While conservative approaches do exist for the treatment of os odontoideum, this form of management remains somewhat limited. However, the neurosurgeon retains a number of techniques at hand, with differing levels of success and technical feasibility, to treat the malformation when surgical intervention is recommended.

## REFERENCES


1. Visocchi M, Di Rocco C. Os odontoideum syndrome: pathogenesis, clinical patterns and indication for surgical strategies in childhood. Adv Tech Stand Neurosurg. 2014; 40:273-93.
2. Matsui H, Imada K, Tsuji H. Radiographic classification of Os odontoideum and its clinical significance. Spine (Phila Pa 1976). 1997;22:1706-9.
3. Perrini P, Montemurro N, Iannelli A. The contribution of Carlo Giacomini (1840-1898): the limbus Giacomini and beyond. Neurosurgery. 2013;72:475-81; discussion 481-2.
4. Wang S, Wang C. Acquired os odontoideum: a case report and literature review. Childs Nerv Syst. 2012;28:315-9.
5. Klimo P, Kan P, Rao G, et al. Os odontoideum: presentation, diagnosis, and treatment in a series of 78 patients. J Neurosurg Spine. 2008;9:332-42.
6. Ogata T, Morino T, Hino M, et al. Cervical myelopathy caused by atlantoaxial instability in a patient with an os odontoideum and total aplasia of the posterior arch of the atlas: a case report. J Med Case Rep. 2012;6:171.
7. Klimo P, Coon V, Brockmeyer D. Incidental os odontoideum: current management strategies. Neurosurg Focus. 2011; 31:E10.

8. Arvin B, Fournier-Gosselin M-P, Fehlings MG. Os odontoideum: etiology and surgical management. Neurosurgery. 2010;66:22-31.
9. Fielding JW, Griffin PP. Os odontoideum: an acquired lesion. J Bone Joint Surg Am. 1974;56:187-90.
10. Vickers ED. Atlantoaxial anomalies with particular emphasis on os odontoideum. J Manipulative Physiol Ther. 1990; 13:471-6.
11. Muhleman M, Charran O, Matusz P, et al. The proatlas: a comprehensive review with clinical implications. Childs Nerv Syst. 2012;28:349-56.
12. Fielding JW, Hensinger RN, Hawkins RJ. Os Odontoideum. J Bone Joint Surg Am. 1980;62:376-83.
13. McHugh BJ, Grant RA, Zupon AB, et al. Congenital os odontoideum arising from the secondary ossification center without prior fracture. J Neurosurg Spine. 2012;17:594-7.
14. Kirlew KA, Hathout GM, Reiter SD, et al. Os odontoideum in identical twins: perspectives on etiology. Skeletal Radiol. 1993;22:525-7.
15. Fagan AB, Askin GN, Earwaker JWS. The jigsaw sign. A reliable indicator of congenital aetiology in os odontoideum. Eur Spine J. 2004;13:295-300.
16. Al Kaissi A, Chehida F Ben, Ghachem M Ben, et al. Atlanto-axial segmentation defects and os odontoideum in two male siblings with opsismodysplasia. Skeletal Radiol. 2009; 38:293-6.
17. McKay SD, Al-Omari A, Tomlinson LA, et al. Review of cervical spine anomalies in genetic syndromes. Spine (Phila Pa 1976). 2012;37:E269-77.
18. Ali FE, Al-Bustan MA, Al-Busairi WA, et al. Cervical spine abnormalities associated with Down syndrome. Int Orthop. 2006;30:284-9.
19. Pueschel SM, Scola FH, Tupper TB, et al. Skeletal anomalies of the upper cervical spine in children with Down syndrome. J Pediatr Orthop. n.d.;10:607-11.
20. Pizzutillo PD, Herman MJ. Cervical spine issues in Down syndrome. J Pediatr Orthop. n.d.;25:253-9.
21. Taggard DA, Menezes AH, Ryken TC. Treatment of Down syndrome-associated craniovertebral junction abnormalities. J Neurosurg. 2000;93:205-13.
22. Ashraf J, Crockard HA, Ransford AO, et al. Transoral decompression and posterior stabilisation in Morquio's disease. Arch Dis Child. 1991;66:1318-21.
23. Sherk HH, Dawoud S. Congenital os odontoideum with Klippel-Feil anomaly and fatal atlanto-axial instability. Report of a case. Spine (Phila Pa 1976). n.d.; 6:42-5.
24. Morgan MK, Onofrio BM, Bender CE. Familial os odontoideum. Case report. J Neurosurg. 1989;70:636-9.
25. Winer N, Kyndt F, Paumier A, et al. Prenatal diagnosis of Larsen syndrome caused by a mutation in the filamin B gene. Prenat Diagn. 2009;29:172-4.
26. Campbell RM. Spine deformities in rare congenital syndromes: clinical issues. Spine (Phila Pa 1976). 2009; 34: 1815-27.
27. Too CW, Tang PH. Imaging findings of chronic subluxation of the os odontoideum and cervical myelopathy in a child with Beare-Stevenson cutis gyrata syndrome after surgery to the head and neck. Ann Acad Med Singapore. 2009;38:832-4.
28. Ain MC, Chaichana KL, Schkrohowsky JG. Retrospective study of cervical arthrodesis in patients with various types of skeletal dysplasia. Spine (Phila Pa 1976). 2006;31:E169-74.
29. Shetty GM, Song HR, Unnikrishnan R, et al. Upper cervical spine instability in pseudoachondroplasia. J Pediatr Orthop. n.d.;27:782-7.
30. Matsui Y, Yasui N, Kimura T, et al. Genotype phenotype correlation in achondroplasia and hypochondroplasia. J Bone Joint Surg Br. 1998;80:1052-6.
31. Ferrante L, Acqui M, Celli P, et al. Achondroplasia: unusual bone abnormalities of the cervical spine. Neurosurg Rev. 1992;15:143-5.
32. Yukata K, Katoh S, Sairyo K, et al. Os odontoideum in achondroplasia: a case report. J Pediatr Orthop B. 2008;17:103-5.
33. Crockard HA, Stevens JM. Craniovertebral junction anomalies in inherited disorders: part of the syndrome or caused by the disorder? Eur J Pediatr. 1995; 154: 504-12.
34. Schuler TC, Kurz L, Thompson DE, et al. Natural history of os odontoideum. J Pediatr Orthop n.d.;11:222-5.
35. Stillwell WT, Fielding JW. Acquired os odontoideum. A case report. Clin Orthop Relat Res. 1978;135:71-3.
36. Clements WD, Mezue W, Mathew B. Os odontoideum—congenital or acquired —That's not the question. Injury 1995; 26:640-2.
37. Sakaida H, Waga S, Kojima T, et al. Os odontoideum associated with hypertrophic ossiculum terminale. Case report. J Neurosurg. 2001;94:140-4.
38. Hammerstein J, Russo S, Easton K. Atlantoaxial dislocation in a child secondary to a displaced chondrum terminale. A case report. J Bone Joint Surg Am. 2007; 89:413-7.
39. Holt RG, Helms CA, Munk PL, et al. Hypertrophy of C-1 anterior arch: useful sign to distinguish os odontoideum from acute dens fracture. Radiology. 1989; 173:207-9.
40. Kawaguchi Y, Iida M, Seki S, et al. Os odontoideum with cervical mylopathy due to posterior subluxation of C1 presenting sleep apnea. J Orthop Sci. 2011;16:329-33.
41. Kasliwal MK, Traynelis VC. Hypertrophic posterior arch of atlas causing cervical myelopathy. Asian Spine J. 2012;6: 284-6.
42. Okada K, Sato K, Abe E. Hypertrophic dens resulting in cervical myelopathy: histologic features of the hypertrophic dens. Spine (Phila Pa 1976). 2000;25:1303-7.
43. Choit RL, Jamieson DH, Reilly CW. Os odontoideum: a significant radiographic finding. Pediatr Radiol. 2005;35:803-7.
44. Rowland LP, Shapiro JH, Jacobson HG. Neurological syndromes associated with congenital absence of the odontoid process. AMA Arch Neurol Psychiatry. 1958; 80:286-91.
45. Chrobak K, Larson R, Stern PJ. Varied clinical presentation of os odontoideum: a case report. J Can Chiropr Assoc. 2014;58:268-72.
46. Buyukkaya A, Yazgan O, Yazgan S, Ozel MA. Characteristic imaging findings of os odontoideum. Spine J. 2014;14 (12):3052-3.
47. Park JS, Cho DC, Sung JK. Feasibility of C2 translaminar screw as an alternative or salvage of C2 pedicle screws in atlantoaxial instability. J Spinal Disord Tech. 2012; 25:254-8.
48. Hadley M. Os odontoideum. Neurosurgery. 2002:50(3 Suppl):S148-55.

49. Sabat D, Arora S, Kumar V, et al. Os odontoideum complicating craniovertebral junction tuberculosis: a case report. Spine (Phila Pa 1976). 2011;36:E814-8.
50. Spierings EL, Braakman R. The management of os odontoideum. Analysis of 37 cases. J Bone Joint Surg Br. 1982; 64:422-8.
51. Haid RW. C1-C2 transarticular screw fixation: technical aspects. Neurosurgery. 2001;49:71-4.
52. Grob D, Crisco JJ, Panjabi MM, et al. Biomechanical evaluation of four different posterior atlantoaxial fixation techniques. Spine (Phila Pa 1976). 1992;17:480-90.
53. Stulík J, Vyskocil T, Sebesta P, et al. [Harms technique of C1-C2 fixation with polyaxial screws and rods]. Acta Chir Orthop Traumatol Cech. 2005;72:22-7.
54. Harms J, Melcher RP. Posterior C1-C2 fusion with polyaxial screw and rod fixation. Spine (Phila Pa 1976). 2001;26: 2467-71.
55. Menezes AH. Pathogenesis, dynamics, and management of os odontoideum. Neurosurg Focus. 1999;6:e2.
56. Visocchi M, La Rocca G, Della Pepa GM, et al. Anterior video-assisted approach to the craniovertebral junction: transnasal or transoral? A cadaver study. Acta Neurochir (Wien). 2014;156:285-92.
57. Kansal R, Sharma A, Kukreja S. An anterior high cervical retropharyngeal approach for C1-C2 intrafacetal fusion and transarticular screw insertion. J Clin Neurosci. 2011; 18:1705-8.

Chapter 13

# Atlantoaxial Dislocations

*Shenglin Wang, Chao Wang*

## INTRODUCTION

The atlantoaxial joint comprises C1 (the atlas), C2 (the axis), and affiliated ligaments, which combine to permit complex movements of the cervical spine while continually providing sufficient mechanical strength to stabilize the head. Articulation of this joint accounts for over 50% of all cervical rotations occurring between the odontoid process of C2 and C1 and the transverse ligament.[1,2]

An atlantoaxial dislocation (AAD) is defined as a loss of the normal position of the first and second vertebral articulation (Figs. 13.1A and B). In normal patients, a number of predominant conditions prevent this C1-C2 dislocation: (1) the unique position of the odontoid process, which projects through the ring of the atlas ventrally; (2) the dorsal transverse atlantal ligament; and (3) the C1-C2 lateral mass joints.[3] Patients predisposed to AAD often display disruption of the integrity of the odontoid or the transverse atlantal ligament.[4-6] Atlantoaxial dislocations are often associated with complex deformities of the craniovertebral junction (CVJ) and are significant risk factors for downstream neurological symptoms and deterioration. Severe AAD has been associated with the onset of a number of serious pathological conditions, including upper cervical myelopathy, respiratory failure, and even death.[7,8]

All acute AAD resulting from C1 or C2 fractures should be reduced by traction and treated according to the treatment strategy for original fractures. However, chronic AAD retains multiple etiologies and specialized treatment algorithms. In this chapter, we will specifically present and summarize our clinical experience of chronic atlantoaxial disorders.

## ETIOLOGY AND CLASSIFICATIONS

The cause of AAD is commonly multifactorial. Nevertheless, the etiology of the disorder can be broadly divided into congenital, developmental, inflammatory, timorous, or traumatic categories (Table 13.1). As previously mentioned, any disruption of the various structures that stabilize the atlantoaxial joint would predispose a patient to AAD.

The distribution of these different etiologies varies across countries and territories. In our institution's clinical

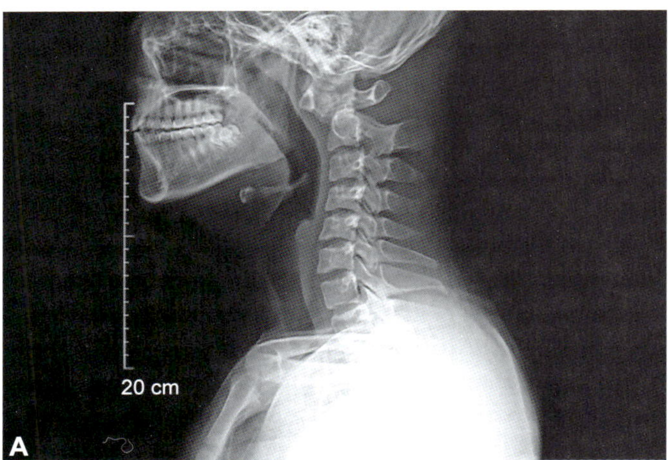


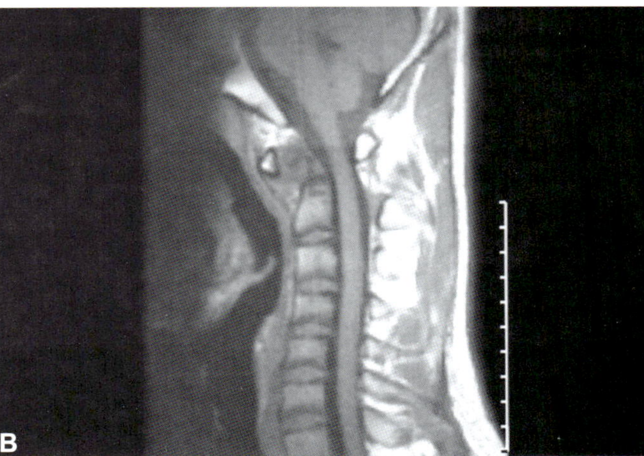


**Figs. 13.1A and B:** (A) Atlantoaxial dislocation (AAD); (B) Magnetic resonance imaging showing spinal compression from AAD.

**Table 13.1:** Etiology of the atlantoaxial dislocation in the literature.

**Congenital or developmental deformities**
Occipitalization of the atlas
Block vertebra C2-C3
- Spondyloepiphyseal dysplasia
- Down syndrome
- Morquio syndrome
- Goldenhar syndrome
- Os odontoideum

**Inflammations (or infections)**
Rheumatoid arthritis
Ankylosis spondylitis
- Grisel syndrome
- Tuberculosis
- Bacteria

**Tumors**
Primary
- Metastatic

**Trauma**
Transverse ligament loosen
Os odontoideum
- Fracture of the odontoid

**Table13.2:** Etiologies of atlantoaxial dislocation in 1,106 cases at our institution (1998–2012).

| *Diagnosis* | *Cases* | *Percentage* |
|---|---|---|
| Os odontoideum | 503 | 45.5 |
| Atlas occipitalization | 241 | 21.8 |
| Transverse ligament loosen | 90 | 8.1 |
| Atlas occipitalization and block vertebra C2-C3 | 86 | 7.8 |
| Rheumatoid arthritis | 49 | 4.4 |
| Old odontoid fracture, nonunion | 36 | 3.3 |
| Ankylosis spondylitis | 11 | 1.0 |
| Down syndrome | 8 | 0.7 |
| Block vertebra C2-C3 | 8 | 0.7 |
| Atlas occipitalization and os odontoideum | 7 | 0.7 |
| Block vertebra C2-C3 and os odontoideum | 5 | 0.5 |
| Unknown | 62 | 5.6 |
| Total | 1106 | 100 |

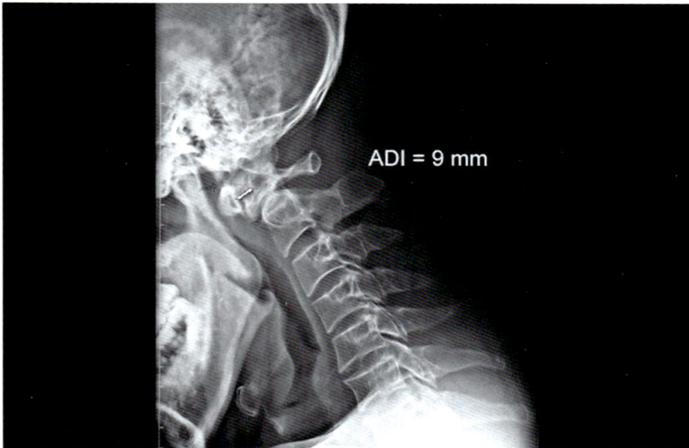


**Fig. 13.2:** Atlantodental interval measurement.

practice from 1998 to 2012, the predominant cause of chronic AAD was os odontoideum (45.5%, Table 13.2). The second most common source was occipitalization of the atlas (21.8%). In many cases, the origin of AAD could not be clearly defined (unknown, 5.6%). Of note, the presence of tumor or acute fracture at the CVJ excluded patients from this series.

## DIAGNOSIS

Atlantoaxial dislocation is defined by means of radiographic measurements of the atlantoaxial joint articulation using the atlantodental interval (ADI). The ADI is a small slit-like space between the posterior aspect of the anterior atlas ring and the anterior aspect of the odontoid process (Fig. 13.2). The ADI is normally constant in length during cranial movement, and generally does not exceed 3 mm for adults and 5 mm for children.[3,9-11] Atlantoaxial dislocation can be successfully diagnosed in patients with an ADI >3 mm in adults >18 years of age and >5 mm in children.[12] Dynamic flexion and extension radiographs of the cervical spine permit the measurement of the ADI and the determination of whether or not the atlantoaxial joint reduces itself in these positions.[13] Occasionally, patients fail to have full ability for movement and thus the diagnosis of AAD can be overlooked (Figs. 13.3A to D). In our institution, the extreme flexion and extension lateral radiographs had been used for the diagnosis of AAD. Prior to these radiographs, patients were taught how to display the full movements required for the dynamic images.

In the case of patients with incomplete odontoid processes (such as with os odontoideum or old odontoid fractures), comparable criteria were adopted for diagnosing AAD: measuring the distance between the inferior rim of C1's anterior arch and the remaining attached part of the odontoid or C2 anterior-superior edge (Fig. 13.4).[13]

Computed topographic (CT) scans can further confirm the ADI length and the concomitant osseous deformities. Thin-slice scanning for the CVJ, especially using

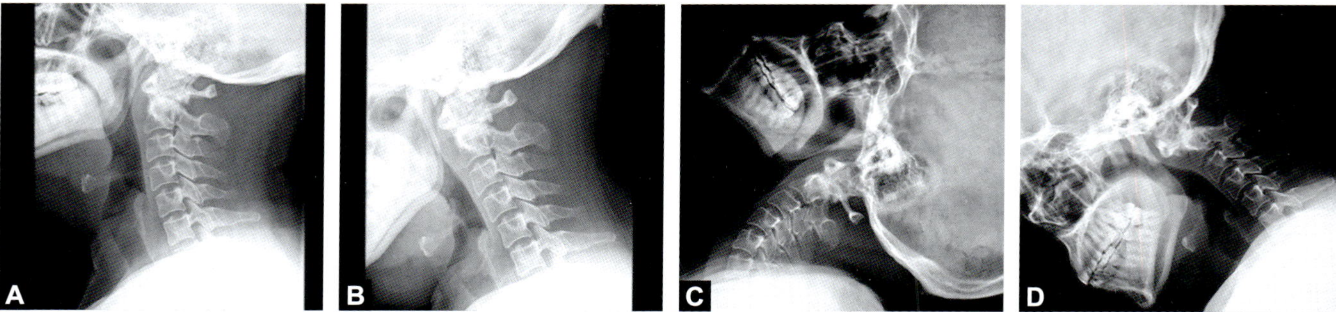


**Figs. 13.3A to D:** (A) X-ray of extension; (B) Flexion (the patient did not have full movement and atlantoaxial dislocation cannot be found); (C and D) X-ray of full extension and flexion showed an abnormal atlantodental interval.

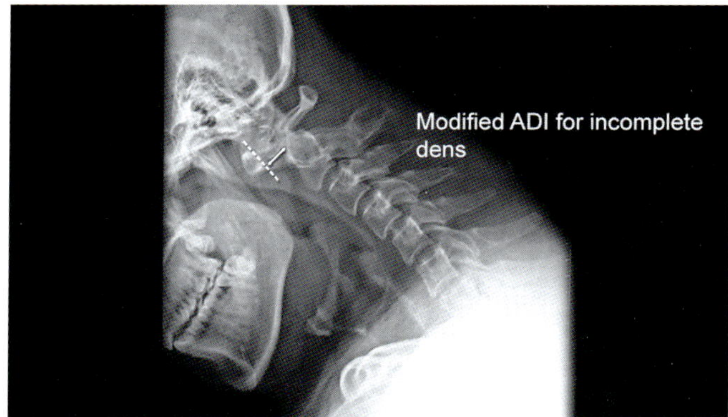


**Fig. 13.4:** For patients with incomplete odontoid, modified atlantodental interval is the distance between the inferior rim of C1 anterior arch and the remaining attached part of the odontoid or C2 anterior-superior edge.

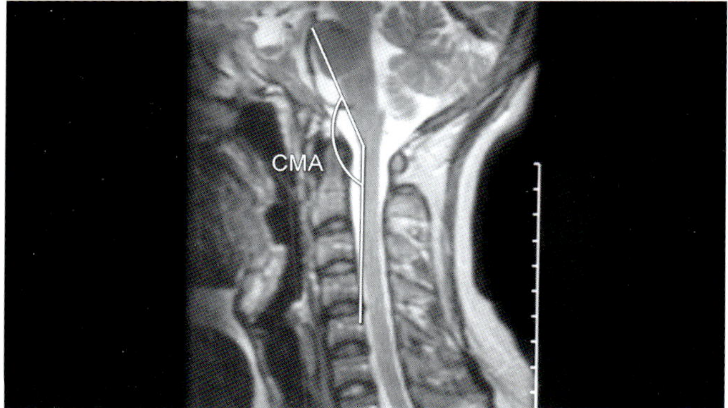


**Fig. 13.5:** The cervicomedullary angle measurement.

reconstructive CT, can reveal osseous structures and the position of the vertebral artery (VA). The surgical decisions, approaches, and trajectory of the screws, to some degree, rely on an accurate preoperative CT. In the setting of AAD with rotatory fixation, ADI should be solely measured on the axial CT image because measurements on the lateral plain radiograph are unreliable for the torticollis cases.

Magnetic resonance imaging (MRI) is also a useful diagnostic tool in that it can reveal the compression of the spinal cord and brain stem. The cervicomedullary angle (CMA) is the angle subtended by the lines drawn parallel to the ventral surfaces of the medulla and upper cervical cord on MRI (Fig. 13.5). Cervicomedullary angle values have been used effectively to evaluate the amount of compression in the upper cervical cord, brain stem, and medulla, as well as the amount of subsequent postoperative decompression. The normal CMA values range from 139.0° to 175.5°, with an average value of 158.46°, and a 95% confidence interval from 144.8° to 172.1°.[14] A decreased CMA value refers to compression of one of the above-mentioned structures. It has been previously reported that there is a strong correlation between CMA values < 135° and clinical evidence of myelopathy and/or brain stem compression.[15]

## PATHOLOGICAL CHANGES IN AAD DEVELOPMENT

Every AAD originates from instability, but some forms of atlantoaxial instability will progress into dislocation. Chronic AAD arises from the gradual progression of several events. As the majority of cases present with anterior displacement, this cascade can be illustrated using a model of anterior atlas dislocation. Indeed, loss of either odontoid or transverse atlantal ligament integrity can result in an unstable atlantoaxial joint. Several nodes are derived from the subsequent consecutive process. In the early stages of the condition, the relative motion between C1 and C2 is increased and the C1-2 facets remain horizontal. Alterations to the facet joints represent an important aspect of chronic AAD development. During head flexion, the atlas slides anteriorly along the horizontal facets. However, in extension, the atlas can revert to its normal position or may even exceed this orientation due to posterior subluxation (Node I: instability, Figs. 13.6A and B). In the second stage of the condition, repetitive atlas sliding and compression remodels C1-2 facets such that they become increasingly vertically sloped, followed by subsequent degeneration of the facet joints. The atlas slides distantly along the sloped C1-2 facets, while the C1-2 motion begins to decrease. The muscles, ligaments, and capsules of the atlantoaxial joint become shortened and eventually contracted. With time, extension of the head can no longer achieve atlantoaxial reduction, resulting in a subaxial lordosis to achieve global balance.[16] In many cases, however, skeletal traction under general anesthesia has the potential to open the sloped C1-2 lateral mass joints and to achieve complete reduction (Node II: reducible dislocation, Figs. 13.7A to D). In the third stage, marked by severe anterior sliding of the atlas

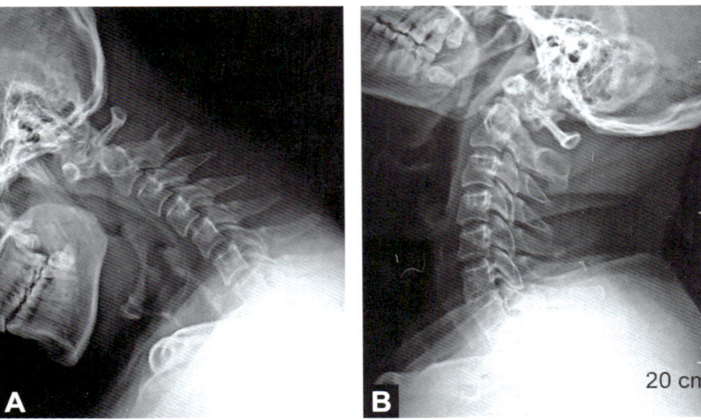


**Figs. 13.6A and B:** During flexion of head, the atlas slides anteriorly (A). However, the atlas can revert to its normal position in extension, or even exceed its normal position to posterior subluxation (B).

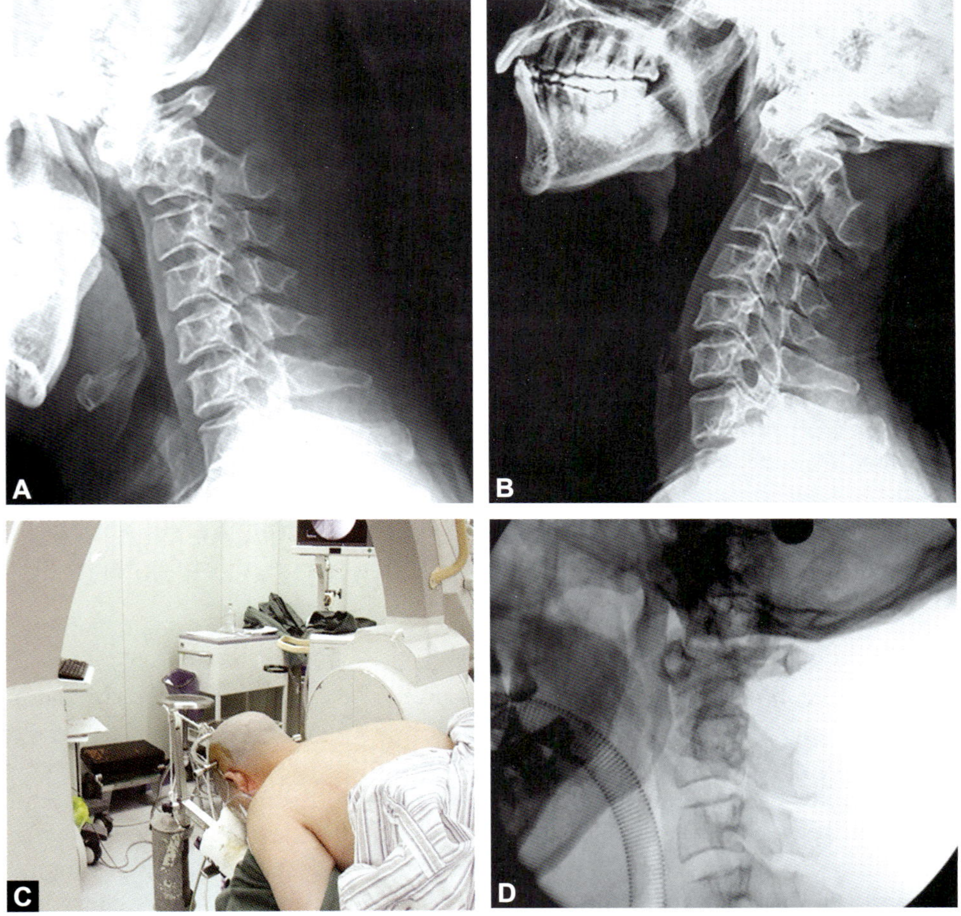


**Figs. 13.7A to D:** The patient had a fixed atlantoaxial dislocation on the radiographs of flexion (A) and extension (B). Using skeletal traction under general anesthesia (C), complete reduction was achieved (D).

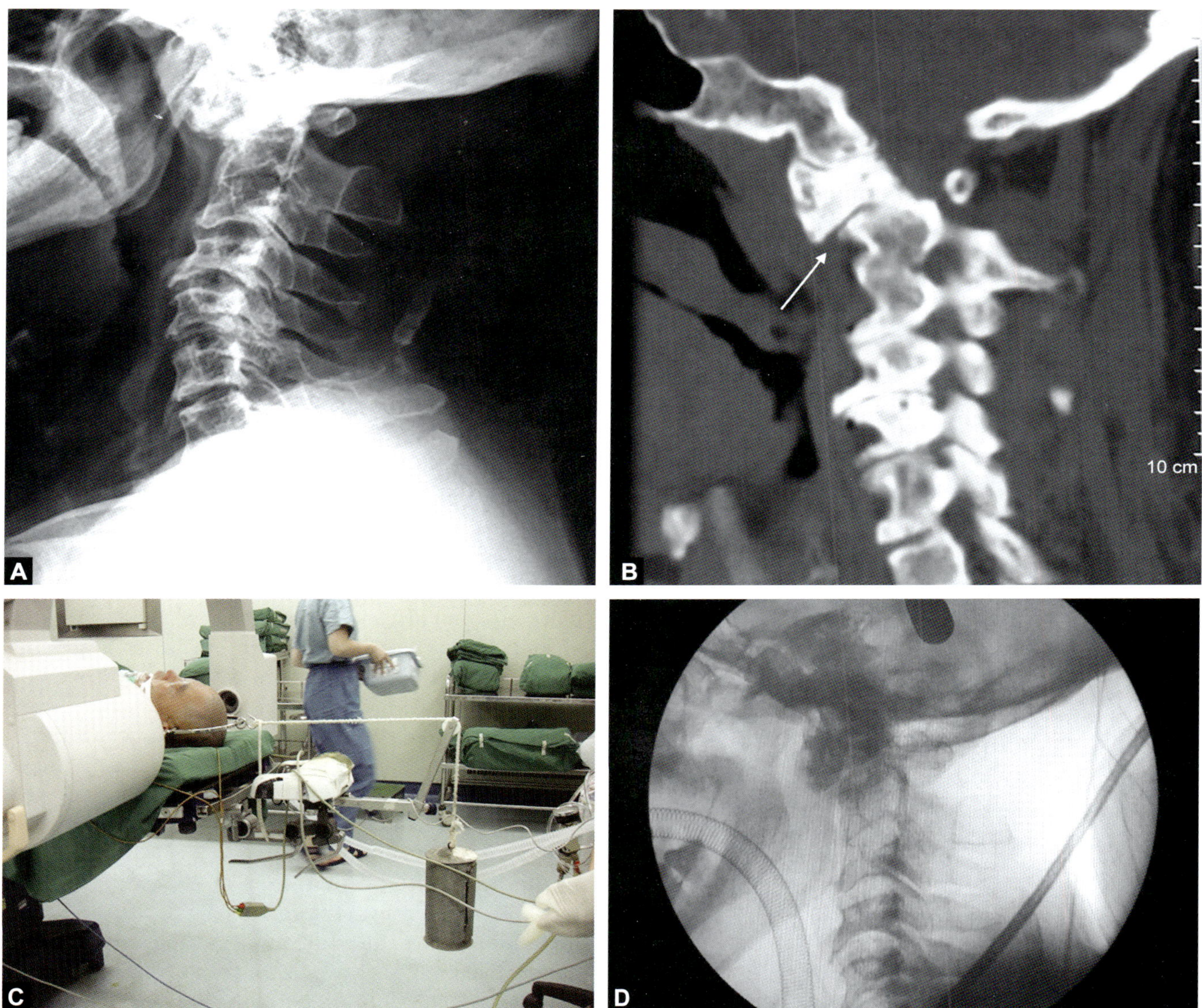


**Figs. 13.8A to D:** (A) Atlantoaxial dislocation (AAD) was confirmed by X-ray; (B) The facet orientation becomes sloped severely and degeneration occurred; (C) Skeletal traction under general anesthesia; (D) C-arm confirmed incomplete reduction (irreducible AAD).

and collapse of the facets resulting in a fixed atlas, little motion exists between C1 and C2. The advanced combination of AAD and subaxial hyperlordosis is referred to as a swan neck deformity, wherein the muscles, ligaments, and capsules of the atlantoaxial joint are even further contracted and shortened.[16] With further degeneration, the facet orientation becomes sloped severely, with the potential to obtain a complete vertical orientation (Fig. 13.8B, arrow).[17] In this setting, skeletal traction under general anesthesia cannot achieve a complete reduction (Node III: irreducible dislocation, Figs. 13.8A to D). In the final stage of the AAD, motion disappears completely, and a bony fusion occurs between the C1 and C2 lateral mass joint (Node IV: bony dislocation, Figs. 13.9A to D). These four stages of the pathologic dislocation represent self-remodeling processes in AAD. Based on these presented pathologic intervals, we have designed a novel classification for chronic AAD, as follows.

## Resulting Pathology of the Lower Cervical Spine

Destabilization of the upper cervical spine results in compromised sagittal balance and subsequent compensation

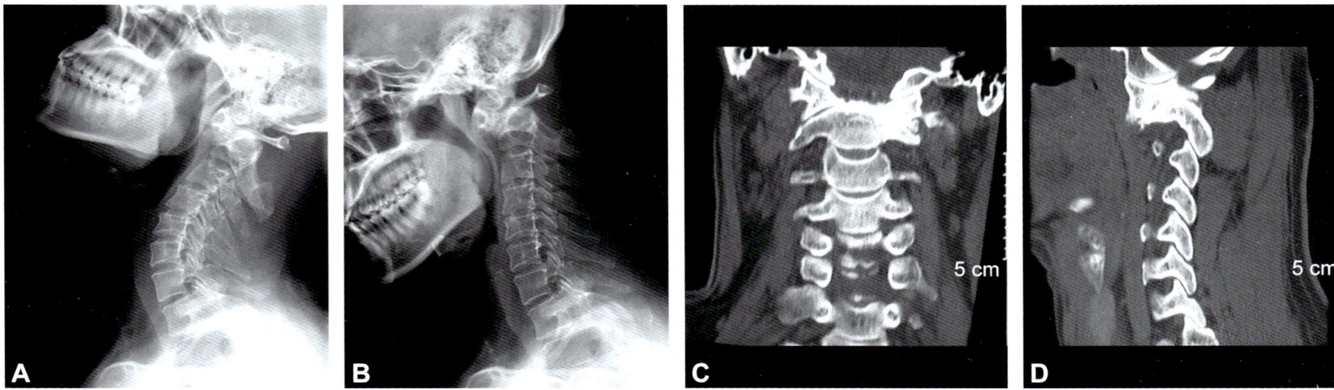


**Figs. 13.9A to D:** In the last stage, the motion between C1 and C2 disappears completely (A and B), while a bony fusion occurs between the C1 and C2 lateral mass joint (C and D).

**Table 13.3:** Clinical presentation in 1,106 cases.

| *Symptom and signs* | *Cases* | *Percentage* |
|---|---|---|
| Short neck | 104 | 9.4 |
| Neck pain | 373 | 33.7 |
| Neck movement restriction | 295 | 26.7 |
| Vertigo | 49 | 4.4 |
| Extremities weakness | 712 | 64.4 |
| Numbness | 688 | 62.2 |
| Pyramidal signs | 709 | 64.1 |
| Sphincter disturbances | 282 | 25.5 |
| Lower cranial nerve dysfunction | 33 | 3.0 |
| Respiratory distress | 12 | 1.1 |
| Total | 1106 | 100 |

of the lower cervical spine, which may lead to subaxial pathology and deformities.[9,18-20] When AAD causes diminished lordosis at the C0-C2 segment, the subaxial cervical region is observed to compensate with increased lordosis so that balance is maintained.[20] Kyphosis at the occipito-axial segment together with extreme hyperlordosis subaxially can occur in some patients with end-stage disease, resulting in swan-neck deformity.[9]

## CLINICAL PRESENTATION

The clinical presentation of AAD may range from minor axial neck pain to death. Overall, AAD encompasses four forms of symptoms: (1) restricted neck movement and/or pain of the CVJ area from the stimulation of instability or neurological compression; (2) signs and symptoms due to cervical myelopathy, including weakness, numbness, pyramidal signs, and sphincter disturbances; (3) lower cranial nerves and brain stem involvement, including ataxia, articulation disorder, swallowing disturbance, nystagmus, diplopia, vertigo, and tinnitus; and (4) respiratory difficulties from myelopathy or brain stem lesions. Clinical presentation of the 1,106 cases in our series is summarized in Table 13.3.

In our clinical practice, a standardized functional scoring criteria for CVJ compressive disease has been used for AAD (Table 13.4). In this scoring criterion, the JOA score for cervical myelopathy was quoted. It is especially useful for the assessment of preoperative and postoperative function in AAD.

The neurological compression of AAD with an intact odontoid comes from the odontoid (Fig. 13.10A). However, AAD cases with unfused odontoids display spinal compression beginning at the posterior top of the C2 vertebral body (Fig. 13.10B). Regardless of the etiology, the clinical consequences of AAD have clear potential for neurological compromise.

Some patients may have an acute presentation after acute, minor trauma if he or she has a congenital and asymptomatic yet unstable atlantoaxial joint.[21] The symptoms may also present as relapsing and remitting episodes due to the motion of day-to-day life.[13,22,23]

## SURGICAL CLASSIFICATION AND TREATMENT STRATEGY

Based on the pathologic stages of AAD previously presented, a surgical classification and treatment strategy has been designed.[12] The classification system is based on the results of three tests as outlined below:

**Table 13.4:** A standardized functional score for craniovertebral junction compressive disease.

| *Criterion* | *Points* |
|---|---|
| **1. Cervical myelopathy (from Japanese Orthopedic Association)** | (17) |
| **Motor function (upper extremity)** | |
| Paralysis | 0 |
| Fine motor function massively decreased | 1 |
| Fine motor function decelerated | 2 |
| Discreet weakness in hands or proximal arm | 3 |
| Normal function | 4 |
| **Motor function (lower extremity)** | |
| Unable to walk | 0 |
| Need walking aid on flat floor | 1 |
| Need handrail on stairs | 2 |
| Able to walk without walking aid, but inadequate | 3 |
| Normal function | 4 |
| **Sensory (upper extremity/lower extremity/ trunk)** | (6) U/ L/ T |
| Apparent sensory loss | 0 / 0 / 0 |
| Minimal sensory loss | 1 / 1 / 1 |
| Normal function | 2 / 2 / 2 |
| **Bladder function** | |
| Urinary retention | 0 |
| Severe dysfunction | 1 |
| Mild dysfunction | 2 |
| Normal function | 3 |
| **2. Lower cranial nerves or brain stem involvement** including three groups: Articulation disorder, swallowing disturbance, and visual disturbance (nystagmus, diplopia, blurred vision, etc.) | (3) |
| | A/ S/ V |
| Severe symptoms (restriction of function of daily life) | 0 / 0 / 0 |
| Mild symptoms (no restriction of function of daily life) | 0.5 / 0.5 / 0.5 |
| None | 1 / 1 / 1 |
| **3. Respiratory difficulty** | (2) |
| Respiration failure, need assistant respiration | 0 |
| Dyspnea or with cough weakness | 1 |
| None | 2 |
| Total score | 0-22 |

The recovery rate shows the changes of the scores, taking improvement, worsening and no changes of the scores into consideration. It is assessed by the following formula: Recovery rate = (postoperative score – preoperative score)/(total score–preoperative score).

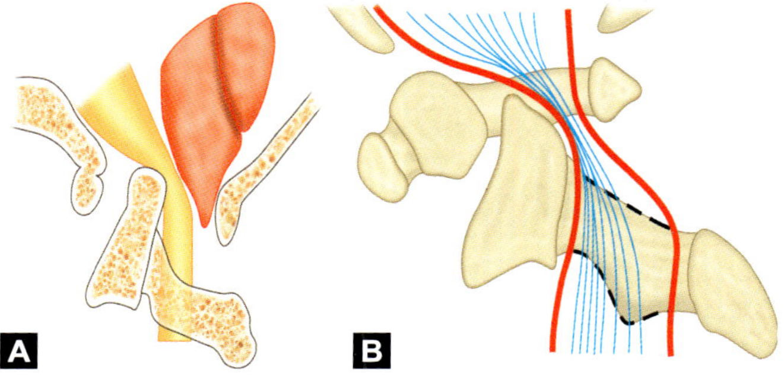


**Figs. 13.10A and B:** (A) The neurological compression of atlantoaxial dislocation (AAD) with an intact odontoid comes from the odontoid; (B) AAD cases with the nonunion odontoid have the spinal compression from C2 vertebral body.

1. Dynamic lateral X-ray: if atlantoaxial reduction can be achieved on the flexion or extension X-rays, the patients were classified as "Type I: Instability" (*see* Figs. 13.6A and B). If the patients could not achieve full reduction on the dynamic X-rays, they were then further evaluated according to the following steps.
2. Reconstructive CT: the presence of a bony fusion between C1 and C2 on a reconstructive CT scan was given a classification of type IV, i.e. a "Bony Dislocation" (BD, *see* Figs. 13.7A to D). Only cases without evidence of a C1-2 bony fusion would then undergo the following step.
3. Skeletal traction test under general anesthesia: the Gardner-Wells cranial traction was performed in the operating room under general anesthesia, using one sixth of the body weight. Fluoroscopic guidance was used with a gradual incremental increase in traction weight. A 15°–20° head high position provided counter traction. Following full muscle paralysis after 10 minutes, reducibility was judged using the C-arm. Individuals with a complete reduction were classified as "Type II: Reducible Dislocation" (RD, *see* Figs. 13.8A to D). If this was not the case, they were classified as "Type III: Irreducible Dislocation" (ID, *see* Figs. 13.9A to D). After the test, the soft tissues and ligaments of the CVJ were loosened by the traction and the atlantoaxial joint was rendered more unstable. Therefore, our recommendation is that the following treatment procedures be performed immediately, and the traction should be carefully maintained and monitored during the procedure, from the supine to prone position. The surgical classification is summarized in Flowchart 13.1.

**Flowchart 13.1:** The surgical classification of atlantoaxial dislocation. Note the three tests (blue squares) determining the classification.

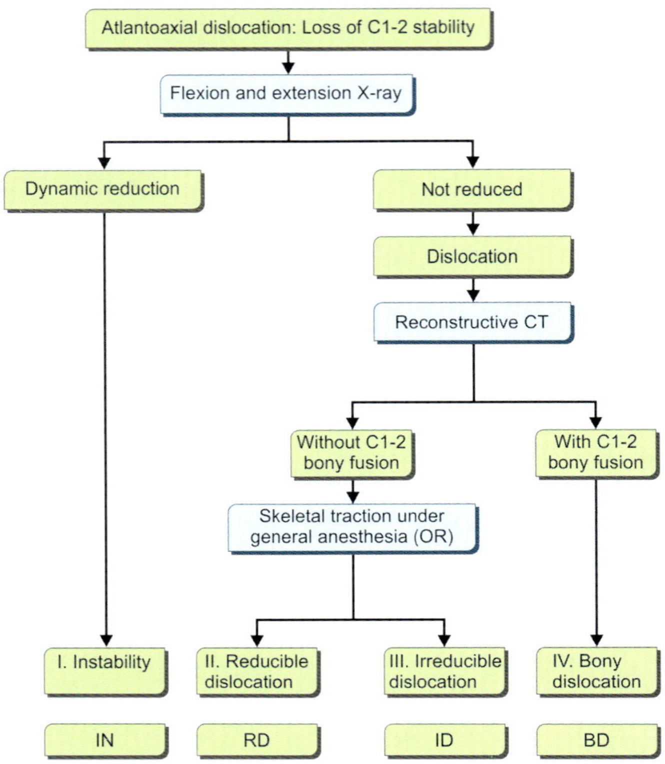


## SURGICAL TREATMENT: THE DECISION TREE AND TECHNIQUES

The goal of treatment for AAD includes reduction, decompression and reconstruction (fixation and fusion). Reduction is the fundamental step of the treatment goal. The principle of atlantoaxial fixation and fusion in AAD is using the shortest fixation and sacrificing the adjacent joint as little as possible. Flowchart 13.2 summarizes the decision tree in our series of 1,106 cases during a 14-year period.

### Posterior Reduction and Fixation

Type I and II AAD cases are relatively easily fixed in the reduced position by using a posterior approach. For those two categories of instability, four techniques of short segment fixation were introduced:

#### *Transarticular C1-C2 Fixation (Modified Magerl Technique, Fig. 13.11)*

Patients without occipitalization and swan-neck deformity underwent this surgical technique.[24] First, the patient was intubated in the supine position, then turned prone with a Mayfield head holder. To expose the posterior arch of the atlas and the lamina of C2, a midline incision was made. The lower edge of the conjunction of C2 lamina and lateral mass was the screw entry point. A 2.0 mm hand drill was inserted through the isthmus, exiting the articular mass of C2 located at the posterior one third of its superior articular surface while not entering the C1 lateral mass. The drill was switched to a 3.0 mm bit. If necessary, to achieve full reduction the C2 spinous process was pushed ventrally or dorsally. The drill was then driven into the C1 lateral mass while a second drill was inserted into the contralateral side. Two 3.5 mm full-threaded cortical titanium screws (length: 38–42 mm) were inserted across the C1-C2 joints. An additional cable was not utilized between the C1 arch and C2 lamina. From the posterior iliac crest, cancellous autografts were harvested. The lamina of C2 and the posterior arch of C1 were decorticated with a high-speed burr. The bone graft was morselized and then placed between C1 and C2.

#### *C1 Lateral Mass Screw and C2 Pedicle Screw Fixation (Goel[25] and Harms[26] Technique)*

This surgical technique was for cases without occipitalization even if a swan-neck deformity was present (Figs. 13.12A and B). Skeletal traction using 1/6 body weight lasted throughout the procedure. Using a midline incision, the posterior arch of the atlas and the lamina of C2 were exposed. The venous plexus and nerve roots of C2 were pulled caudally, thereby exposing the junction between the lateral mass and the inferior edge of the C1 arch. A starting point was opened with a burr hole while the lateral mass of C1 was visualized and palpated. The trajectory was determined with C-arm guidance. The lateral mass of C1 was prepared with a 2.5 mm drill. After tapping, a 3.5 mm screw (usually 30 mm in length) was inserted. Then, the vessels and nerve roots of C2 were retracted cephalad to expose and palpate the superior-medial surface of the C2 pedicle. The C2 pedicle screw (diameter, 3.5 mm; length, 26–28 mm) was inserted according to Abumi's technique.[27] Two reconstruction plates between C1 and C2 were placed. Atlantoaxial fixation was achieved as the locking caps were tightened down to the plate. The bone plating and postoperative treatment were the same as for the above-mentioned procedure.

Occasionally, the fixation between C1 and C2 is not available, such as in cases of C1 arch dysplasia or C1 screw placement failure, and a salvaged occipitocervical fixation can be used, as described below. However, the morselized bone graft should be placed between C1 and C2 (the shortest fusion).

**Flowchart 13.2:** Decision tree of atlantoaxial dislocation (AAD) cases (1,106 cases in Peking University Third Hospital). Note the conversion from irreducible to reducible AAD by a transoral release (blue arrow).

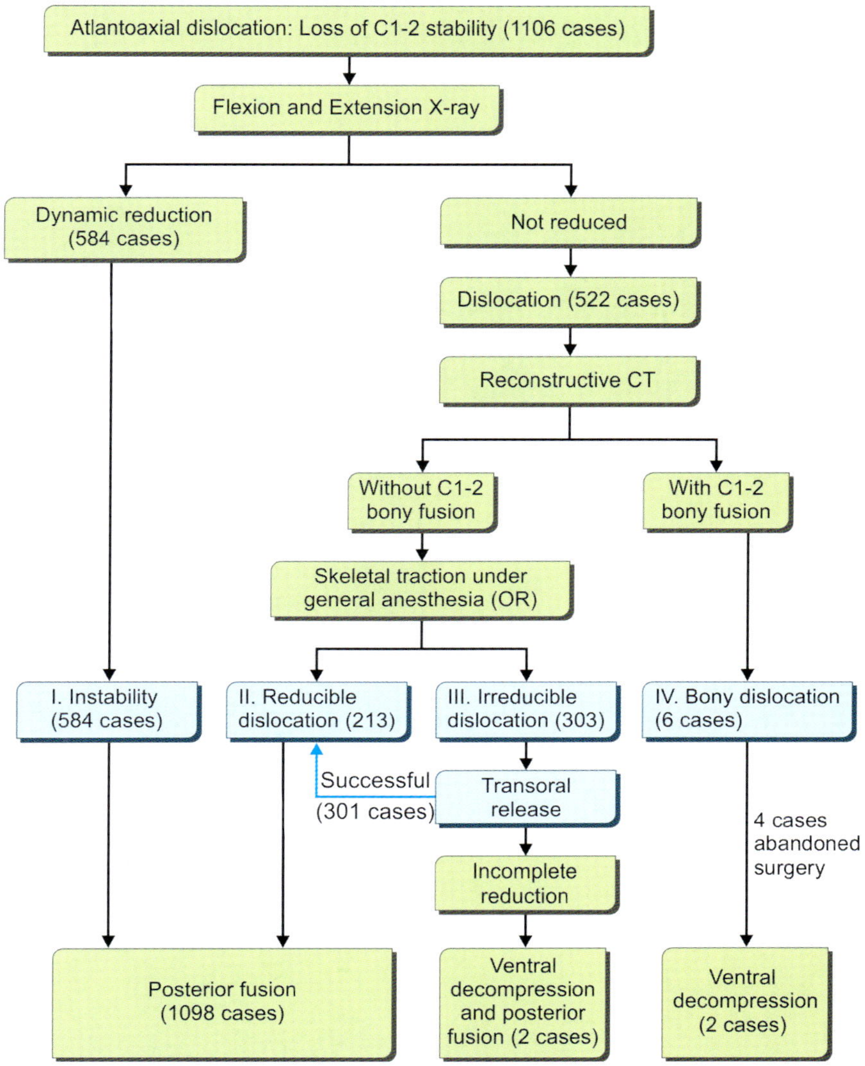


### *Occiput to C2 Fixation Using C2 Pedicle Screws (Abumi's Technique)*[27]

This technique was implemented for cases in which patients had occipitalization of the atlas or dysplasia of C1 posterior arch (Figs. 13.13A and B). C2 pedicle screws were placed as previously described. The occiput and C2 were connected by two reconstruction plates. Six 3.5 mm bicortical screws were placed into the occiput. With tightening the locking caps of the C2 screws, Oc-C2 fixation was achieved. The C2 lamina and occiput were decorticated with a burr, followed by the placement of morselized ilic grafts (Fig.13.13B). In the salvage surgery the grafts were placed between the C1 arch and C2 lamina.

### *C1-C2 or Occiput to C2 Fixation Using C2 Laminar Screw*

If patients had a high-riding VA or an osseous anomaly of the C2 pedicle, C2 laminar screws (LS) were used for C1–C2 or occipitocervical fixation using Wright's technique (Figs. 13.14A and B).[28] The high-speed drill was used to open an entry point at the C2 spinous process and lamina junction. A hand drill was carefully drilled into contralateral lamina, with the drill visually aligned along the angle of the exposed contralateral laminar surface. To avoid any breakthrough into the spinal canal, the trajectory was kept slightly less than the down slope of the lamina. A polyaxial screw (26–30 mm) was then carefully inserted along the same trajectory, which was subsequently connected

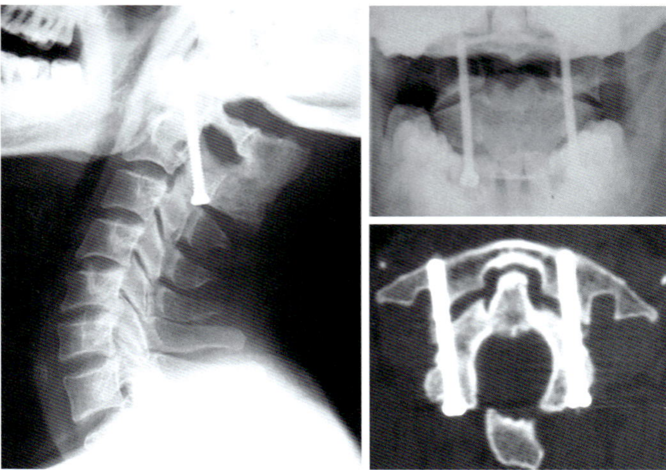

**Fig. 13.11:** Modified transarticular C1-C2 fixation technique. We abandon the cable of C1-C2 laminar.

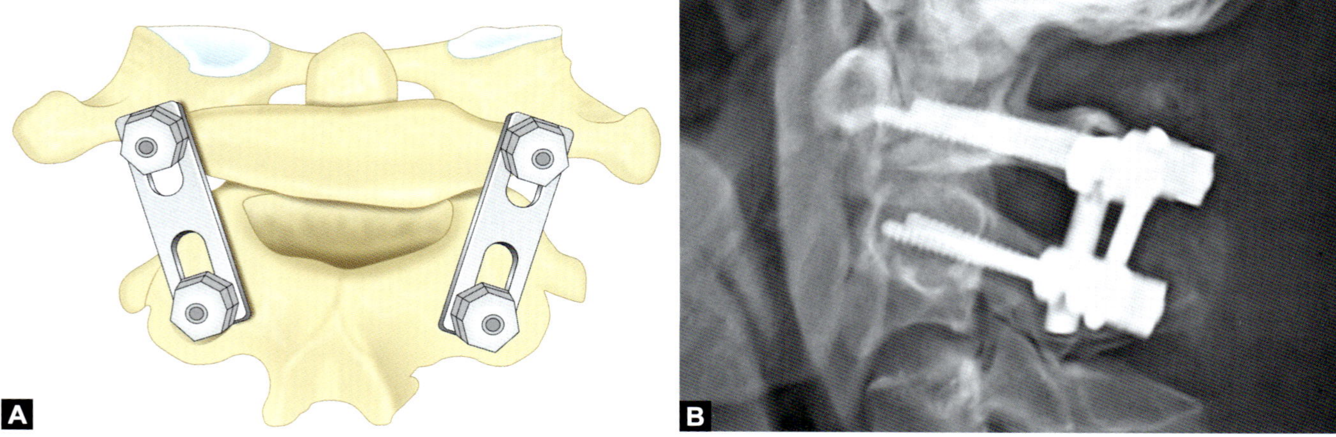


**Figs. 13.12A and B:** C1 lateral mass screw and C2 pedicle screw fixation. (A) Line drawing of the screws and plates. (B) Lateral radiograph of the technique.

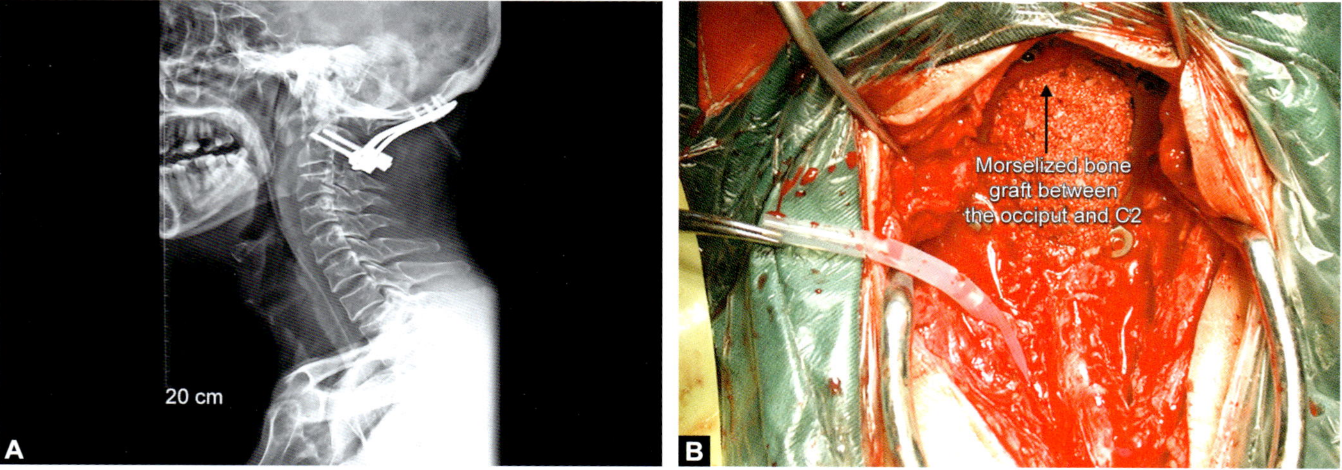


**Figs. 13.13A and B:** (A) Occiput to C2 fixation using C2 pedicle screws (Abumi's technique). (B) Intraoperative image (note the morselized bone graft).

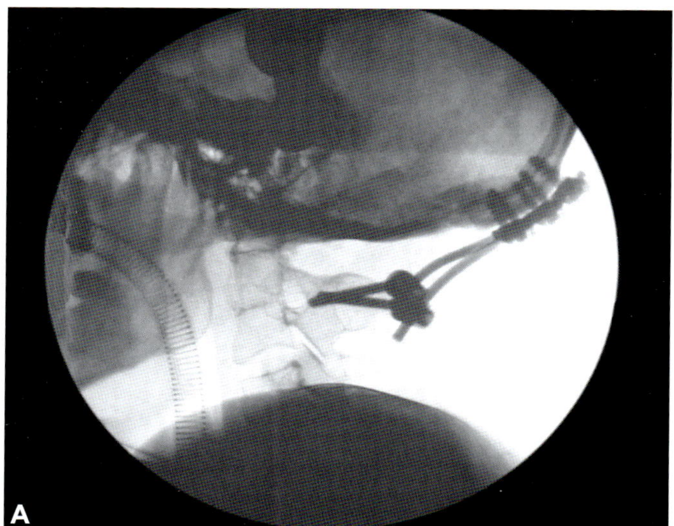


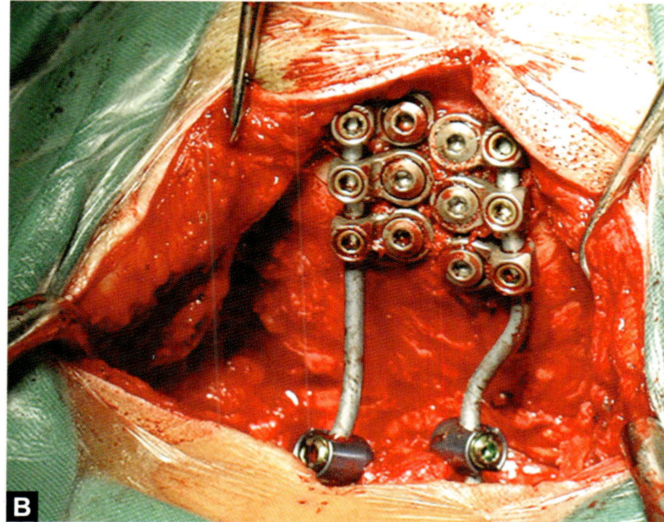


**Figs. 13.14A and B:** (A) Occiput to C2 fixation using bilateral C2 laminar screws. (B) An intraoperative image.

with the C1 or occipital screws using a rod. Due to the polyaxial screws and acute bending of titanium rods required to connect the laminar fixation points, the instrumentation was biomechanically inferior compared to that of pedicle screws.[29] We used a postoperative halo-vest for supplemental stability for the cases with bilateral C2 LS placement.

## Transoral Atlantoaxial Joint Release: A Conversion from Irreducible to Reducible AAD

The transoral atlantoaxial joint release provides a conversion from irreducible to reducible dislocation.[30] We have abandoned transoral odontoidectomies and propose neural decompression by odontoid reduction in the setting of irreducible AAD. Patients with Type III (irreducible dislocation) underwent the following procedure:

After intubation, while the patient remained in the supine position, a nasogastric feeding tube was placed. Throughout the procedure, skull traction was maintained. The head of the surgical bed was tilted 15–30°. The oropharynx was prepared using a povidone-iodine solution. With the assistance of a tongue blade, a transoral retractor was inserted. Two rubber catheters were then passed through the nostril and sutured to the uvula. To push the uvula and soft palate from the operative field, the catheter was pulled. A midline retropharyngeal incision was made from the superior aspect of C1 to the bottom of C2. The atlantoaxial vertebrae were exposed subperiosteally. The bilateral longus coli muscles, longus capitis muscles, and anterior longitudinal ligament were dissected just caudal to the anterior ring of C1 (Figs. 13.15A to D). In the setting of occipitalization, the caudal half of atlantal anterior ring was also removed. To cleanse the bilateral C1/2 lateral joints cavity, a Kerrison rongeur was used. The apical and alar ligaments were detached along the odontoid process. To obtain further reduction, the tip of the curette could be placed at the tip of the odontoid process and pulled inferiorly and anteriorly (Fig. 13.15D). The release procedure was deemed complete when the dens could be easily levered up to contact the C1 anterior arch by a curette. This means the anatomic reduction of the AAD has been achieved. Using C-arm, full reduction of C1 and C2 was confirmed. The operative site was irrigated with a povidone-iodine solution thoroughly. The wound at the posterior pharynx was closed with a single layer of interrupted sutures.

After the conversion from an irreducible to a reducible AAD, the previous posterior techniques were performed immediately.

## Transoral Odontoidectomy

If a patient had been classified as type IV (bony dislocation), the odontoidectomy was performed by a transoral approach, as described by Menezes et al.[31] In the setting of incomplete reduction after transoral release, patients also needed a transoral odontoidectomy followed by posterior fusion (Figs. 13.16A and B).

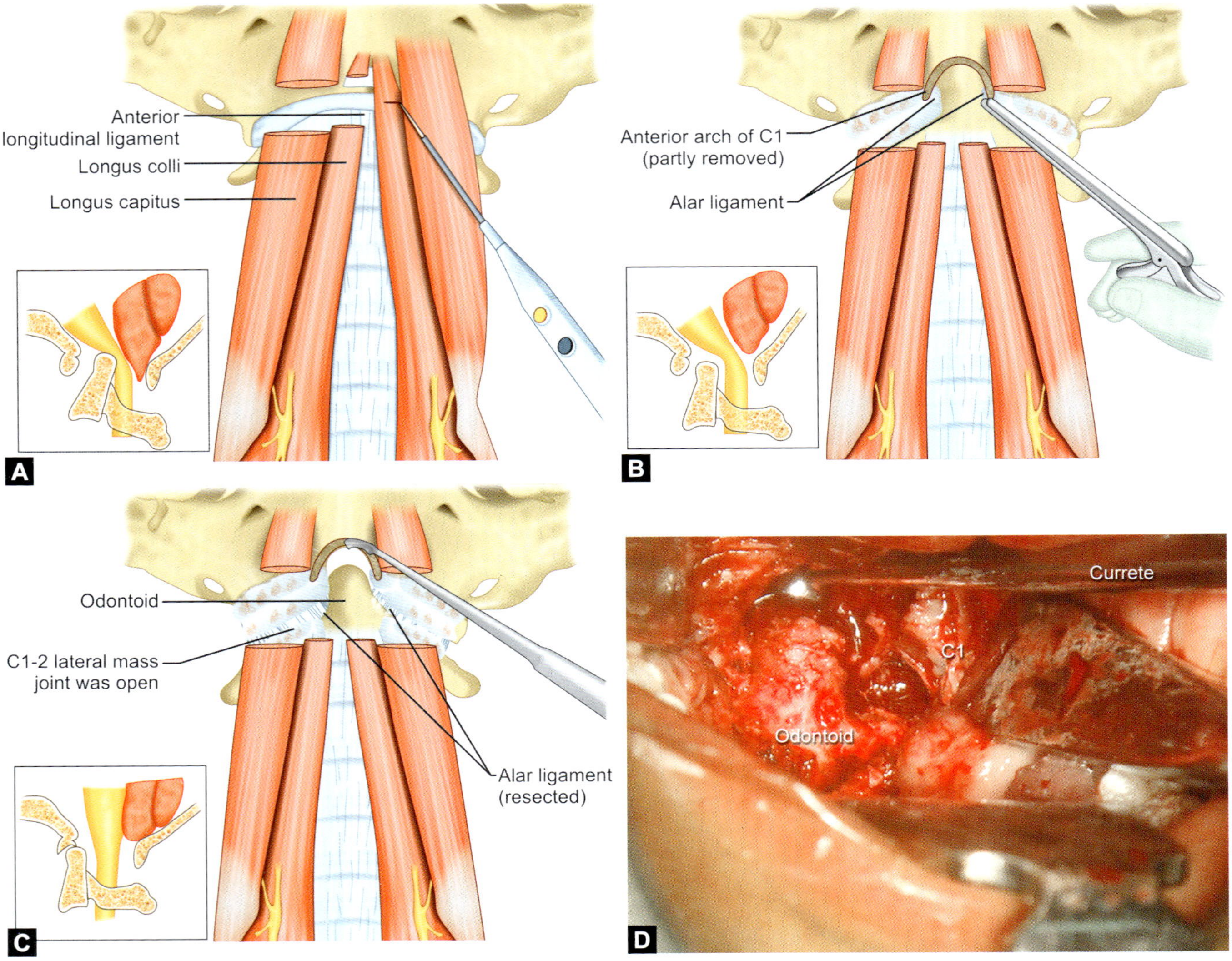

**Figs. 13.15A to D:** Patients with a type III (irreducible dislocation) underwent transoral atlantoaxial joint release. (A) The bilateral longus colli muscles, longus capitis muscles, and anterior longitudinal ligament were dissected. (B) After the bilateral C1/2 lateral joints cavity was cleansed, the apical and alar ligaments were detached along the odontoid process. (C) The tip of the curette could be placed at the tip of the odontoid process and pulled inferiorly and anteriorly to get further reduction. (D) An intraoperative image at the end of the procedure.

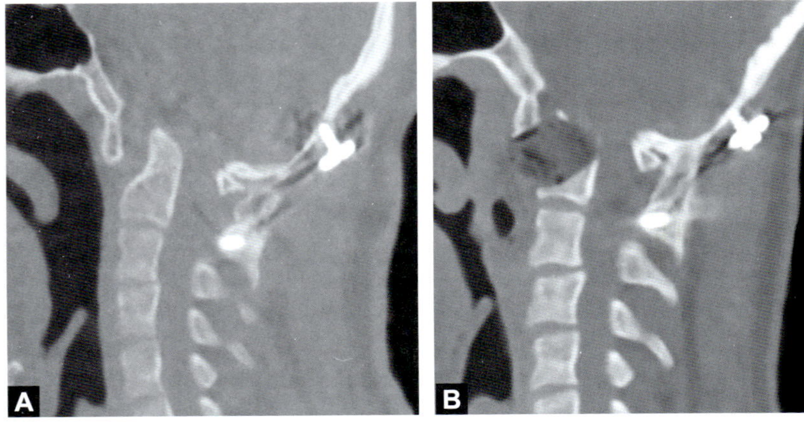


**Figs. 13.16A and B:** Because of an incomplete reduction after transoral release, transoral odontoidectomy, and posterior fusion were performed.

**Table 13.5:** Complications in 1,106 cases.

| *Complications* | | *Cases* |
|---|---|---|
| During the surgery | Vertebral artery (VA) injury during the transoral approach | 3 (2 died) |
| | VA injury during the posterior approach | 4 |
| | Cerebrospinal fluid leakage | 6 |
| Postoperative: Early stage | Incision infection | 14 |
| | Hematosepsis | 5 |
| | Neurological deterioration | 6 |
| | Hyposmia | 5 |
| | Swallow dysfunction | 12 |
| | Deep vein thrombosis | 5 |
| | Pulmonary embolism | 2 (1 died) |
| | Ischemic stroke | 2 |
| | Respiratory distress | 4 (3 died) |
| Postoperative: Late stage | Instrumentation failure or fusion failure | 12 |
| | Revision | 10 |
| | Delayed deep infection | 5 |
| | Undesired addition fusion (Oc-C1 or C2-3) | 4 |
| | Subaxial kyphosis | 2 |
| Total | | 100 |

### Postoperative Treatments

Patients were allowed out of bed after drain removal at 48 hours. No external fixation such as cast or orthosis was needed after surgery. This was saved for the cases with bilateral C2 LS using a halo-vest. For the patients who received the transoral surgical approach, oral feeding was not allowed until the 7th postoperative day.

All patients underwent postoperative X-ray and reconstructive CT and MRI of the cervical spine at 5–7 days and 4–6 months, respectively. X-rays were taken at 12 months and annually thereafter. The patients with myelopathy had MRI at follow-up at 1 and 2 years.

## SURGICAL COMPLICATIONS AND PITFALLS

Surgical complications vary from procedure to procedure. Broadly, complications can be divided into three types based on the period of time during which they develop: during surgery, in the early postoperative stage, and in the late postoperative stage. During surgery, VA and spinal cord injuries are the most destructive issues. Fortunately, these severe complications are rare. Of note, skeletal traction during the procedure can protect the instable atlantoaxial joint and reduce the rate of intraoperative spinal cord injuries. In our practice, traction with one-sixth of the body weight is safe and effective.

In our series of 1,106 cases, the overall complication rate was 9%. Readers can find the details in Table 13.5.

### Pitfalls

1. When implementing a transoral approach, VA injury is fatal. One patient experienced severe bleeding when we removed the posterolateral capsules of the left C1-C2 lateral mass joint. The estimated blood loss was 2000 mL for the procedure. We hypothesized that the reason for VA injury was "too much lateral" release. We controlled the bleeding with immediate hemostatic tamponade, and an intraoperative VA angiography confirmed a left VA injury. Subsequently, a left VA embolization using spring coils was then performed in the operating room. After this, the remaining portion of the procedure was performed and the bleeding in the transoral incision was completely resolved. However, after completion of the surgical procedures, the patient failed weaning of sedation and attempt at extubation. The patient was unarousable without independent breathing activity. Postoperative CT found a large infarction in the brain stem, and the patient expired 35 hours after the surgery. A second patient had severe bleeding during dissection of the right longus coli muscle, with an estimated blood loss of

700 mL. Hemostatic tamponade was performed and a VA angiography confirmed right VA injury. Then spring coils were placed in the operating room. This patient awoke and recovered uneventfully after surgery, with no symptoms of cerebral ischemia. We share the opinion with Peng et al.[32] that immediate angiography should be performed and endovascular techniques such as coil embolization be used for controlling the potentially fatal bleeding.

2. Four cases experienced postoperative respiratory failure in our series. All four patients had symptoms of preoperative respiratory difficulty, including dyspnea on exertion, less so at rest, and as a result they were unable to work. One case had preoperative dyspnea with high carbon dioxide levels (arterial blood sample revealed $PaCO_2 > 50$ mm Hg) and required intermittent respirator support. Postoperatively, all four patients required prolonged ventilation with a respirator. Three of the four patients died postoperatively from pneumonia and carbon dioxide retention at 3 days, 2 weeks, and 6 weeks, respectively. Poor preoperative pulmonary function was associated with fatality in three of the four cases. In conclusion, patients with preoperative respiratory difficulty require careful assessment prior to surgery.
3. There are various explanations for instrumentation failure or fusion failure. First, in the setting of severe irreducible AADs, large stress exists on the hardware. Full release of the atlantoaxial joint may decrease the instrumentation failure rate. Second, the instrumentation of polyaxial screws is biomechanically inferior compared to that of single-axial screws. Hence, a halo-vest should be considered in the setting of bilateral C2 LS placement. Third, the instrumentation of cervical lateral mass, laminar, or pars screws is biomechanically inferior compared to that of pedicle screws. C2 pedicles are always the first option for C2 fixation.
4. Hematosepsis is one of the serious complications of a transoral procedure. Two kinds of antibiotics for aerobic and anaerobic bacteria should be used perioperatively. One case in our series had delayed meningitis 1 month after surgery.

## PROGNOSIS AND THE SURGICAL OUTCOMES

Because of the rarity of cases, the natural history of AAD was not available in the literature. However, to our knowledge, most AAD cases can result in subsequent neurological deficit, and the vast majority of untreated cases will experience progressive neurological deterioration. In clinical practice, some cases of late-stage AAD have even been found to suffer from respiratory failure, which significantly increases mortality. In addition, AADs of late stage and irreducible deformity will face more challenging surgical procedures and more complications. Any severe and irreducible dislocation is from an unstable atlantoaxial joint. In this sense, surgery should be recommended for all patients with AAD, even for those who are asymptomatic.

In our series of 1,106 cases, 709 cases (64%) had preoperative cervical myelopathy. In the average 48 months' follow-up, neurological improvement was seen in 84.7% (601/709) of the patients with myelopathy. About 15% of the patients had an unsatisfied recovery or even deterioration. Several factors may contribute to a low recovery rate: elderly patients, later period of the myelopathy (or with myelopathy hand), and amyelotrophy on the MRI.

## KEY POINTS

- Loss of the normal position of the first and second vertebral articulation signifies the presence of an AAD.
- A total of 1,106 patients in our institution were retrospectively studied.
- A novel surgical classification and treatment strategy for AADs were described in this chapter.
- The goal of treatment for AAD includes reduction, decompression and reconstruction. Reduction represents the fundamental step of the treatment goal.
- The principle of atlantoaxial fixation and fusion in AAD is using the shortest fixation and sacrificing the adjacent joint as little as possible.
- Neurological improvement was seen in 84.7% of patients with myelopathy. The overall complication rate was 9%.
- Surgery should be recommended for all patients with AAD, even for those who are asymptomatic.

## REFERENCES


1. Wasserman BR, Moskovich R, Razi AE. Rheumatoid arthritis of the cervical spine—clinical considerations. Bull NYU Hosp Jt Dis. 2011;69(2):136-48.
2. Klimo P Jr, Rao G, Brockmeyer D. Congenital anomalies of the cervical spine. Neurosurg Clin North Am. 2007;18(3): 463-78.
3. Greenberg AD. Atlanto-axial dislocations. Brain. 1968; 91(4):655-84.

4. Gholve PA, Hosalkar HS, Ricchetti ET, et al. Occipitalization of the atlas in children. Morphologic classification, associations, and clinical relevance. J Bone Joint Surg Am. 2007;89(3):571-8.
5. Cremers MJ, Bol E, de Roos F, et al. Risk of sports activities in children with Down's syndrome and atlantoaxial instability. Lancet. 1993;342(8870):511-4.
6. Lourie H, Stewart WA. Spontaneous atlantoaxial dislocation. A complication of rheumatoid disease. N Engl J Med. 1961;265:677-81.
7. Kumar R, Kalra SK, Mahapatra AK. A clinical scoring system for neurological assessment of high cervical myelopathy: measurements in pediatric patients with congenital atlantoaxial dislocations. Neurosurgery. 2007;61(5):987-93; discussion 93-4.
8. Reddy KR, Rao GS, Devi BI, et al. Pulmonary function after surgery for congenital atlantoaxial dislocation: a comparison with surgery for compressive cervical myelopathy and craniotomy. J Neurosurg Anesthesiol. 2009;21(3):196-201.
9. Passias PG, Wang S, Kozanek M, et al. Relationship between the alignment of the occipitoaxial and subaxial cervical spine in patients with congenital atlantoaxial dislocations. J Spinal Disord Tech. 2011;26(1):15-21.
10. Fielding JW, Hawkins J, Ratzan SA. Management of atlantoaxial instability. Bull N Y Acad Med. 1976;52(7):752-60.
11. Fielding JW, Hawkins RJ, Ratzan SA. Spine fusion for atlantoaxial instability. J Bone Joint Surg Am. 1976;58(3):400-7.
12. Wang S, Wang C, Yan M, et al. Novel surgical classification and treatment strategy for atlantoaxial dislocations. Spine (Phila Pa 1976). 2013;38(21):E1348-56.
13. Wadia NH. Myelopathy complicating congenital atlanto-axial dislocation. (A study of 28 cases). Brain. 1967;90(2):449-72.
14. Wang S, Wang C, Passias PG, et al. Interobserver and intraobserver reliability of the cervicomedullary angle in a normal adult population. Eur Spine J. 2009; 18(9):1349-54.
15. Bundschuh C, Modic MT, Kearney F, et al. Rheumatoid arthritis of the cervical spine: surface-coil MR imaging. AJR Am J Roentgenol. 1988;151(1):181-7.
16. Passias PG, Wang S, Zhao D, et al. The reversibility of swan neck deformity in chronic atlantoaxial dislocations. Spine (Phila Pa 1976). 2013;38(7):E379-85.
17. Yin YH, Yu XG, Zhou DB, et al. Three-dimensional configuration and morphometric analysis of the lateral atlantoaxial articulation in congenital anomaly with occipitalization of the atlas. Spine (Phila Pa 1976). 2012;37(3):E170-3.
18. Subin B, Liu JF, Marshall GJ, et al. Transoral anterior decompression and fusion of chronic irreducible atlantoaxial dislocation with spinal cord compression. Spine (Phila Pa 1976). 1995;20(11):1233-40.
19. Matsunaga S, Onishi T, Sakou T. Significance of occipitoaxial angle in subaxial lesion after occipitocervical fusion. Spine (Phila Pa 1976). 2001;26(2):161-5.
20. Yoshimoto H, Ito M, Abumi K, et al. A retrospective radiographic analysis of subaxial sagittal alignment after posterior C1-C2 fusion. Spine (Phila Pa 1976). 2004; 29(2):175-81.
21. Yang SY, Boniello AJ, Poorman CE, et al. A review of the diagnosis and treatment of atlantoaxial dislocations. Global Spine J. 2014;4(3):197-210.
22. Salunke P, Behari S, Kirankumar MV, et al. Pediatric congenital atlantoaxial dislocation: differences between the irreducible and reducible varieties. J Neurosurg. 2006;104(2 Suppl):115-22.
23. Bhagwati SN, Deopujari CE, Parulekar GD. Trauma in congenital atlanto-axial dislocation. Childs Nerv Syst. 1998;14(12):719-21.
24. Wang C, Yan M, Zhou H, et al. Atlantoaxial transarticular screw fixation with morselized autograft and without additional internal fixation: technical description and report of 57 cases. Spine (Phila Pa 1976). 2007;32(6):643-6.
25. Goel A, Desai KI, Muzumdar DP. Atlantoaxial fixation using plate and screw method: a report of 160 treated patients. Neurosurgery. 2002;51(6):1351-6; discussion 6-7.
26. Harms J, Melcher RP. Posterior C1-C2 fusion with polyaxial screw and rod fixation. Spine (Phila Pa 1976). 2001;26 (22):2467-71.
27. Abumi K, Takada T, Shono Y, et al. Posterior occipitocervical reconstruction using cervical pedicle screws and plate-rod systems. Spine (Phila Pa 1976). 1999; 24(14):1425-34.
28. Wright NM. Posterior C2 fixation using bilateral, crossing C2 laminar screws: case series and technical note. J Spinal Disord Tech. 2004;17(2):158-62.
29. Finn MA, Fassett DR, McCall TD, et al. The cervical end of an occipitocervical fusion: a biomechanical evaluation of 3 constructs. Laboratory investigation. J Neurosurg Spine. 2008;9(3):296-300.
30. Wang C, Yan M, Zhou HT, et al. Open reduction of irreducible atlantoaxial dislocation by transoral anterior atlantoaxial release and posterior internal fixation. Spine (Phila Pa 1976). 2006;31(11):E306-13.
31. Menezes AH. Surgical approaches: postoperative care and complications "transoral-transpalatopharyngeal approach to the craniocervical junction". Childs Nerv Syst. 2008;24 (10):1187-93.
32. Peng CW, Chou BT, Bendo JA, et al. Vertebral artery injury in cervical spine surgery: anatomical considerations, management, and preventive measures. Spine J. 2009;9(1):70-6.

Chapter 14

# Basilar Invagination

*Andrew J Grossbach, Arnold H Menezes*

## INTRODUCTION

Basilar invagination occurs when the vertebral column ascends into the skull base. Basilar invagination results from a defect in primary development. As basilar invagination is the result of an underlying developmental anomaly, it is primarily a radiologic finding (Figs. 14.1A and B).[1] It can result from basiocciput (clivus) hypoplasia, incomplete ring of C1 with spreading of the lateral masses, achondroplasia, or atlanto-occipital assimilation.[1-3] The terms basilar impression, platybasia, and cranial settling are often confused with basilar invagination. Basilar impression refers to the secondary acquired form of invagination, as opposed to the primary developmental form (Figs. 14.2A and B). This can be secondary to rheumatoid arthritis (RA), osteomalacia, Paget's disease, tumor, infection, rickets, Ehlers-Danlos syndrome, Marfan syndrome, hyperparathyroidism, osteogenesis imperfecta, Hurler syndrome, or other diseases.[3] Platybasia refers to an abnormally obtuse basilar angle when measured from the plane of the clivus to the plane of the anterior skull base. Platybasia in and of itself is of no consequence; however, it can often be associated with basilar invagination. Cranial settling is a form of basilar impression in cases of RA (Figs. 14.3A and B).[4]

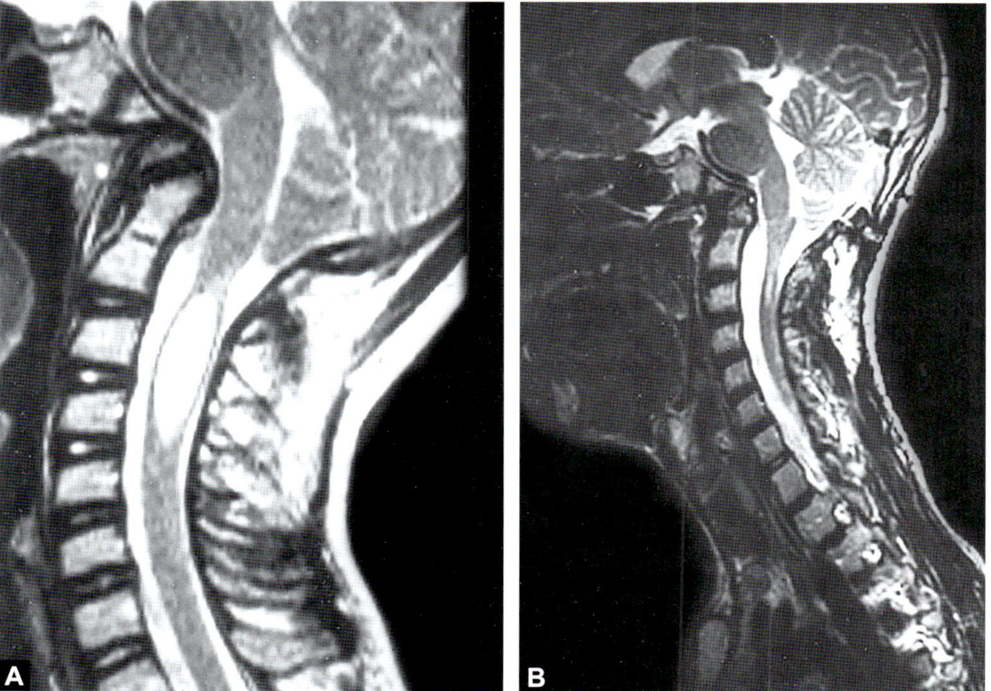


**Figs. 14.1A and B:** (A) Preoperative sagittal T2-weighted magnetic resonance imaging (MRI) showing basilar invagination with atlas assimilation and cervical syringomyelia. (B) Postoperative sagittal T2 MRI after ventral medullary decompression and posterior occipitocervical fusion. Note the resolution of the syrinx.

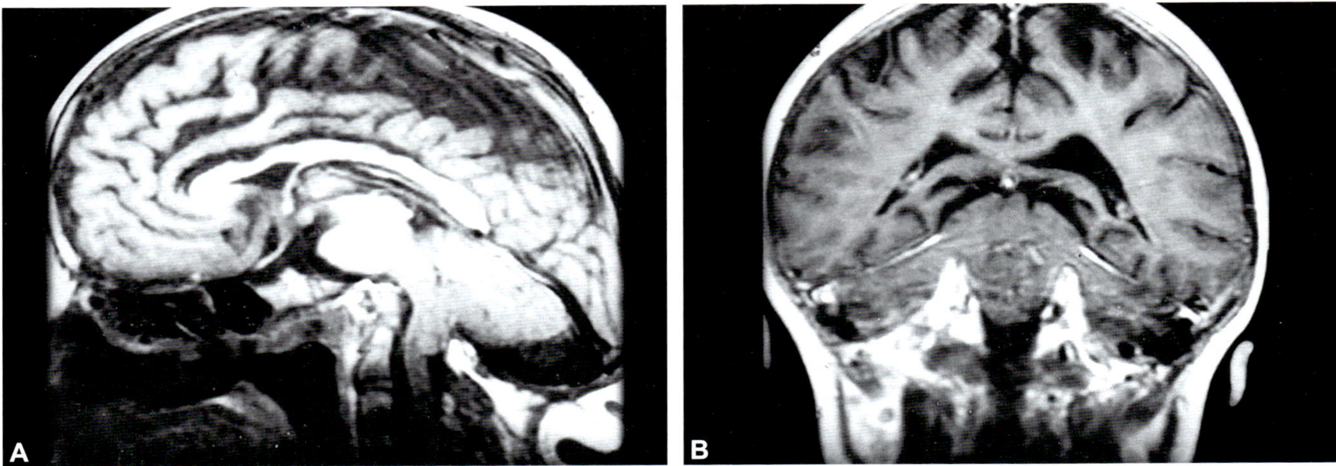


**Figs. 14.2A and B:** Sagittal (A) and coronal (B) T1-weighted magnetic resonance imaging scans showing basilar impression in the setting of osteogenesis imperfecta. The entire skull base has ascended.

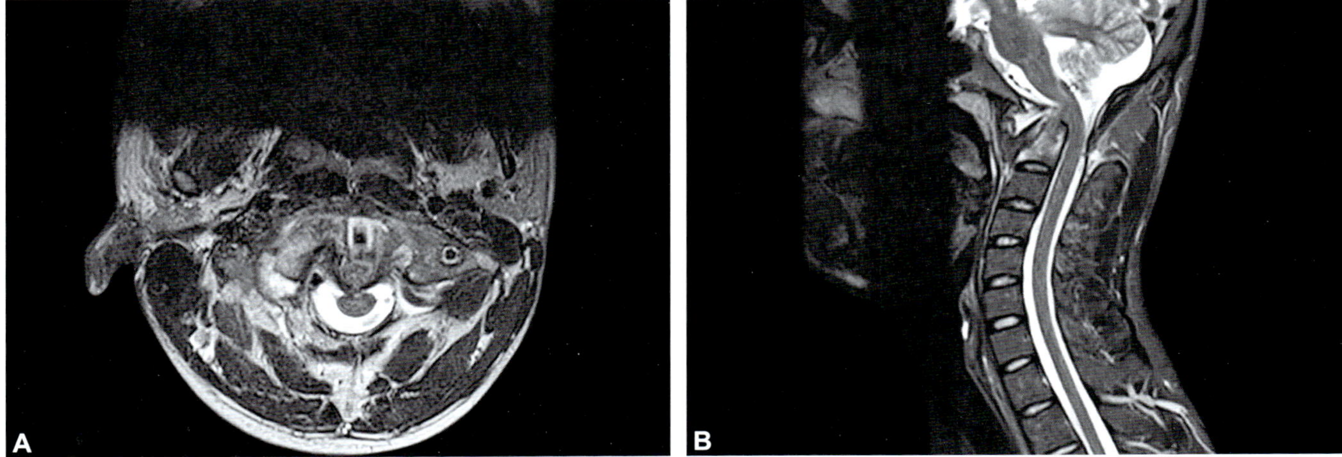


**Figs. 14.3A and B:** Axial (A) and sagittal (B) T2-weighted magnetic resonance imaging reveals cranial settling with destruction of the odontoid in advanced rheumatoid arthritis. The ventral cervicomedullary junction is markedly compressed.

There are two types of basilar invagination: an anterior or ventral form and a paramesial form. In the anterior form, there is a shortening of the basiocciput. The clivus may be small and horizontally oriented. This is often associated with platybasia. The posterior fossa contents become crowded, often leading to hindbrain herniation syndrome. In the paramesial form, there is hypoplasia of the occipital condyles so the clivus becomes dorsally displaced into the posterior fossa. However, despite the differences in these two forms, there is often a combination of features present, and a distinction between them is not clinically relevant.

## ASSOCIATED CONDITIONS

Basilar invagination is often associated with other craniovertebral abnormalities. This can include assimilation of the atlas, remnants of the occipital vertebrae, blocked vertebrae, short neck, or other vertebral anomalies.[5,6] Basilar invagination is also associated with Chiari I malformation (CM1) and syringohydromyelia in up to 35% of patients. Syringobulbia and hydrocephalus are less common findings.[1] These conditions occur more often in the anterior or ventral form of basilar invagination. Treatment of the underlying condition can often lead to resolution of the syringohydromyelia (*see* Fig. 14.1B).

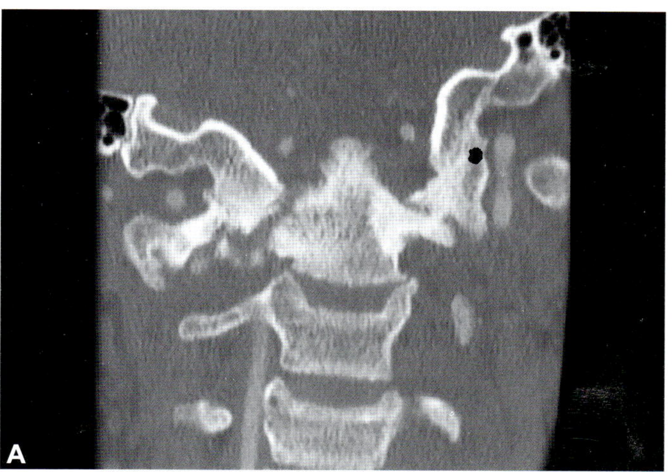

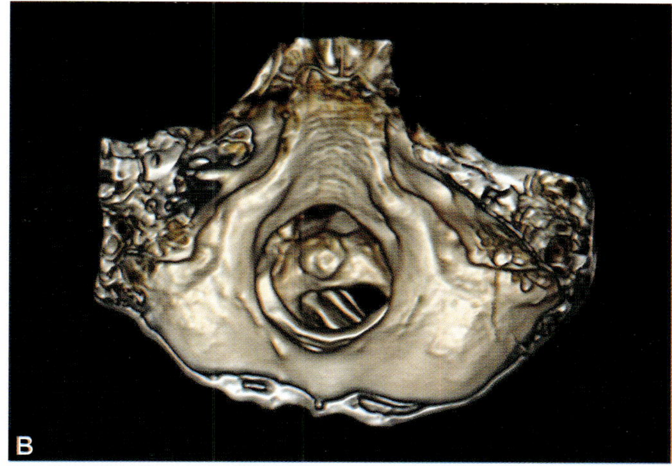

**Figs. 14.4A and B:** (A) Coronal computed tomography (CT) scan showing destruction of lateral masses of C1 secondary to advanced rheumatoid arthritis. (B) Three-dimensional CT reconstruction looking out the foramen magnum in the same patient. Note that the position of the odontoid has migrated posteriorly, greatly reducing the diameter of the canal.

The most common cause of basilar impression is RA. The cervical spine is the most0 commonly affected spinal site in RA patients due to the large number of synovial joints. Complications in the cervical spine from RA include cranial settling, atlantoaxial dislocation, subaxial subluxation, and rheumatoid granulation tissue. Vertical penetration of the dens into the cranial base is secondary to loss of bone in the lateral masses of the atlas (Figs. 14.4A and B). The destructive changes to the craniovertebral junction may be so severe that the occipital condyles come to rest upon the lateral masses of the axis, completely displacing the anterior and posterior arches of the atlas.[7]

## PRESENTATION

Symptoms of basilar impression may be hard to delineate. Although basilar invagination is congenital, often patients do not become symptomatic until early adulthood.[1] Presentation can be fairly acute. Minor trauma may precipitate symptoms. In their series, Goel et al. report that 48% of patients with basilar invagination had an associated trauma that led to presentation when they had no associated CM1. Oddly, no patients with both basilar invagination and a CM1 had a trauma preceding their presentation.[8] Patients with both basilar invagination and a CM1 tended to have a more gradual onset of progressive symptoms.

Symptoms of basilar invagination, which can generally be attributable to compression of the ventral brain stem, often include motor and sensory disturbances. De Barros et al. report that 85% showed symptoms of paresthesias and weakness in the upper extremities. As discussed, basilar impression may often be associated with CM1, and the symptoms often overlap. Both basilar impression and hindbrain herniation can cause symptoms secondary to the dysfunction of the lower cranial nerves. This most often includes the trigeminal (V), glossopharyngeal (IX), vagus (X), and hypoglossal (XII) nerves. Other common findings include headache and neck pain.[6] In a large series by Menezes, 90% of patients with cranial settling presented with occipital or suboccipital pain.[9] Additionally, patients may present with diplopia, nystagmus, or signs of vascular compromise such as vertigo, blackouts, syncope, or rarely, sudden death. Long track signs are often present, including hyper-reflexia and Babinski response. Neurogenic bladder may also be present in severe cases.

Goel et al. reported on 190 surgically treated patients with basilar invagination, 88 of whom had no associated CM1. Of those without an associated CM1, patients presented with weakness (100%), neck pain (59%), posterior column dysfunction (39%), bowel and bladder disturbance (28%), and paresthesias (25%). Physical exam findings included torticollis (69%), restricted neck movements (59%), low hairline (48%), webbed neck (47%), and short neck (41%).[1,8] In patients with an associated CM1, the most common signs and symptoms included weakness (94%), paresthesias (79%), posterior column and spinothalamic tract disturbance (56%), and ataxia (47%). Common physical exam findings included short neck (50%), webbed neck (38%), and low hairline (37%).[1,8]

## DIAGNOSIS

Despite the typical presenting symptoms and the array of associated conditions, there are no pathognomonic findings that lead to the diagnosis of basilar invagination. Suspicion should be high in cases of neurologic dysfunction, which should lead to radiographic investigation.

Basilar invagination can be difficult to assess with standard radiographic techniques. Several measurement schemes have been developed to help classify and diagnose basilar invagination. In 1939 Chamberlain described a line, now known as the Chamberlain line, that extended from the dorsal marginal hard palate to the posterior lip of the foramen magnum, or opisthion.[10] This line can be difficult to use, as the opisthion may be difficult to identify on plain lateral radiographs. Furthermore, the opisthion may be abnormally invaginated in cases of basilar impressions. The McGregor line is similar; however, this line extends from the hard palate to the most caudal point of the occipital curve of the skull.[11] This line may be easier to identify on plain radiographs. If the position of the tip of the odontoid process is >4.5 mm above this line, it is considered to be abnormal. A third commonly used reference line is the McRae line, which defines the opening of the foramen magnum.[12] McRae noted that if the tip of the odontoid process lies below the opening of the foramen magnum, the patient is likely to be asymptomatic.

There are several criticisms of these craniometric lines. First of all, the hard palate is not actually part of the skull base. It may vary in position regardless of abnormalities of the craniovertebral junction. Furthermore, the length of the odontoid itself may complicate these measurements. There are also reports of poor intraobserver reliability and reproducibility using radiologic criteria.[13]

More recently, the use of computed tomography (CT) scans and magnetic resonance imaging (MRI) has largely replaced the need to rely on plain radiographs for diagnosis of basilar invagination. These radiologic techniques allow the direct visualization of the pathology along with the ability to assess any neurologic compression. Furthermore, MRI can identify concurrent pathology, including the CM1, syringomyelia, and hydrocephalus. Using MRI, a retrospective review of 200 adults showed the odontoid peg to be an average of 1.2 mm (median 1.5 mm, SD 3 mm) below Chamberlain's line; 0.9 mm (median 1.1, SD 3 mm) below the McGregor line; and 4.6 mm (median 4.8, SD 2.6) below the McRae line.[14] Any penetration above the McRae line is considered abnormal, as is >3 mm above Chamberlain's line and >4.5 mm above the McGregor line, although exact criteria vary.

When obtaining CT and/or MRI studies, the importance of flexion-extension views should be kept in mind. Flexion-extension studies allow for the assessment of craniovertebral instability as well as neural compression not seen in neutral views. Furthermore, these studies may help determine if the pathology is reducible, which has a large impact on surgical planning.

Three-dimensional CT reconstructions may also be of benefit as they allow further preoperative assessment of the often complex bony anatomy that can accompany basilar invagination.[1]

## INDICATIONS

Pathology located at the craniovertebral junction poses a technical challenge to surgeons. Recent advances in techniques and surgical equipment have improved access to this region; however, there still exists a steep learning curve. Ventral pathology, such as in the case of basilar invagination, remains the most technically challenging area to access.

Basilar invagination can lead to progressive neurologic dysfunction and even death if left untreated. The indications for treatment of basilar invagination include intractable pain, progressive deformity, myelopathy, and brain stem dysfunction. Mild basilar invagination may be followed clinically and radiographically for signs of progression.[1] The goals of surgical treatment include decompression of the brain stem, cervical spinal cord, and cranial nerves, ensuring adequate vertebrobasilar circulation, as well as stabilization of the craniovertebral junction. Before a surgical strategy can be developed, it must be determined whether the pathology is reducible or irreducible.[15,16] Once the underlying condition is addressed, syringohydromyelia often improves (Figs. 14.5A and B).

To determine reducibility, patients should undergo dynamic imaging with flexion-extension MRI or CT scan. Furthermore, patients are placed in an MRI-compatible crown-halo for axial traction. Typically, traction is applied at about 7 lbs, which is gradually increased as needed over the course of 4–5 days to a maximum of around 12 lbs. A repeat MRI study is obtained in traction to access for appropriate reduction. If adequate reduction is achieved, traction in left in place and the patient is taken

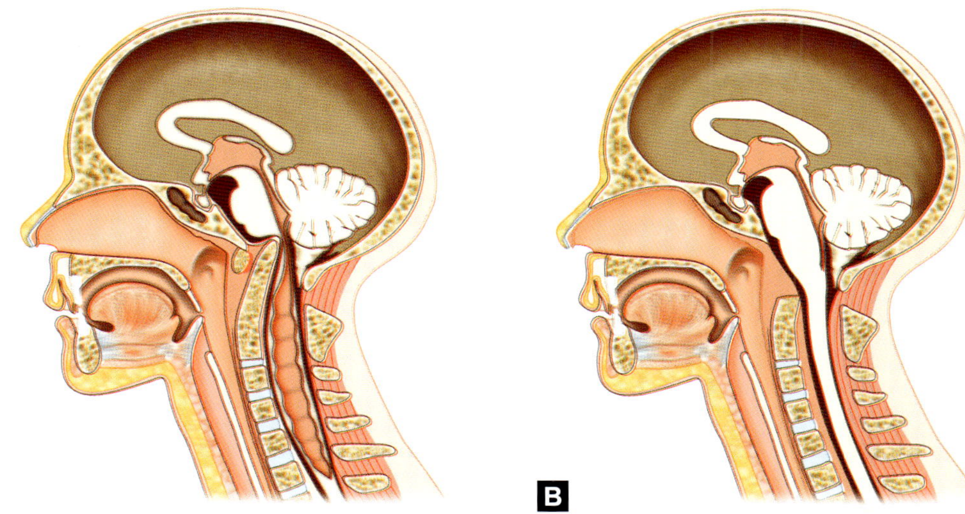


**Figs. 14.5A and B:** (A) Schematic drawing of basilar invagination with compression of the cervicomedullary junction causing syringomyelia. (B) After ventral decompression with removal of the odontoid. Note the resolution of the syringomyelia.

to the operating room (OR) for a posterior only procedure involving an occipitocervical fusion with or without posterior decompression.[17] Recently, an additional method to achieve reduction has been utilized including crown-halo traction in the setting of general anesthesia and neuromuscular blockade in the OR using intraoperative CT to access for adequate reduction.[15] Irreducible lesions necessitate an anterior approach to remove the offending structures causing compression on the brain stem and cervicomedullary junction combined with posterior fixation.[17] There are several approaches that can accomplish this, including the transoral, transpharyngeal approach that offers quick, direct access to the pathology.

## TRANSORAL, TRANSPHARYNGEAL APPROACH

The transoral, transpharyngeal approach is used to treat midline, ventral, irreducible pathology. This approach was first described by Kanavel in 1917.[18] However, it was not until many years later that the technique was redescribed by Scoville and Sherman in 1951 for platybasia repair[19] and by Fang and Ong in 1962 for addressing infectious etiology.[20] The procedure remained rife with complications, including meningitis and cerebrospinal fluid (CSF) leaks, until Menezes and Crockard, who showed the procedure could be done safely with minimal complications, popularized it.[21,22]

Prior to undertaking a transoral, transpharyngeal approach, several factors must be taken into consideration. First of all is nutritional status. Lower cranial nerve dysfunction secondary to basilar invagination may contribute to a poor nutritional status. This may in turn lead to poor wound healing and/or inhibit bony fusion. If nutritional status is in question, preoperative nutritional supplementation may be beneficial. Another factor to take into consideration when utilizing this approach is dental hygiene. Dental carries and gingivitis should be addressed prior to surgery, as these can act as a source of infection. Preoperative nasopharyngeal as well as oropharyngeal cultures are taken. No additional antibiotic therapy is needed if the results indicate normal flora. Nystatin rinses and Peridex chlorhexidine gargles should be performed three times a day, and Mupirocin nasal ointment is used in the nasal passages for 2 days prior to the operative procedure. Additionally, limited access to the area of pathology due to variations in patient anatomy may be a relative contraindication. For example, patients who cannot open their mouths >25 mm between their upper and lower teeth may require extended exposure with a midline glossotomy or transmandibular approach.

The transoral, transpharyngeal approach offers access from the lower third of the clivus rostrally to the C2/3 disk space caudally. Variations in anatomy may reduce the available exposure. Splitting of the soft palate may be necessary to improve rostral access in some situations. Likewise, a median glossotomy may be necessary to improve caudal access. If access down to C4 is indicated, a mandibulotomy can be used. The condylar canals of the

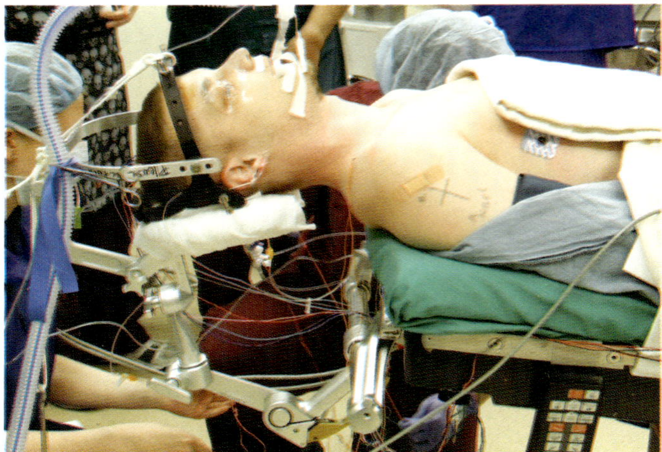

**Fig. 14.6:** Preoperative positioning of the patient. Note the placement of crown-halo traction and the use of intraoperative somatosensory-evoked potentials.

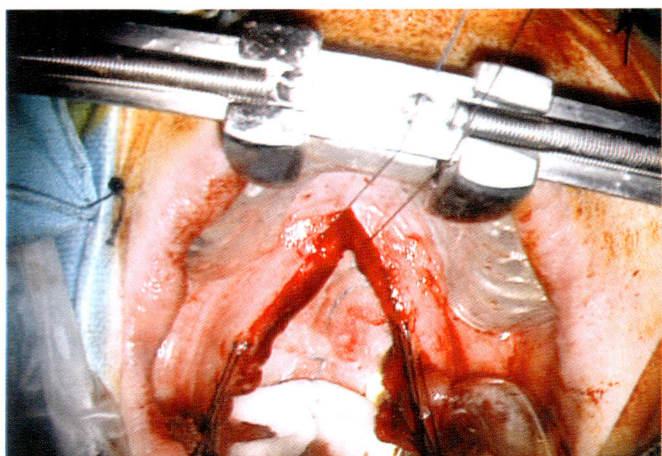

**Fig. 14.7:** A midline incision is made in the soft palate exposing the posterior oropharyngeal wall.

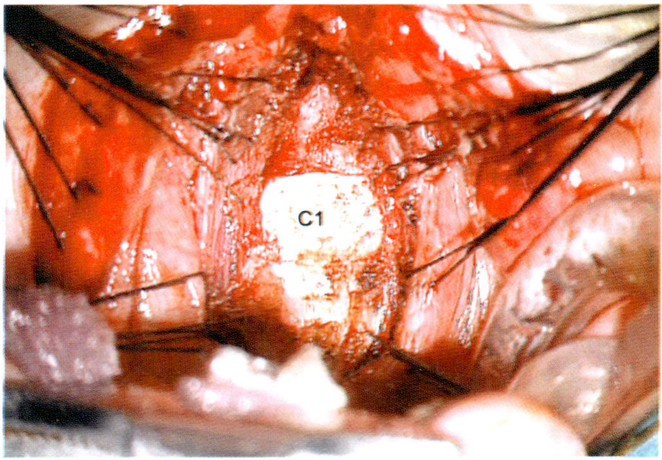


**Fig. 14.8:** Exposure of the anterior arch of C1.

hypoglossal nerve, the Eustachian tubes, and the vertebral arteries before they enter into the intradural space limit the lateral extent of exposure.

If possible, patients are intubated using awake, fiberoptic oral intubation to limit possible neurologic injury. Some patients may require preoperative tracheotomy if they have compromised pulmonary function, as can be the case with brain stem compression and lower cranial nerve dysfunction.[1] If not already present, a crown-halo is placed and the patient is placed in gentle traction (Fig. 14.6). In pediatric patients, the halo is secured using four pins (for patients aged 8–16 years), six pins (for patients aged 6-8 years), or eight pins (for patients <6 years). Pins are tightened to 6-8 lbs of pressure (for patients aged 8–16 years), 4-5 lbs of pressure (for patients aged 6-8 years), or 1-lb of pressure (for patients <6 years).[1] The endotracheal tube is secured to the skin laterally overlying the mandible. A throat pack is used to occlude the laryngopharynx, and oral preparation is carried out with 10% providence-iodine and hydrogen peroxide. For self-retaining retraction, the Dingman mouth retractor with tongue blade is used.

Once adequate retraction is obtained, the posterior pharyngeal wall is topically anesthetized and incised in the midline (Fig. 14.7). An operative microscope is used for visualization. The pharyngeal wall is then retracted laterally. The longus colli muscles and longus capitis are then detached from their medial origin on the ventral surface of the cervical vertebra. This exposes the anterior arch of C1 and the underlying dens process (Fig. 14.8). A high-speed electric drill with a diamond burr is used to remove the anterior arch of C1 (Fig. 14.9) and core out the dens process (Figs. 14.10 and 14.11). Once the dens have been adequately shelled out, the outer shell can be removed using a curette.

If necessary, the inferior portion of the clivus can be removed using a diamond burr and fine Kerrison rongeurs. The cruciate ligament should be visualized after removal of the dens, with the tectorial membrane behind it. Cervical traction is maintained during the procedure as removal of the dens increases the instability at the craniovertebral junction.

Closure of the wound often is the most challenging portion of the procedure. The longus colli and longus

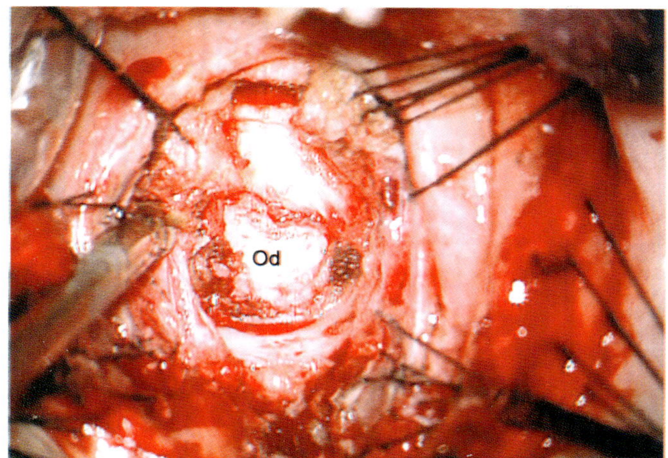


Fig. 14.9: Odontoid process after removal of anterior arch of C1.

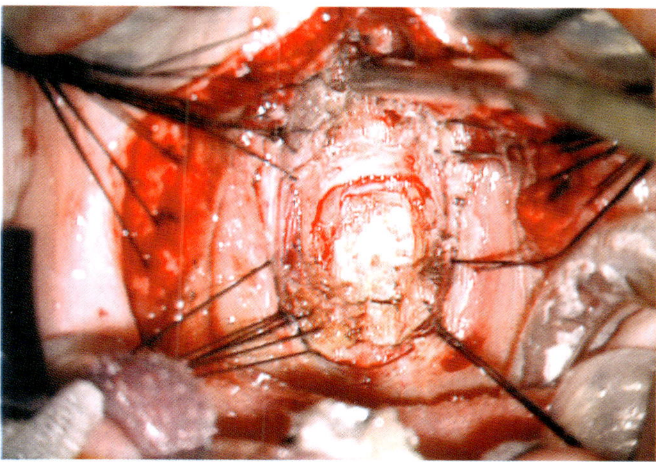

Fig. 14.10: View after odontoid process has been cored out using a high-speed drill.

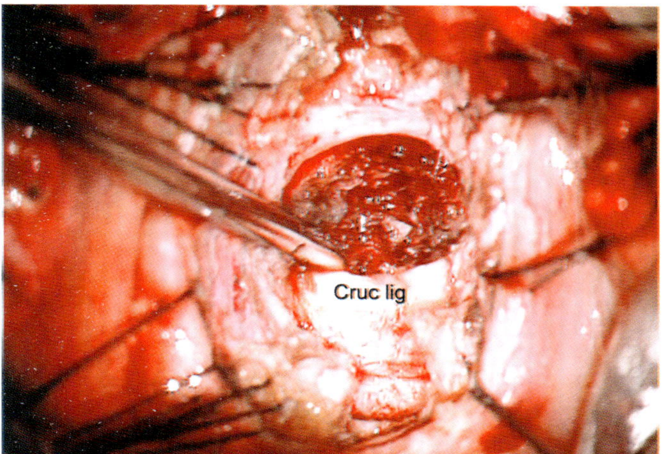


Fig. 14.11: Visualization of the cruciate ligament (Cruc lig) after removal of the superior portion of the odontoid process.

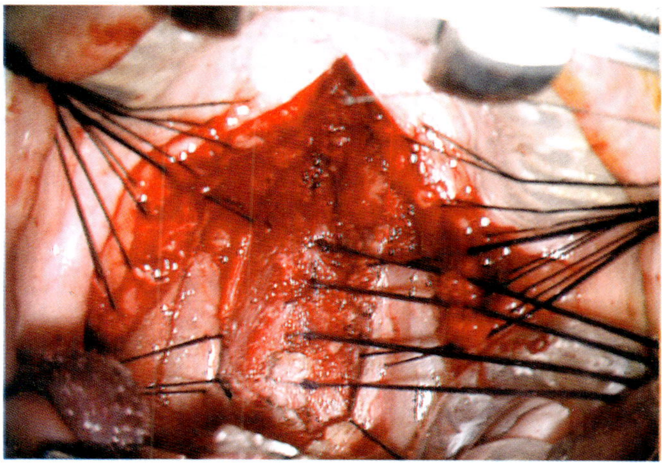

Fig. 14.12: Layered closure of the posterior pharyngeal musculature and pharyngeal mucosa.

capitis muscles are reapproximated (Fig. 14.12) and, subsequently, the posterior pharyngeal musculature and the posterior pharyngeal mucosa. The soft palate, if split, is closed in two layers. To aid in postoperative nutrition, a nasogastric tube is placed in the operative room under direct visualization to avoid damaging the soft palate or posterior pharynx.

Postoperative care in these patients is of utmost importance. Nasogastric tube feedings are maintained for 5 days postoperatively, at which time a clear liquid diet is started and slowly advanced. Care must be taken to avoid any hard foods that may injure the surgical site. Endotrachial intubation is maintained until swelling of the oral tissues, including the tongue, has receded.

Transoral, transpalatal decompression must be accompanied by a dorsal stabilizing procedure (Figs. 14.13A and B).

## COMPLICATIONS

Although there have been great strides made to reduce complications from the transoral, transpharyngeal approach, there are several possible complications of this procedure. These include velopharyngeal incompetence, hypernasal speech, dental injury, vertebrobasilar artery injury, CSF leak, airway obstruction, wound dehiscence, dysphagia, meningitis, pharyngeal cellulitis, mandibular dislocation, and injury to the temporomandibular

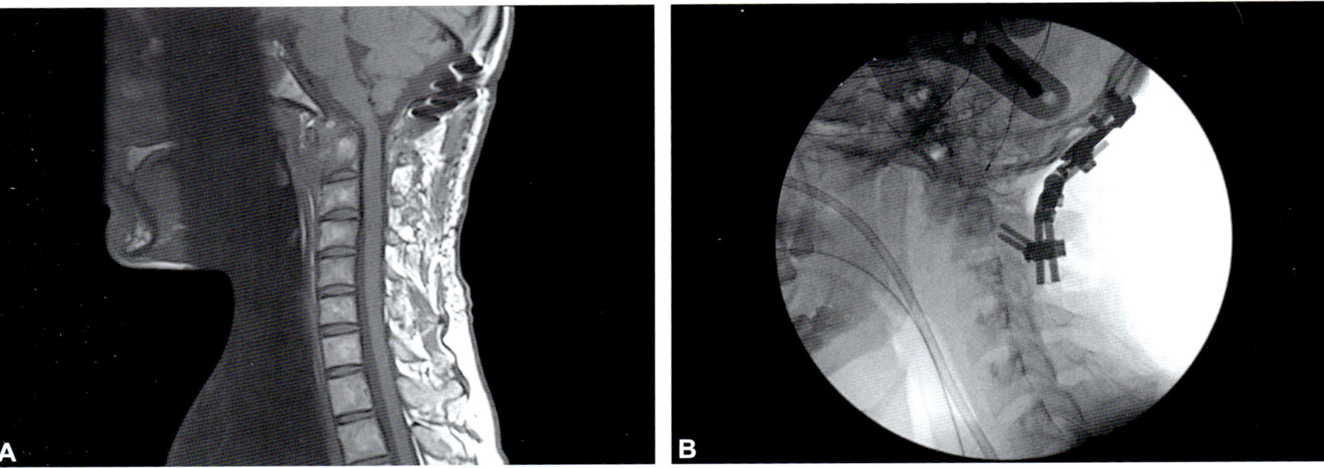


**Figs. 14.13A and B:** (A) Sagittal T1 magnetic resonance imaging showing improvement in cranial settling and cervicomedullary compression after transoral odontoidectomy and posterior instrumentation. (B) Lateral fluoroscopy showing occipitocervical instrumentation.

joint.[16,17,23-29] Preoperative vascular studies can help delineate the vertebrobasilar circulation, thus aiding in preoperative planning. If there is injury to the vertebrobasilar system, formal angiography should be employed. If a CSF leak is encountered, primary closure should be attempted. If closure is not possible, a dural graft and sealant is used. Lumbar subarachnoid drainage can also aid in sealing a CSF leak. Deep wound infections usually need operative drainage; however, superficial infections may be managed with percutaneous drainage and antibiotics. The jaw should always be checked postoperatively to ensure there is no mandibular dislocation.

## REFERENCES


1. Smith JS, Shaffrey CI, Abel MF, et al. Basilar invagination. Neurosurgery. 2010; 66(no. Supplement): A39-A47.
2. Menezes AH. Craniocervical developmental anatomy and its implications— Springer. Childs Nerv Syst. 2008;24 (10):1109-22.
3. Smoker WR. Craniovertebral junction: normal anatomy, craniometry, and congenital anomalies. RadioGraphics. 1994;14(2):255-77.
4. El-Khoury GY, Wener MH, Menezes AH, et al. Cranial settling in rheumatoid arthritis. Diagn Radiol. 1980;137:637-42.
5. Albright AL, Pollack IF, Adelson PD. Priniciples and Practice of Pediatric Neurosurgery, 2nd edition. New York: Thieme; 2011.
6. Caetano de Barros M, Farias W, Ataide L, et al. Basilar impression and Arnold-Chiari malformation. A study of 66 cases. J Neurol Neurosurg Psychiatry. 1968;31 (6):596-605.
7. Winn HR. Youmans Neurological Surgery, 6th edition. Philadelphia: Elsevier Health Sciences;, 2011.
8. Goel A, Bhatjiwale M, Desai K. Basilar invagination: a study based on 190 surgically treated patients. J Neurosurg. 1998; 88(6):962-8.
9. Menezes AH, VanGilder JC, Clark CR, et al. Odontoid upward migration in rheumatoid arthritis. J Neurosurg. 1985;63(4):500-9.
10. Chamberlain WE. Basilar impression (platybasia): a bizarre developmental anomaly of the occipital bone and upper cervical spine with striking and misleading neurologic manifestations. Yale J Biol Med. 1939;11(5):487.
11. McGregor M. The significance of certain measurements of the skull in the diagnosis of basilar impression. Br J Radiol. 1948;21(244):171-81.
12. McRae DL. Bony abnormalities in the region of the foramen magnum: correlation of the anatomic and neurologic findings. Acta Radiol Old Ser. 1953;40(2-3):335-54.
13. Riew KD, Hilibrand AS, Palumbo MA, et al. Diagnosing basilar invagination in the rheumatoid patient the reliability of radiographic criteria. J Bone Jt Surg. 2001;83(2):194-200.
14. Cronin CG, Lohan DG, Ni Mhuircheartigh J, et al. MRI evaluation and measurement of the normal odontoid peg position. Clin Radiol. 2007;62(9):897-903.
15. Dahdaleh NS, Dlouhy BJ, Menezes AH. Application of neuromuscular blockade and intraoperative 3D imaging in the reduction of basilar invagination. J Neurosurg Pediatr. 2012;9(2):119-24.
16. Menezes AH. Surgical approaches: postoperative care and complications transoral-transpalatopharyngeal approach to the craniocervical junction. Childs Nerv Syst. 2008;24(10): 1187-93.
17. Menezes AH, VanGilder JC. Transoral-transpharyngeal approach to the anterior craniocervical junction. J Neurosurg. 1988;69(6):895-903.
18. Kanavel AB. Bullet located between the atlas and the base of the skull: technique of removal through the mouth. Surg Clin Chic. 1917; 1:361-6.

19. Scoville WB, Sherman IJ. Platybasia: report of ten cases with comments on familial tendency, a special diagnostic sign, and the end results of operation. Ann Surg. 1951;133(4): 496-502.
20. Fang HSY, Ong G. Direct anterior approach to the upper cervical spine. J Bone Joint Surg Am. 1962;44(8):1588-604.
21. Menezes AH, Traynelis VC, Gantz BJ. Surgical approaches to the craniovertebral junction. Clin Neurosurg. 1994;41: 187-203.
22. Crockard HA. The transoral approach to the base of the brain and upper cervical cord. Ann R Coll Surg Engl. 1985;67(5):321.
23. Di Lorenzo N, Fortuna A, Guidetti B. Craniovertebral junction malformations. J Neurosurg. 1982;57(5):603-8.
24. Kingdom TT, Nockels RP, Kaplan MJ. Transoral-transpharyngeal approach to the craniocervical junction. Otolaryngol Head Neck Surg. 1995;113(4):393-400.
25. Shaha AR, Johnson R, Miller J, et al. Transoral-transpharyngeal approach to the upper cervical vertebrae. Am J Surg. 1993;166(4):336-40.
26. Yang S, Gao Y. Clinical results of the transoral operation for lesions of the craniovertebral junction and its abnormalities. Surg Neurol. 1999;51(1):16-20.
27. Cantarella G, Mazzola RF, Benincasa A. A possible sequela of transoral approach to the upper cervical spine. Velopharyngeal incompetence. J Neurosurg Sci. 1998;42(1):51-5.
28. Hadley MN, Spetzler RF, Sonntag VKH. The transoral approach to the superior cervical spine. J Neurosurg. 1989; 71(1):16-23.
29. Spetzler PRF, Hadley MN, Sonntag VKH. The transoral approach to the anterior superior cervical spine. A review of 29 cases. In: Isamat PDF, Jefferson DA, Loew PDF, et al. (Eds). Proceedings of the 8th European Congress of Neurosurgery, Barcelona, September 6–11, 1987. Vienna: Springer; 1988. pp. 69-74.

Chapter 15

# Congenital Anomalies of the Cervical Spine

*Peter G Passias, Cyrus M Jalai, Nancy Worley*

## INTRODUCTION

Congenital abnormalities of the cervical spine can occur as separate, isolated incidences, or they may present as a syndrome of two or more anomalies.[1] Symptoms typically present at birth and vary from nonexistent to neurologic symptoms and pain.[1] It is of the utmost importance that patients see a doctor for a thorough diagnosis at first recognition, as other associated anomalies are often left unnoticed until a later date.[1] Being able to treat such abnormalities early is helpful. Congenital abnormalities of the cervical spine include Klippel-Feil syndrome (KFS), occipitalization of the atlas, atlantal anomalies, achondroplasia, basilar invagination, iniencephaly, posterior C2 arch anomalies, odontoid anomalies, and others.[1]

## KLIPPEL-FEIL SYNDROME

### Embryology

Two weeks after conception, gastrulation occurs, producing mesenchymal cells.[2] The bilaminar disk becomes a trilaminar disk, and development of the primitive streak, germ layers, and notochord occurs.[3] During segmentation, the paraxial mesoderm divides into somites, which later subdivide into the sclerotome, myotome, and dermatome.[2] During resegmentation of the sclerotome, the somites join to form the vertebral body.[2] Defects in genes responsible for segmentation and resegmentation in the cervical area can prevent somites or their mesenchyme from properly dividing and forming the vertebral body.[2,3] Failure to divide can be accompanied by growth plate loss and can lead to the development of KFS.[3]

### Clinical Presentation

Klippel-Feil syndrome is characterized by congenital synostosis, or fusion, of two or more cervical vertebrae.[2] Klippel-Feil syndrome arises from a defect in cervical spinal segmentation.[2,3] It occurs in 1 out of every 40,000–42,000 births.[2,4] Slightly more females than males have KFS, with a predominance in females of 3:2.[2] The stereotypical triad of signs associated with KFS is a lowered posterior hairline with a shortened neck and limited neck mobility.[2] However, only approximately half of all patients with KFS present with all three of these signs.[2] A wide range of symptoms and anomalies has been associated with KFS, including hearing impairment, heart problems, synkinesia, renal problems (such as unilateral renal agenesis, horseshoe kidney, ectopic kidney, and renal malrotation), congenital scoliosis, Sprengel's deformity, basilar impression, occipitocervical synostosis, odontoid anomalies, cervical ribs, genitourinary issues, and rib anomalies.[2,5-7] However, neck pain, neurologic symptoms, and difficulty with neck movement are the most common reasons that lead patients with KFS to see a doctor.[2]

### Assessment and Diagnosis

The fusion of cervical vertebrae can be identified on anteroposterior, lateral, and open-mouth odontoid cervical radiographs.[1] Cervical instability can be identified on flexion and extension radiographs.[1] In cases in which there may be potential issues involving compression of the brain stem or spinal cord, including instability and stenosis, magnetic resonance imaging should be performed.[1] Finally, computed tomography may be used to view pathological bony anatomy.[2]

In patients diagnosed with KFS, additional radiographs of the thoracic and lumbar spine are recommended in order to catch any potential associated anomalies.[1,4] Scoliosis, for example, was reported in 60–70% of patients with KFS.[4,8] Because embryologic development of the heart, kidneys, and inner ear occurs concurrently with embryologic development of the cervical spine, patients with KFS may also present with associated anomalies involving the aforementioned organ systems.[2] About

3.5–4.2% of patients with KFS have also reported incidences of cardiovascular problems.[4,9,10] Sprengel's has been reported as a wide range of frequency, from rare occurrences to 30% incidence.[4,11,12] Wildervanck syndrome has been reported in patients with KFS.[4,13,14] Thus, audiologic, cardiac, renal, and neurologic testing should be performed.[2,6]

Diagnosis of KFS in children can be appreciably more difficult than in adults, as certain abnormalities in adults are occasionally normal in children. For example, pseudosubluxation of cervical vertebrae can be normal in children while pathologic in adults.[2,15] Children with juvenile rheumatoid arthritis can have fusions that appear to be KFS, but are not.[2,4] Additionally, as children grow, their cervical spine may appear to have no synostosis, but instead narrowed space between vertebral bodies that will eventually fuse.[2]

## Classifications of KFS

The first classifications of KFS into three different types were based purely on anatomical features of the diagnosis, including the extent of fusion and its location.[2] Type I was characterized by many cervical vertebrae fusions[2-4] and occasionally upper thoracic vertebral fusions as well.[3,4] Type II described cervical fusions occurring only at one or two interspaces.[2,3] Type III consisted of cervical spine fusions in addition to lower lumbar spine fusions.[2,3] More recent studies have characterized those classifications further, having found correlations between specific types of KFS and genetic inheritance patterns as well as other anomalies. Type I has been reported to be most frequently autosomal recessive and associated with syndromic abnormalities and a scoliotic curve.[2] Type II has been shown to be most commonly autosomal dominant and to have associations with Sprengel's and cervical ribs. Type III is usually autosomal recessive and associated with a scoliotic curve.[2] Classification has been further enhanced based upon cervical spine kinematics.[2,16] Assessment of lateral flexion-extension radiographs led Pizzutillo et al. to conclude that KFS associated with upper cervical segment hypermobility puts patients at risk for neurological problems, while lower cervical segment hypermobility leads to greater risk for degenerative problems.[2,16] Pizzutillo et al. thus provide a new classification system that takes radiographic evaluation into account: Class I characterizes no impairment in cervical range of motion, Class II characterizes upper cervical hypermobility, Class III is lower cervical hypermobility, and Class IV comprises a combination of both Class II and III.[16]

## Conservative Treatment

In addition to presenting with a wide range of signs and symptoms, patients with KFS experience an array of severities of those symptoms. Fusions that are stable tend to be asymptomatic and are usually discovered on radiographs. Theiss et al. and Rouvreau et al. both reported a very small incidence of patients with KFS with stable fusions who presented with symptoms at 10- to 12.5-year follow-up.[2,17,18] If patients with stable fusions begin to experience symptoms, conservative treatment is indicated and may include limiting certain activities, use of a brace, and traction.[2,5,6]

## Operative Treatment

Patients with symptomatic unstable fusions most often experience radiculopathy or myelopathy.[2,19] Symptomatic instability can arise from fusion of C2-C3 and occipitocervical synostosis. In cases of instability and/or presentation of neurological symptoms, operative treatment is recommended, the goal of which is to correct the instability. Occipitocervical, atlantoaxial, and subaxial arthrodesis are the surgeries typically performed.[2] When performing an occipitocervical arthrodesis, which is usually achieved through a posterior approach, surgeons have several options, including the use of autogenous graft, optional use of an occipital periosteal flap, and internal fixation can be executed with wires, rings, or plates and screws.[2] In the case of atlantoaxial arthrodesis, various factors determine the technique. If posterior components are intact, wires are usually used for fusion.[2] If the C1 arch is not intact or is compromised, or if there is limited space for wires, screws are used for fixation.[2] Afterward, immobilization is maintained with the use of a halo ring and vest.[2]

## REFERENCES

1. Klimo P Jr, Rao G, Brockmeyer D. Congenital anomalies of the cervical spine. Neurosurg Clin North Am. 2007;18:463-78.
2. Tracy MR, Dormans JP, Kusumi K. Klippel-Feil syndrome: clinical features and current understanding of etiology. Clini Orthop Relat Res. 2004;(424):183-90.
3. Kaplan KM, Spivak JM, Bendo JA. Embryology of the spine and associated congenital abnormalities. Spine J. 2005;5:564-76.

4. Thomsen MN, Schneider U, Weber M, et al. Scoliosis and congenital anomalies associated with Klippel-Feil syndrome types I-III. Spine. 1997;22:396-401.
5. Copley LA, Dormans JP. Cervical spine disorders in infants and children. Am Acad Orthop Surg. 1998;6:204-14.
6. Herman MJ, Pizzutillo PD. Cervical spine disorders in children. Orthop Clin North Am. 1999;30:457-66, ix.
7. Manaligod JM, Bauman NM, Menezes AH, et al. Cervical vertebral anomalies in patients with anomalies of the head and neck. Annals Otol Rhinol Laryngol. 1999;108:925-33.
8. Hensinger RN, Lang JE, MacEwen GD. Klippel-Feil syndrome; a constellation of associated anomalies. J Bone Joint Surg Am. 1974;56:1246-53.
9. Brill CB, Peyster RG, Keller MS, et al. Isolation of the right subclavian artery with subclavian steal in a child with Klippel-Feil anomaly: an example of the subclavian artery supply disruption sequence. Am J Med Genet. 1987;26:933-40.
10. Morrison SG, Perry LW, Scott LP 3rd. Congenital brevicollis (Klippel-Feil syndrome) and cardiovascular anomalies. Am J Dis Child. 1968;115:614-20.
11. Bavinck JN, Weaver DD. Subclavian artery supply disruption sequence: hypothesis of a vascular etiology for Poland, Klippel-Feil, and Mobius anomalies. Am J Med Genet. 1986;23:903-18.
12. Greenspan A, Cohen J, Szabo RM. Klippel-Feil syndrome. An unusual association with Sprengel deformity, omovertebral bone, and other skeletal, hematologic, and respiratory disorders. A case report. Bull Hosp Jt Dis Orthop Inst. 1991; 51:54-62.
13. Daniilidis J, Demetriadis A, Triaridis C, et al. Otological findings in cervico-oculo-auditory dysplasia. J Laryngol Otol. 1980;94:533-44.
14. Corsello G, Carcione A, Castro L, et al. Cervico-oculo-acusticus (Wildervanck's) syndrome: a clinical variant of Klippel-Feil sequence? Klin Padiatr. 1990;202:176-9.
15. Dormans JP. Evaluation of children with suspected cervical spine injury. J Bone Joint Surg Am. 2002;84-A:124-32.
16. Pizzutillo PD, Woods M, Nicholson L, et al. Risk factors in Klippel-Feil syndrome. Spine. 1994;19:2110-6.
17. Theiss SM, Smith MD, Winter RB. The long-term follow-up of patients with Klippel-Feil syndrome and congenital scoliosis. Spine. 1997;22:1219-22.
18. Rouvreau P, Glorion C, Langlais J, et al. Assessment and neurologic involvement of patients with cervical spine congenital synostosis as in Klippel-Feil syndrome: study of 19 cases. J Pediatr Orthop B. 1998;7:179-85.
19. Xue X, Shen J, Zhang J, et al. Klippel-Feil syndrome in congenital scoliosis. Spine (Phila Pa 1976). 2014;39(23):E1353-8.

# Section 4

# Surgical Management

Chapter 16

# Surgical Management of Cervical Spondylotic Myelopathy: Anterior Techniques

*Michael Gerling, Nancy Worley*

## INTRODUCTION

Cervical spondylotic myelopathy (CSM) is a progressive degenerative disease. Generally, patients with mild CSM are managed with nonoperative treatment, while patients with moderate to severe CSM are treated surgically. Surgical treatments are categorized based on surgical approach as either an anterior or posterior approach. Anterior approaches include anterior cervical discectomy and fusion (ACDF), corpectomy, hybrid discectomy–corpectomy, and cervical disk arthroplasty (CDA). Posterior approaches include laminoplasty, laminectomy, and laminectomy and fusion.

A surgeon's decision between an anterior and posterior surgical approach in the context of CSM is based upon the extent and location of the pathology as well as cervical sagittal alignment, and thus the decision must be individualized for each patient.[1] Although there are no randomized controlled studies comparing anterior to posterior approaches for the treatment of CSM, data exist that demonstrate efficacy of anterior approaches that are performed in the right clinical context. Shamji et al. found an anterior approach to be associated with fewer complications and cost compared to a posterior approach.[1,2] Fehlings et al. found similar results.[3]

An anterior approach should be utilized over a posterior approach in cases of cervical kyphosis as a posterior approach will only increase tension and provides no outlet for decompression if kyphosis worsens.[4,5] A goal of surgery should be to correct sagittal alignment, which is more easily accomplished in a kyphotic spine through an anterior approach than a posterior approach as lordotic spacers may be inserted to aid in re-establishing cervical lordosis.[4,6] An anterior approach should be used to address ventral degenerative changes, including herniated disks and anteriorly localized osteophytes, as it provides the best access for decompression.[6] There is debate about whether or not ossification of the posterior longitudinal ligament that extends into four or more levels should be treated via a posterior surgical procedure or an anterior corpectomy.[6,7]

## ANTERIOR CERVICAL DISCECTOMY AND FUSION

### Indications

Indications for multilevel discectomies include compression due to bone spurs[6] or disk herniation without osteophytes,[8] and compression of one, two, or three disks.[9] Anterior cervical discectomy and fusions address pathology at the disk level. Damage adjacent to the disk (s) should be repaired with another surgical technique.[10] In the right circumstances, based on the extent of the pathology and its effect on the anatomy of the cervical spine, multilevel discectomies are desirable for treating CSM because they generally result in less intraoperative bleeding than corpectomies.[1] Additionally, with ACDFs, there is greater potential for segmental fixation and sagittal realignment.[1]

### Technique

A standard Smith-Robinson approach via the carotid triangle allows access to the C2-T1 spinal segments. An incision may be made either transversely or obliquely, depending on the target levels. Anatomical landmarks include the hyoid bone, or C3; the thyroid cartilage, or the C4-5 interspace; and the cricothyroid membrane, or C5-6 level. The platysma is then incised either transversely or longitudinally. Blunt dissection is performed along the medial border of the sternocleidomastoid muscle, and both sides of the longus colli muscle are identified. The carotid sheath and associated vessels are retracted laterally. Midline structures, including the esophagus, trachea, and thyroid gland, are retracted medially. Fluoroscopy is used to verify the level, and the retractor blades are carefully inserted underneath the longus colli muscle.

Discectomies are performed through the anterior longitudinal ligament and anterior annulus, and the intervertebral disk is completely removed. A small curette or Kerrison rongeur is used to remove the disk or bony spur. After decompression, the end plates are prepared for fusion. An appropriately sized bone graft or cage is applied, followed by plate fixation. Sagittal plane defects can be repaired with the use of lordotic spacers between vertebrae.[6]

## Complications

Vulnerable anatomic structures in an anterior procedure are the vertebral artery, recurrent laryngeal nerve (RLN), esophagus, carotid sheath, and cervical sympathetic chain. Excessive retraction while performing ACDF can result in RLN injury, which may present as hoarseness, cough, and airway problems.[11] Recurrent laryngeal nerve palsy has a reported prevalence after ACDF of 0.2–16.7%.[11-21] Short-term dysphagia is a common complication reported after an anterior surgical procedure, with a reported prevalence ranging from 2% to 67%.[11,22-24] It has been reported that dysphagia occurs more frequently in patients who have undergone a three-level ACDF compared to those who had a one- or two-level ACDF, which is explained by the fact that greater retraction and dissection is necessary when there are more levels surgically involved.[11] Persistent dysphagia is also a reported complication, although it is much less common than short-term dysphagia, with varying reported incidence. In one study, the reported rate was 12.5% at 1-year postoperatively,[25] while another study reported 21% incidence at 2-year postoperatively.[11,26]

Wound hematoma is another complication associated with ACDF, with a reported prevalence ranging 1–11%,[11,14,27,28] and it is resolved either conservatively or surgically.[11] Cerebrospinal fluid leak is another associated complication with a reported rate of 0.3–1.8%,[11,18] and it can be managed by implementing a drain system and wound closure.[11] Esophageal injury, with a reported rate of 0.3%,[11] can sometimes be fatal and should be repaired surgically and with antibiotics.[11] Worsening of myelopathy can also occur and is best managed with physical therapy.[11,26] Fountas et al. identified 0.2% of patients with worsening of myelopathy postoperatively.[11]

Emery et al. reported that pseudoarthrosis with related neck pain and myelopathy is a complication associated with ACDFs more often than with corpectomies.[8] However, there are still other studies that report pseudoarthrosis to be a complication equally associated with both types of surgeries. In the case of ACDFs, studies have shown that as the number of disk levels surgically involved increases, so does the risk of pseudoarthrosis as well as the risk of needing a future revision surgery.[10] In two- and three-level ACDFs, use of a locking plate can aid fusion and help prevent nonunion.[10,29,30] According to Wang et al., in a study analyzing outcomes of patient undergoing two-level ACDFs with or without plating, 0% of patients with addition of plating experienced pseudoarthrosis compared to 25% without plating.[29]

## Evidence

Ebersold et al. reported good results in patients with CSM who were treated with anterior discectomy and fusion.[31] In the few patients who experienced neurologic compromise, all had other concurrent diagnoses in addition to CSM.[31]

# CORPECTOMY

## Indications

While discectomies have been shown to be safe and efficacious in cases of CSM only affecting disks on one, two, or three levels, there was a need for another strategy to surgically manage CSM affecting four levels[7] as well as disk herniations associated with large osteophytes, excess disk material, and/or retrovertebral disease involving ossification of the posterior longitudinal ligament behind the vertebral body.[8,1] In these cases, corpectomy is indicated. An additional indication for corpectomies is kyphosis, where it is necessary for the spine to be straightened out to relieve compression.[10]

Advantages of a corpectomy include the opportunity for better decompression than ACDF, which is crucial in the case of any retrovertebral disease contributing to narrowing of the canal behind the vertebral body.[1] With a corpectomy, in addition to repairing the compression of the disk, compression adjacent to the disk due to osteophytes or an ossified posterior longitudinal ligament behind the vertebral body can be resolved.[9] The entire vertebral body can be eliminated in order to achieve decompression, whereas it is dangerous to try to reach around the back of the vertebral body in order to gain access to the posterior longitudinal ligament when performing an ACDF.[9] Cervical spondylotic myelopathy has a multifactorial etiology, and corpectomy can be beneficial as it addresses more than one factor all at once.[32]

### Technique

A standard Smith-Robinson approach is performed. After exposing the disks, discectomies are executed directly above and below each affected vertebral body with a bur. A bur or rongeur is used to form a channel in the center of the vertebral body, which is extended to the posterior cortex. Contact with the lateral walls should be avoided so that the vertebral artery is not injured. Bleeding should be controlled with bone wax. A curette or Kerrison rongeur is used to remove the cortex. After decompression, a curette is used to remove end-plate cartilage. The strut graft is measured, and fixation is achieved with a plate.

### Complications

Vertebral artery injury can result from removal of the uncinate process during removal of osteophytes.[6] Mummaneni reported a higher risk of graft failure with corpectomies than with ACDFs.[33] Airway problems, vertebral artery injury, and radiculitis are complications associated with corpectomies.[9,32] Rates of C5 palsy following corpectomy have been reported to range from 3.1% to 8.5%.[6] There has been a reported rate of 3.5% of RLN injury in those with corpectomies.[6,34-37] As with ACDF, the literature has shown that the risk of complications increases with an increased number of levels surgically involved.[9]

### Evidence

Kimura et al. performed a study in which they evaluated the outcomes of patients undergoing anterior cervical corpectomy and fusion (ACCF) to C2 (ACCF-C2) for cervical myelopathy.[38] They reported that, although a challenging technique, ACCF-C2 was effective in treating patients with cervical myelopathy with extensive ossification of the posterior longitudinal ligament, stenosis, and kyphosis.[38]

Bernard and Whitecloud performed subtotal corpectomies on patients with CSM and found that patients achieved good functional outcomes with no incidence of pseudoarthrosis.[39] Yonenobu et al. and Okada et al. both performed similar studies on patients who underwent subtotal corpectomy and fusion for CSM, reporting high rates of neurologic improvement and few patients with decline.[40,41] Neither of these studies analyzed pain. Saunders et al. performed a study analyzing patients with subtotal corpectomy for CSM and reported high rates of neurologic improvement and low rates of deterioration, and although there was a 48% complication rate, such complications were primarily minor and manageable.[32]

## CERVICAL DISK ARTHROPLASTY

### Indications

Cervical disk arthroplasty, or total disk replacement, was developed as an alternative to ACDF that would potentially be able to preserve cervical motion while also reducing pain in patients with CSM.[42] It has also been proposed that this newer surgical technique, which is similarly performed through an anterior approach, might have the potential to prevent what is thought to be adjacent-segment disk degeneration brought about after ACDF by reducing the stress on adjacent-level disks.[42] It is not clear whether or not the latter complication occurs as a result of ACDF or if it is a natural progression of CSM that would occur regardless of operative or nonoperative treatment.[43]

### Technique

A standard Smith-Robinson technique is used as in ACDF and ACCF. Discectomy is performed, and the end plates are prepared. The vertebral body is kept intact in order to avoid postoperative implant slippage. Any posterior osteophytes are eradicated. The posterior annulus fibrosus is released to leave adequate space for the implant. A trial is used to assess the amount of disk space available. Keel channels are formed in the vertebral bodies above and below the disk space. A milling or chiseling technique may be used to create channels. The implant is inserted. Any necessary cuts in the vertebral bodies are made, and then the artificial disk is inserted.

### Contraindications

As CDA is a newer technique, more studies should be conducted to assess the complications. Cervical disk arthroplasty has many associated contraindications, including osteoporosis, instability, degeneration of facet joints, immobile segments, deformity, cancer, renal failure, rheumatoid arthritis, and the use of preoperative corticosteroids.

## COMPARISON OF TECHNIQUES

### ACDF, Corpectomy, and Discectomy-Corpectomy

In a systematic review, Shamji et al. reported that in their comparison of ACDF, corpectomy, and hybrid discectomy-corpectomy, all three techniques showed improvement in patient clinical outcomes and radiographic outcomes in terms of sagittal realignment.[1] Furthermore, all three appear to have similar risks for nonunion, dysphagia, and infection.[1] There may be fewer cases of C5 palsy development in patients who undergo multiple discectomies compared to the other two techniques.[1] Shamji et al. put forth several recommendations for indications of surgical treatment of CSM.[1] When limited or no retrovertebral disease is present, multiple discectomies should be performed. In the presence of extensive retrovertebral disease, a hybrid discectomy-corpectomy should be performed in lieu of multiple corpectomies.[1] There is no overwhelming conclusion in the literature about the superiority of corpectomy compared to hybrid discectomy-corpectomy in terms of clinical outcomes and sagittal alignment.[1] Finally, Shamji et al. found no evidence for the efficacy of immobilization techniques that have been used in the past following anterior procedures.[1]

## ACDF Versus ACCF

Huang et al. performed a meta-analysis comparing the outcomes of ACDF to ACCF in patients with CSM at two levels.[44] They reported that ACDF was associated with more advantages compared to ACCF.[44] Specifically, patients treated with ACDF experienced less bleeding and shorter surgery time as well as superior cervical correction.[44] Han et al. however, performed a similar meta-analysis, reporting that while patients treated with ACDF achieved better lordosis and experienced fewer complications than those treated with ACCF, there is not enough strong evidence to conclude that ACDF is superior to ACCF in the treatment of CSM.[45]

## ACDF Versus Anterior Cervical Hybrid Decompression and Fusion (ACDHF) Versus ACCF

Guo et al. compared the efficacy of three-level ACDF, ACDHF, and two-level ACCF.[46] Fusion rates were similar for all three groups.[46] However, ACDF was superior to ACDHF and ACCF in terms of segmental angle and C2-C7 angle improvement, less operation time, and lowest complication rate.[46] Guo et al. recommend ACDF as the treatment that should be used whenever possible, with ACHDF as the first alternative followed by ACCF as the last alternative.[46]

## Single-Level Corpectomy Versus Two-Level ACDF

Park et al. performed a retrospective review of prospectively collected data analyzing the results of single-level corpectomy with two-level discectomy with anterior plating.[47] They reported that the two procedures had similar results with regard to sagittal alignment, cervical lordosis, graft subsidence, and adjacent-level ossification.[47] Wang et al. found similar results.[48]

## Plate Fixation in Two-Level and Three-Level ACDF and Corpectomy

Fraser and Hartl performed a meta-analysis in which they analyzed fusion rates for patients with degenerative disk disease at one, two, and three levels who had undergone ACD, ACDF, ACDF with an anterior plate (ACDFP), corpectomy, and corpectomy with a plate.[49] They reported that the use of an anterior cervical plate increases the rate of fusion significantly for one- , two- , and three-level disease.[49] Furthermore, there was no difference in the efficacy of fusion for disease at two levels for patients who had undergone ACD with a plate or corpectomy with a plate. However, at three levels of disease, corpectomy with a plate had higher rates of fusion than discectomy performed with a plate.[49]

## Anterior Cervical Discectomy and Fusion Versus Cervical Disk Arthroplasty

Tracey et al. compared the outcomes of single-level ACDF to single-level CDA and reported that the CDA group had similar rates of symptom relief and return to preoperative activity level, with the CDA group's rates only slightly higher.[42] Tracey et al. concluded that CDA is a reasonable alternative to ACDF.[42]

Burkus et al. conducted a prospective randomized study comparing the outcomes of CDA with the Prestige disk to ACDF in 2002.[50,51] The CDA group returned to work earlier.[50] Motion was preserved at both the site of surgery as well as at the disk spaces at adjacent levels.[50] After a 2-year follow-up period, similar results were reported with the use of the Bryan disk.[52,53] There was no difference in dysphagia occurrence in either the Burkus et al. study[50] or in an earlier study by Mcafee et al.[54]

Phillips et al. performed a prospective randomized clinical trial comparing the results of ACDF and CDA with porous coated motion and found that the CDA group had better Neck Disability Index (NDI) scores, higher patient satisfaction, greater range of motion, less dysphagia, and higher overall success rates 2 years after surgery than the ACDF group.[55] Improvement in pain and function, neurological outcomes, occurrence of adverse events and revision surgeries were found to be similar in the two groups after 2 years.[55]

Davis et al. performed a prospective, randomized clinical trial comparing the results of ACDF with Mobi-C CDA for degenerative disk disease at two levels and found there were significantly more revision surgeries and device-related adverse events in the ACDF group than the CDA group.[56] There was also better range of motion, less neurological deterioration, and less adjacent-segment degeneration in the CDA group.[56] Finally, the CDA group had higher overall success rates.[56]

Ding et al. performed a retrospective analysis comparing CDA with ACDF specifically in the treatment of CSM.[57] Ding et al. reported that both groups showed improvement in Short Form Health Survey Physical Component Summary (SF-36 PCS) and Mental Component Summary (SF-36 MCS) scores as well as NDI scores, but that the CDA group had significantly greater score improvement at each follow-up appointment.[57] The CDA group did not experience any changes in their range of motion; however, the ACDF group experienced significantly decreased range of motion.[57] Finally, the CDA group had fewer complications.[57]

## CONCLUSION

Cervical spondylotic myelopathy is a condition that requires subjective review by a surgeon in order to determine the best method of treatment; treatment should be individualized and may vary from patient to patient as the cause of CSM is multifactorial. For those patients who undergo surgical treatment, a surgeon must make a decision between an anterior and a posterior surgical approach. In 2011, Liu et al. found that after a 5-year follow-up period, anterior and posterior surgical approaches had equal efficacy.[1,58] In 2014, Liu et al. had inconclusive results.[59]

If an anterior approach is decided upon, there are several options available, including ACDF, corpectomy, and CDA.

Anterior cervical discectomy and fusion, the oldest technique of the three, is typically indicated for CSM affecting disks at one, two, or three levels without retrovertebral disease. Corpectomy is indicated for CSM with retrovertebral disease and additional pathology that extends to anatomy adjacent to the disks. There is debate over which technique is associated with a higher rate of pseudoarthrosis. Adjacent segment degeneration is another topic of controversy. One school of thought is that fusions accelerate degenerative changes at adjacent segments. Hilibrand et al., however, showed that these changes could be attributable to the typical progressive degeneration strictly related to the natural course of CSM.[43]

Cervical disk arthroplasty is a newer surgical technique used for the treatment of CSM, and it has been shown to preserve cervical range of motion as well as prevent the progression of adjacent-segment disk degeneration. While CDA has been shown to be as effective as, if not more effective than, ACDF, it is a significantly more expensive procedure and is associated with many more contraindications than ACDF.[42] Qureshi et al. performed an analysis that compared the cost-effectiveness of CDA to ACDF and reported that both procedures are cost-effective; however, they found that CDA would need to retain functionality for at least 14 years before it can be considered more cost-effective than ACDF.[60]

There is a need for more prospective, randomized, controlled clinical trials comparing the long-term effects of ACDF, corpectomy, and CDA. In the meantime, when treating patients with CSM, surgeons must use their best judgment and take into consideration the location and extent of the disease as well as the state of the patient's cervical sagittal alignment in order to devise the most appropriate treatment strategy for each individual.

## REFERENCES

1. Shamji MF, Massicotte EM, Traynelis VC, et al. Comparison of anterior surgical options for the treatment of multilevel cervical spondylotic myelopathy: a systematic review. Spine. 2013;38:S195-209.
2. Shamji MF, Cook C, Pietrobon R, et al. Impact of surgical approach on complications and resource utilization of cervical spine fusion: a nationwide perspective to the surgical treatment of diffuse cervical spondylosis. Spine J. 2009;9:31-8.
3. Fehlings MG, Smith JS, Kopjar B, et al. Perioperative and delayed complications associated with the surgical treatment of cervical spondylotic myelopathy based on 302 patients from the AOSpine North America Cervical Spondylotic Myelopathy Study. J Neurosurg Spine. 2012;16:425-32.

4. Klineberg E. Cervical spondylotic myelopathy: a review of the evidence. Orthop Clin North Am. 2010;41:193-202.
5. Sodeyama T, Goto S, Mochizuki M, et al. Effect of decompression enlargement laminoplasty for posterior shifting of the spinal cord. Spine. 1999;24:1527-31; discussion 31-2.
6. Siemionow KB, Neckrysh S. Anterior approach for complex cervical spondylotic myelopathy. Orthop Clin North Am. 2012;43:41-52, viii.
7. Shunzhi Y, Zhonghai L, Fengning L, et al. Surgical management of 4-level cervical spondylotic myelopathy. Orthopedics. 2013;36:e613-20.
8. Emery SE, Bohlman HH, Bolesta MJ, et al. Anterior cervical decompression and arthrodesis for the treatment of cervical spondylotic myelopathy. Two to seventeen-year follow-up. J Bone Joint Surg Am. 1998;80:941-51.
9. Emery SE. Cervical spondylotic myelopathy: diagnosis and treatment. J Am Acad Orthop Surg. 2001;9:376-88.
10. Geck MJ, Eismont FJ. Surgical options for the treatment of cervical spondylotic myelopathy. Orthop Clin North Am. 2002;33:329-48.
11. Fountas KN, Kapsalaki EZ, Nikolakakos LG, et al. Anterior cervical discectomy and fusion associated complications. Spine. 2007;32:2310-7.
12. Bulger RF, Rejowski JE, Beatty RA. Vocal cord paralysis associated with anterior cervical fusion: considerations for prevention and treatment. J Neurosurg. 1985;62:657-61.
13. Heeneman H. Vocal cord paralysis following approaches to the anterior cervical spine. Laryngoscope. 1973;83:17-21.
14. Dohn DF. Anterior interbody fusion for treatment of cervical-disk conditions. JAMA. 1966;197:897-900.
15. Morpeth JF, Williams MF. Vocal fold paralysis after anterior cervical diskectomy and fusion. Laryngoscope. 2000;110: 43-6.
16. Jung A, Schramm J, Lehnerdt K, et al. Recurrent laryngeal nerve palsy during anterior cervical spine surgery: a prospective study. J Neurosurg Spine. 2005;2:123-7.
17. Hart AK, Greinwald JH Jr, Shaffrey CI, et al. Thoracic duct injury during anterior cervical discectomy: a rare complication. Case report. J Neurosurg. 1998;88:151-4.
18. Bertalanffy H, Eggert HR. Complications of anterior cervical discectomy without fusion in 450 consecutive patients. Acta Neurochir (Wien). 1989;99:41-50.
19. Flynn TB. Neurologic complications of anterior cervical interbody fusion. Spine. 1982;7:536-9.
20. Netterville JL, Koriwchak MJ, Winkle M, et al. Vocal fold paralysis following the anterior approach to the cervical spine. Ann Otol Rhinol Laryngol. 1996;105:85-91.
21. Riley LH Jr, Robinson RA, Johnson KA, et al. The results of anterior interbody fusion of the cervical spine. Review of ninety-three consecutive cases. J Neurosurg. 1969; 30:127-33.
22. Stieber JR, Brown K, Donald GD, et al. Anterior cervical decompression and fusion with plate fixation as an outpatient procedure. Spine J. 2005;5:503-7.
23. Baron EM, Soliman AM, Gaughan JP, et al. Dysphagia, hoarseness, and unilateral true vocal fold motion impairment following anterior cervical diskectomy and fusion. Ann Otol Rhinol Laryngol. 2003;112:921-6.
24. Frempong-Boadu A, Houten JK, Osborn B, et al. Swallowing and speech dysfunction in patients undergoing anterior cervical discectomy and fusion: a prospective, objective preoperative and postoperative assessment. J Spinal Disord Tech. 2002;15:362-8.
25. Bazaz R, Lee MJ, Yoo JU. Incidence of dysphagia after anterior cervical spine surgery: a prospective study. Spine. 2002;27:2453-8.
26. Riley LH 3rd, Skolasky RL, Albert TJ, et al. Dysphagia after anterior cervical decompression and fusion: prevalence and risk factors from a longitudinal cohort study. Spine. 2005;30:2564-9.
27. Lunsford LD, Bissonette DJ, Zorub DS. Anterior surgery for cervical disc disease. Part 2: Treatment of cervical spondylotic myelopathy in 32 cases. J Neurosurg. 1980;53:12-9.
28. Williams JL, Allen MB Jr, Harkess JW. Late results of cervical discectomy and interbody fusion: some factors influencing the results. J Bone Joint Surg. 1968; 50:277-86.
29. Wang JC, McDonough PW, Endow KK, et al. Increased fusion rates with cervical plating for two-level anterior cervical discectomy and fusion. Spine. 2000;25:41-5.
30. Wang JC, McDonough PW, Kanim LE, et al. Increased fusion rates with cervical plating for three-level anterior cervical discectomy and fusion. Spine. 2001;26: 643-6; discussion 6-7.
31. Ebersold MJ, Pare MC, Quast LM. Surgical treatment for cervical spondylitic myelopathy. J Neurosurg. 1995;82: 745-51.
32. Saunders RL, Bernini PM, Shirreffs TG Jr, et al. Central corpectomy for cervical spondylotic myelopathy: a consecutive series with long-term follow-up evaluation. J Neurosurg. 1991;74:163-70.
33. Mummaneni PV, Kaiser MG, Matz PG, et al. Cervical surgical techniques for the treatment of cervical spondylotic myelopathy. J Neurosurg Spine. 2009;11:130-41.
34. Beutler WJ, Sweeney CA, Connolly PJ. Recurrent laryngeal nerve injury with anterior cervical spine surgery risk with laterality of surgical approach. Spine. 2001;26:1337-42.
35. Ikenaga M, Shikata J, Tanaka C. Radiculopathy of C-5 after anterior decompression for cervical myelopathy. J Neurosurg Spine. 2005;3:210-7.
36. Wada E, Suzuki S, Kanazawa A, et al. Subtotal corpectomy versus laminoplasty for multilevel cervical spondylotic myelopathy: a long-term follow-up study over 10 years. Spine. 2001;26:1443-7; discussion 8.
37. Hashimoto M, Mochizuki M, Aiba A, et al. C5 palsy following anterior decompression and spinal fusion for cervical degenerative diseases. Eur Spine J. 2010; 19:1702-10.
38. Kimura H, Shikata J, Odate S, et al. Anterior corpectomy and fusion to C2 for cervical myelopathy: clinical results and complications. Eur Spine J. 2014;23:1491-501.
39. Bernard TN Jr, Whitecloud TS 3rd. Cervical spondylotic myelopathy and myeloradiculopathy. Anterior decompression and stabilization with autogenous fibula strut graft. Clin Orthop Relat Res. 1987:149-60.
40. Yonenobu K, Hosono N, Iwasaki M, et al. Neurologic complications of surgery for cervical compression myelopathy. Spine. 1991;16:1277-82.

41. Okada K, Shirasaki N, Hayashi H, et al. Treatment of cervical spondylotic myelopathy by enlargement of the spinal canal anteriorly, followed by arthrodesis. J Bone Joint Surg. 1991;73:352-64.
42. Tracey RW, Kang DG, Cody JP, et al. Outcomes of single-level cervical disc arthroplasty versus anterior cervical discectomy and fusion. J Clin Neurosci. 2014;21 (11):1905-8.
43. Hilibrand AS, Carlson GD, Palumbo MA, et al. Radiculopathy and myelopathy at segments adjacent to the site of a previous anterior cervical arthrodesis. J Bone Joint Surg. 1999;81:519-28.
44. Huang ZY, Wu AM, Li QL, et al. Comparison of two anterior fusion methods in two-level cervical spondylosis myelopathy: a meta-analysis. BMJ Open. 2014; 4:e004581.
45. Han YC, Liu ZQ, Wang SJ, et al. Is anterior cervical discectomy and fusion superior to corpectomy and fusion for treatment of multilevel cervical spondylotic myelopathy? A systemic review and meta-analysis. PloS One. 2014; 9:e87191.
46. Guo Q, Bi X, Ni B, et al. Outcomes of three anterior decompression and fusion techniques in the treatment of three-level cervical spondylosis. Eur Spine J. 2011;20:1539-44.
47. Park Y, Maeda T, Cho W, et al. Comparison of anterior cervical fusion after two-level discectomy or single-level corpectomy: sagittal alignment, cervical lordosis, graft collapse, and adjacent-level ossification. Spine J. 2010;10:193-9.
48. Wang JC, McDonough PW, Endow KK, et al. A comparison of fusion rates between single-level cervical corpectomy and two-level discectomy and fusion. J Spinal Disord. 2001;14:222-5.
49. Fraser JF, Hartl R. Anterior approaches to fusion of the cervical spine: a meta-analysis of fusion rates. J Neurosurg Spine. 2007;6:298-303.
50. Burkus JK, Traynelis VC, Haid RW Jr, et al. Clinical and radiographic analysis of an artificial cervical disc: 7-year follow-up from the prestige prospective randomized controlled clinical trial. J Neurosurg Spine. 2014:1-13.
51. Mummaneni PV, Burkus JK, Haid RW, et al. Clinical and radiographic analysis of cervical disc arthroplasty compared with allograft fusion: a randomized controlled clinical trial. J Neurosurg Spine. 2007;6:198-209.
52. Anderson PA, Sasso RC, Riew KD. Comparison of adverse events between the Bryan artificial cervical disc and anterior cervical arthrodesis. Spine. 2008;33: 1305-12.
53. Heller JG, Sasso RC, Papadopoulos SM, et al. Comparison of BRYAN cervical disc arthroplasty with anterior cervical decompression and fusion: clinical and radiographic results of a randomized, controlled, clinical trial. Spine. 2009;34: 101-7.
54. McAfee PC, Cappuccino A, Cunningham BW, et al. Lower incidence of dysphagia with cervical arthroplasty compared with ACDF in a prospective randomized clinical trial. J Spinal Disord Tech. 2010;23:1-8.
55. Phillips FM, Lee JY, Geisler FH, et al. A prospective, randomized, controlled clinical investigation comparing PCM cervical disc arthroplasty with anterior cervical discectomy and fusion. 2-year results from the US FDA IDE clinical trial. Spine. 2013;38:E907-18.
56. Davis RJ, Kim KD, Hisey MS, et al. Cervical total disc replacement with the Mobi-C cervical artificial disc compared with anterior discectomy and fusion for treatment of 2-level symptomatic degenerative disc disease: a prospective, randomized, controlled multicenter clinical trial: clinical article. J Neurosurg Spine. 2013;19:532-45.
57. Ding C, Hong Y, Liu H, et al. Comparison of cervical disc arthroplasty with anterior cervical discectomy and fusion for the treatment of cervical spondylotic myelopathy. Acta Orthop Belg. 2013;79:338-46.
58. Liu T, Xu W, Cheng T, et al. Anterior versus posterior surgery for multilevel cervical myelopathy, which one is better? A systematic review. Eur Spine J.2011;20: 224-35.
59. Liu X, Wang H, Zhou Z, et al. Anterior decompression and fusion versus posteriorlaminoplasty for multilevel cervical compressive myelopathy. Orthopedics. 2014;37:e117-22.
60. Qureshi SA, McAnany S, Goz V, et al. Cost-effectiveness analysis: comparing single-level cervical disc replacement and single-level anterior cervical discectomy and fusion: clinical article. J Neurosurg Spine. 2013;19:546-54.

Chapter 17

# Cervical Laminectomy with or without Fusion

*Hiroyuki Yoshihara*

## INTRODUCTION

Cervical spinal pathologies, such as disk herniations, spondylotic changes, ossification of the longitudinal ligament (OPLL), and ossification of the yellow ligament, cause cervical canal stenosis, which can lead to cervical myelopathy. Cervical absolute stenosis is defined by a canal measuring 10 mm in the anterior/posterior dimension, while relative stenosis denotes a 13-mm canal,[1] and myelopathic symptoms arise when the canal is narrowed to these critical dimensions. Surgical treatment is indicated to decompress the spinal cord when myelopathic symptoms are moderate to severe or progressing rapidly.

Cervical laminectomy is a basic operative technique for the management of cervical myelopathy, by decompressing and expanding the spinal canal posteriorly. Additional posterior stabilization procedures may be necessary for certain cases. There are a variety of fusion techniques such as wiring, lateral mass screw (LMS), and cervical pedicle screw (CPS) fixation. In this chapter, indications, surgical procedures, complications, and clinical outcomes of cervical laminectomy with or without fusion are described.

## INDICATIONS

### Cervical Laminectomy

Cervical laminectomy can treat cases with compression of spinal cord either anteriorly or posteriorly because the procedure can decompress the spinal cord directly and/or indirectly. When the spinal cord is compressed posteriorly, the procedure can remove the posterior elements directly. Indirect decompression can be achieved, allowing the cord to migrate dorsally away from areas of anterior compression by performing multilevel laminectomy.

Multilevel laminectomy is favorably indicated for cases with spinal cord compression extending more than two levels, no radiculopathy, presence of congenital canal stenosis, lordotic alignment, presence of OPLL, and primary posterior compressive pathology.[2-9] Cervical alignment is an important factor to determine a multilevel laminectomy. The presence of a straight or kyphotic alignment, especially if associated with significant ventral pathology, will limit dorsal migration of the spinal cord.[5] In addition, multilevel laminectomy in cases with such alignment can lead to further neurologic compromise because release of the posterior tension band increases the risk of postoperative kyphotic deformity. Hamanishi and Tanaka[10] mentioned a minimum lordosis of 10° required for adequate dorsal migration of the spinal cord. Yamazaki et al.[11] also reported on continued ventral compression after posterior decompression when the lordosis is < 10° and the extent of ventral compression is >7 mm in cases with OPLL.

### Cervical Laminectomy with Fusion

Cervical laminectomy with fusion is indicated for myelopathy cases with instability, loss of cervical alignment, or moderate to severe neck pain. Determining the presence and extent of instability rests on careful assessment of both static and dynamic imaging studies.[12] Reported findings on radiographs that are suggestive of instability include subluxation of > 3.5 mm on static lateral radiographs > 11° of angulation between adjacent segments, and > 4 mm of subluxation on dynamic views.[13] Release of the posterior tension band also needs to be taken into consideration for a fusion procedure because it can lead to an increased potential for a postlaminectomy kyphosis. In particular, young patients have been reported to carry a high risk for the development of a postlaminectomy kyphosis; therefore, a fusion procedure should be considered when performing multilevel laminectomy in such cases.[14-16] In contrast, despite kyphotic alignment of the cervical spine, if it is a flexible kyphosis, multilevel laminectomy and fusion can be a reasonable option by creating cervical lordosis and direct/indirect decompression. Satisfactory relief of neck pain can be expected by the fusion procedure.

In addition to elective cases with cervical myelopathy, laminectomy with or without fusion is also indicated for trauma cases such as spinal cord injury and traumatic central cord syndrome. The role of laminectomy to treat traumatic central cord syndrome in stenotic cases remains unproven;[3] however, the percentage of patients who undergo surgical treatment for traumatic central cord syndrome without bone injury has been increasing in the United States.[17]

There are multiple fusion techniques that can be used, including facet wiring, LMS, and CPS. The evolution of multiaxial screw rod constructs made the screw fixation technique much easier.[18] Both LMS and CPS have been demonstrated to have sufficient stability and high fusion rates.[19-28] Lateral mass screw fixation has become the popular stabilization technique in North America, whereas CPS fixation is a common procedure in some Asian countries. Cervical pedicle screw placement in the midcervical spine (C3-6) is not approved by the Food and Drug Administration due to the inherent risk. Because of the technical difficulty, small size, and morphological variation in the cervical pedicle, the risk of the vertebral artery, nerve root, and spinal cord is considered greater than observed with LMS fixation. However, CPS fixation may serve as a pragmatic solution under unusual circumstances where LMS fixation cannot be achieved, such as trauma and spinal deformity.[12]

## PROCEDURE

### Cervical Laminectomy

The patient is positioned prone, with the head in a Mayfield head holder. A midline incision is made at the posterior cervical spine. Keeping the midline dissection in the avascular fascial plane will help decrease blood loss. A subperiosteal dissection of the underlying ligaments and paracervical muscles exposes the spinous processes as well as lamina of the cervical spine, using monopolar cautery. When the fusion procedure is not planned, the facet capsule needs to be preserved to prevent postoperative cervical kyphosis. Localization can be performed with anatomic landmarks, such as the prominent C2 spinous process; however, confirmation with intraoperative imaging is recommended.

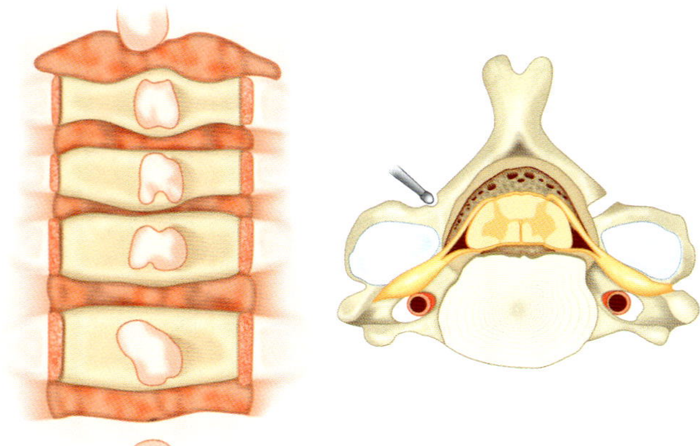

**Fig. 17.1:** Bilateral troughs are drilled at the lamina-facet junction with the drill bit oriented perpendicular to the dorsal surface of the lamina to avoid violation of the lateral mass.
*Source*: Redrawn from Komotar RJ, Mocco J, Kaiser MG. Surgical management of cervical myelopathy: indications and techniques for laminectomy and fusion. Spine J. 2006;6 (6 Suppl):252S-67S.

Bilateral bony troughs are made by using a high-speed drill (matchstick) at the junction of the lamina and bony lateral mass (Fig. 17.1). Care must be taken to hold the drill perpendicular to the dorsal surface of the lamina and not to make the trough lateral to the junction; otherwise, you simply drill deep into the lateral mass without exposing the epidural space. The rostral aspect of the lamina tends to dive deep and requires more extensive drilling to completely disarticulate the lamina. Bleeding from the trough is controlled with bone wax. Continuous irrigation is recommended to avoid thermal injury to the nerve tissues. Once the bony troughs are completed, the spinous processes are elevated with clamps and the ligamentous attachments of the ligamentum flavum within the troughs and between rostral and caudal end laminas and the adjacent lamina are removed using a 1-mm Kerrison rongeur; the entire laminas are then removed. Epidural bleeding is controlled with bipolar cautery and Gelfoam soaked with thrombin. A Hemovac drain is placed to prevent postoperative hematoma, and a multilayer closure is performed.

### Cervical Fusion (C3-7)

Exposure for LMS fixation requires soft-tissue dissection to be extended until the far lateral margin of the facet is identified. To avoid compromise of uninvolved segments, care must be taken to maintain the facet capsule at the rostral and caudal extremes of the intended fusion.

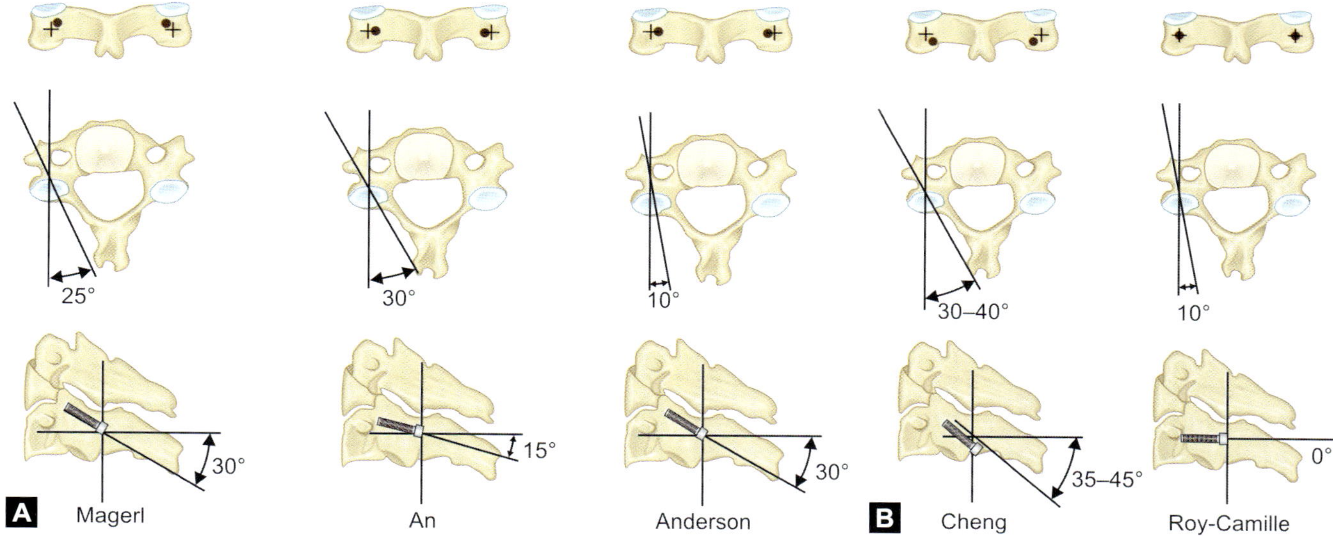


**Figs. 17.2A and B:** Comparison of the entry points and screw trajectories described by various authors. The black dots indicate the entry points for the lateral mass screws. Our modified entry point (Cheng) is 1.5 mm caudal and medial to the center and has a relatively more oblique (30°–40°) and steeper (35°–45°) trajectory aiming toward the superior lateral quadrant of the ventral lateral mass. Roy-Camille's entry point is located right in the center, with a trajectory perpendicular to the sagittal plane. An and Anderson's techniques share a common entry point at the center of lateral mass, whereas Magerl's entry point is 1 mm cranial and medial to the center. The An, Anderson, and Magerl techniques have different trajectories in the sagittal and axial planes, respectively.
*Source*: Redrawn from Wu JC, Huang WC, Chen YC, et al. Stabilization of subaxial cervical spines by lateral mass screw fixation with modified Magerl's technique. Surg Neurol. 2008;70(Suppl 1):25-33.

Placement of screw trajectories prior to decompression maintains familiar landmarks, eases attainment of correct trajectories, and is safer to protect the dura and neural elements. Once the soft-tissue exposure is completed, entry sites for the lateral screws are marked to the dorsal cortical wall using a high-speed drill. Then the lateral mass is cannulated and tapped using a hand-drill. Various LMS insertion techniques have been described in the literature (Figs. 17.2A and B).[27-29] Jeanneret and Magerl[29] described a starting point 1–2 mm medial and superior to the midpoint of the lateral mass with the trajectory aimed 30° superior and 15°–25° lateral. An et al.[30] recommended a starting point 1 mm medial to the lateral mass center and angled 15° cranial and 30° lateral. Anderson et al.[31] described a starting point 1 mm medial to the lateral mass center and aimed 20°–30° cranially and 10°–20° laterally. Overall, LMSs are inserted into the predrilled holes aiming in a superolateral direction (Figs. 17.3A to D). Resection of the spinous process may be necessary to obtain the optimal trajectory. The lateral mass at C7 is somewhat elongated in the rostral-caudal direction and is thinner, so care needs to be taken not to make a fracture of lateral mass, especially for osteoporotic cases, and a violation of the adjacent facet joint. Heller et al.[21] demonstrated 20% higher pullout strength of the bicortical LMS than the unicortical one; however, the bicortical screw has a risk of nerve root injury. Satisfactory placement of the screws is confirmed using intraoperative fluoroscopy.

The entry point of CPS is slightly lateral to the center of the lateral mass and close to the inferior margin of the inferior articular process of the cranially adjacent vertebra.[32] The cortical bone at the entry point is drilled away to expose the dorsal cancellous bone of the pedicle. Then a small pedicle probe is inserted into the pedicle with the help of a lateral image intensifier to confirm the direction and insertion depth. Tapping is performed before insertion of the pedicle screw. The insertion angle of CPS is intended to be 25°–45° medial to the midline in the transverse plane, depending on the level (Figs. 17.4 and 17.5). The intended angle of screw insertion in the sagittal plane is parallel to the upper endplate for the pedicles of C5, C6, and C7, and in a slightly cephalad direction in C3 and C4.[32] Increased accuracy has been observed with direct exposure of the pedicle through a laminoforaminotomy and the addition of fluoroscopy and computer-assisted navigational techniques.[33,34] Richter et al.[35] reported that the rate of pedicle perforation was 3% in the computer-assisted group and 8.6% in the conventional freehand

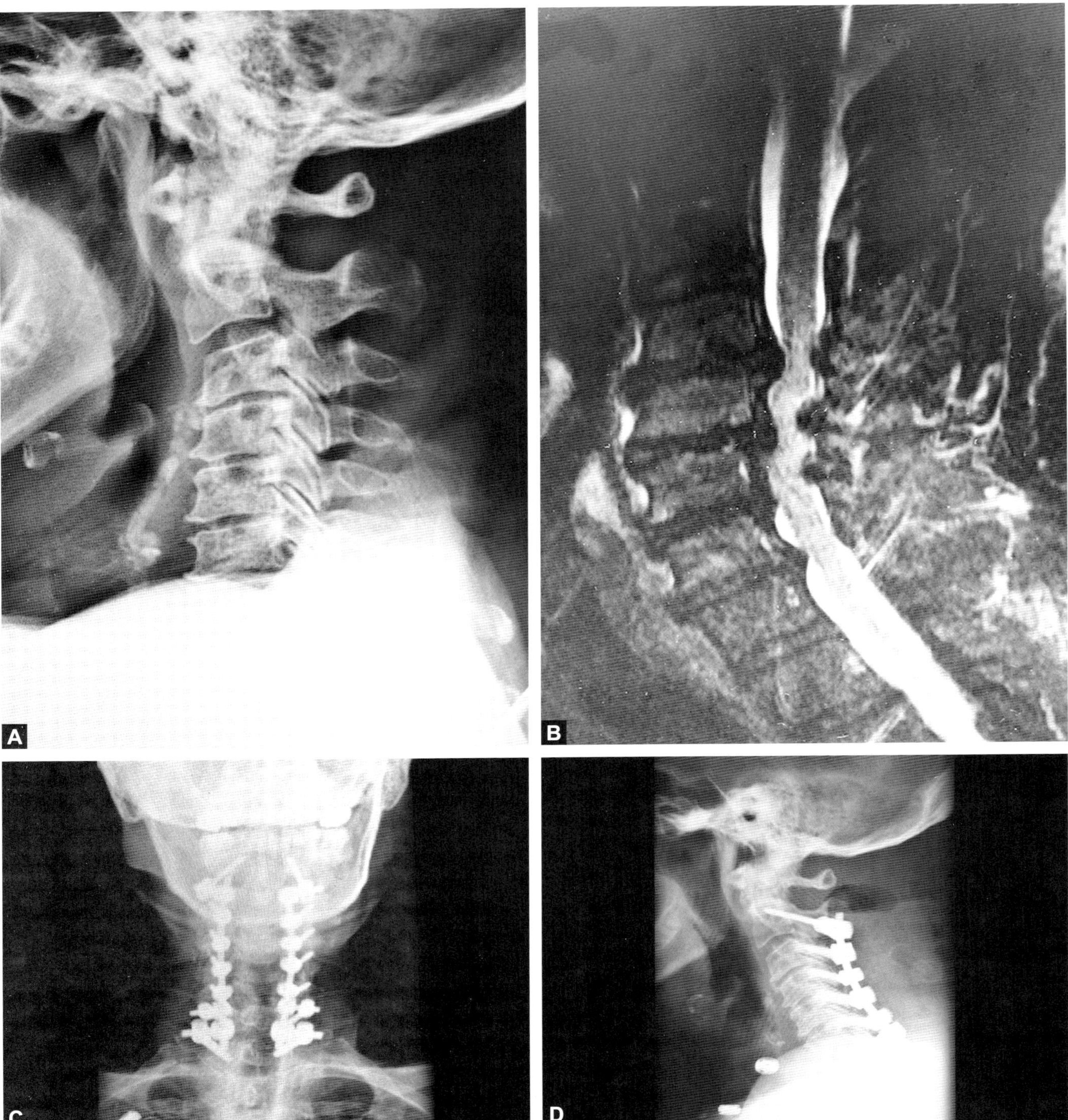


**Figs. 17.3A to D:** A 70-year-old woman with the symptoms of myelopathy hand and gait instability. (A) Lateral X-ray of cervical spine shows spondylotic changes and straight to kyphotic alignment. (B) Sagittal magnetic resonance imaging shows severe cervical stenosis at C3-4, C4-5, and C5-6. (C and D) Cervical laminectomy from C3 to C6 and posterior spinal fusion from C2 to T1 were performed. Lateral mass screws were used from C3 to C6 and pedicle screws were used for C2, C7, and T1.

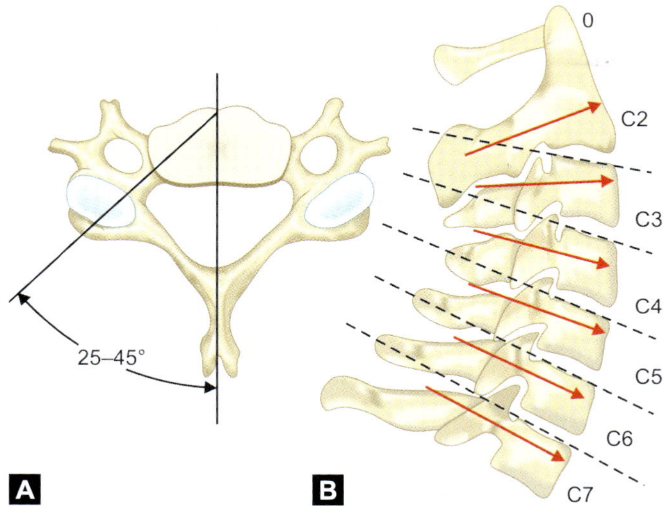


**Figs. 17.4A and B:** The trajectories required for appropriate cervical pedicle screw placement in both the sagittal and axial planes. (A) The insertion angle of the pedicle screw from C3 to C7 was intended to be 25°–45° medial to the midline in the transverse plane. (B) The intended angle of screw insertion in the sagittal plane was parallel to the upper endplate in the C5-C7 pedicles, and was slightly cephalad in C2-C4 because of the pedicle angle of C2 in the sagittal plane.
*Source*: (A) Redrawn from Ladd JE, Heller JG, Silcox HD, et al. Cervical pedicle screws versus lateral mass screws: Anatomic feasibility and biomechanical comparison. Spine. 1997;22:977-82. (B) Redrawn from Abumi K, Kaneda K. Pedicle screw fixation for nontraumatic lesions of the cervical spine. Spine. 1997;22:1853-63.

group. Cervical pedicle screw is more indicated for C7 because of the larger size of pedicle; in addition, the risk of vertebral artery injury is eliminated at C7.

Rods are contoured to make a lordosis and not to make a significant pull-out force to the screws, particularly for LMS. When using CPS at C7 and LMS at C6, an off-set connector may need to be utilized because of the close placement of each screw. A cross-link connector can be used to enhance the construct biomechanical stability and to prevent laminectomy membrane. The lateral masses as well as facet joints are decorticated using a high-speed burr. The bone graft is placed over these surfaces.

## COMPLICATIONS

Similar to other spine surgeries, iatrogenic neurological injuries, hematoma, infection, hardware complications, and pseudarthrosis can occur, although the incidence is not high. There are several complications inherent to cervical laminectomy with or without fusion.

### Cervical Laminectomy

Despite the common postoperative complication after laminoplasty, postoperative upper-extremity palsy has not been reported as much for cervical laminectomy. However, Dai et al.[36] observed that 37 (12.9%) patients

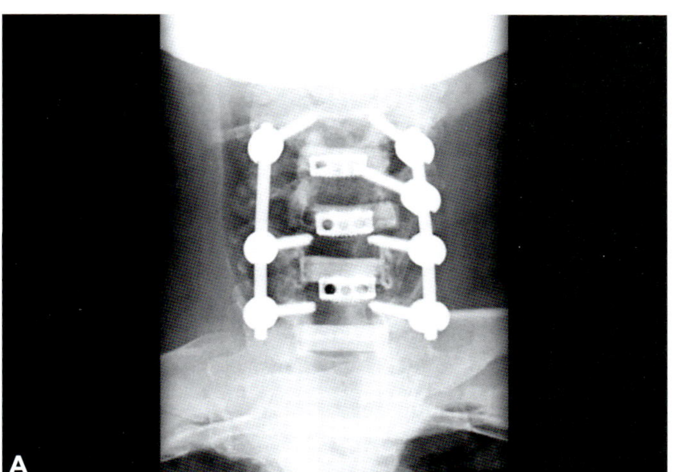


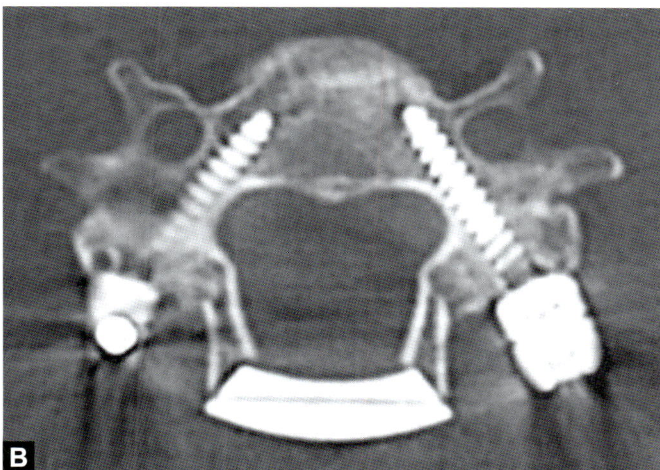


**Figs. 17.5A and B:** A 48-year-old woman suffering from athetoid cervical myelopathy who underwent C3-C6 circumferential fusion with Axon system and SynCage-C. (A) Anteroposterior X-ray film after surgery and (B) Postoperative computed tomography at C6.
*Source*: Reprinted with permission from Yoshimoto H, Sato S, Hyakumachi T, et al. Clinical accuracy of cervical pedicle screw insertion using lateral fluoroscopy: a radiographic analysis of the learning curve. Eur Spine J. 2009;18(9):1326-34.

exhibited new postoperative root deficits involving the C5 and C6 nerve roots following 287 cervical laminectomies.

Postlaminectomy kyphosis is the major concern following laminectomy procedure. The incidence of kyphotic change after multilevel laminectomy has been reported to be between 14% and 47% in larger retrospective series.[37-39] Facet injury, including capsule injury, may be an important contributor to postoperative kyphosis. When the degree of facetectomy approaches 50%, significant kyphosis and resultant instability may ensue.[40,41] A straight or kyphotic alignment of the spine may predict a greater chance of late instability and kyphosis. Younger patients are at an increased risk as a result of incomplete ossification of the vertebral bodies and reduced resistance to the incremental compressive forces that develop with compromise of the posterior tension band.[15,16]

### Cervical Laminectomy with Fusion

Complications relating to instrumentation for cervical fusion include perioperative and late complications. Possible perioperative complications include root injury, spinal cord injury, vertebral artery injury, fracture of lateral mass, facet violation, and malposition requiring postoperative revision or removal.[42] Possible late complications are screw loosening, screw pullout, screw breakage, plate/rod breakage, loss of reduction, pseudarthrosis, and adjacent segment disease requiring operation.[42]

Specific complications associated with LMS fixation include impingement of the traversing nerve root, fracture of lateral mass, and facet violation. The potential for nerve root injury is increased when attempting bicortical purchase. Heller et al.[25] reported nerve root injury in 4 of 78 cases. Fracture of lateral mass can happen when the patient is osteoporotic or the entry point is too close to the bony edge. Facet violation also needs to be taken into account, particularly at the elongated lateral mass of C7.

Insertion of CPS is associated with risks to the vertebral artery, nerve root, and spinal cord. Because of the technical difficulty, small size, and morphological variation in the cervical pedicle, the risk is considered greater than observed with LMS fixation. The reported incidence of pedicle perforation in the previous studies ranged from 1.1% to 29.8%.[43,44] Although the incidence of lateral pedicle perforation was relatively high in previous studies, the actual cases in which a vertebral artery injury was sustained were found to be rare. Reported incidences of vertebral artery injuries were 1 of 180 cases reported by Abumi et al.,[45] 1 of 144 cases by Yukawa et al.,[46] and 2 of 84 cases by Nakashima et al.[47] A recent systematic review article found that vertebral artery injuries are extremely rare with both LMS and CPS techniques, although statistically significantly more common when using CPS.[42] There was no case reported in which spinal cord injury occurred in a procedure using CPS.[42] However, as Yoshimoto et al.[48] reported, the learning curve of CPS and the perforation rate in their study was 12% in the initial 19 cases, and decreased to 7% in the next 18 cases and to 1.1% in the last 15 cases; thus, less experienced surgeons should use such techniques with extreme caution and perhaps with the assistance of more experienced surgeons. Injury to bilateral vertebral arteries might cause serious problems such as cerebral infarction or death. When occlusion of the vertebral artery on one side is seen preoperatively, the insertion of CPS in the remaining side should be avoided.[49] In such cases, CPS fixation on the occluded side and LMS fixation on the remaining side are recommended.[49]

The risk of neurovascular injury is considered greater in CPS, and LMS is considered biomechanically weaker. However, a recent systematic review article reported that perioperative neurovascular and late biomechanical complication rates, including pseudarthrosis, are similarly low for both LMS and CPS techniques.[42]

## CLINICAL OUTCOME

### Cervical Laminectomy

Historically, cervical laminectomies have been a safe direct method for decompressing cervical spinal cord compression causing myelopathy. Most of the studies were retrospective studies published in the 1960s and 1970s.[39] They described success rates ranging from 42% to 92%.[39] Some studies reported a significant incidence of delayed deterioration, with rates as high as 40%.[38,50,51] Good outcomes can be obtained in the lordotic cervical spine for indirect decompression. Adam and Logue[52] found that both a decreased range of motion postoperatively and a lesser degree of change of the spinal curvature were significantly correlated with the good outcome group. Factors that have been shown to correlate with poor outcome after laminectomy for cervical spondylotic myelopathy (CSM) include advanced age (>70 years at the time of the first surgery), severe original myelopathy, and recent trauma.[53-56] Postlaminectomy kyphosis has been mentioned to be correlated with worse clinical outcome.

However, thus far no study has clearly demonstrated a relationship between postlaminectomy kyphosis and deterioration in the quality of life of the patient.[39] Lee et al.[57] reported that long-term outcome of laminectomy for cervical OPLL was satisfactory and the risk of postlaminectomy kyphosis was not high, raising the possibility that the OPLL itself may serve as a support for the spinal column.

Cervical laminectomy procedure has demonstrated comparable immediate postoperative results to anterior procedures for myelopathy patients.[51] For the long-term follow-up, Carol et al.[58] reported that the improvement rate of 68% for the laminectomy group was comparable to the 73% improvement rate in the anterior surgical group at 10 years' follow-up; however, Ebersold et al.[51] reported an inferior outcome of laminectomy procedure compared to anterior procedure.

## Cervical Laminectomy and Fusion

Previous studies demonstrated significant improvement of neurological function in the vast majority of patients (>70%) who underwent laminectomy and fusion for CSM.[59] Long-term improved neurologic status and maintenance of cervical alignment also have been demonstrated.[60] Morio et al.[61] reported that decreased range of motion and better alignment were correlated with better outcomes. Huang et al.[56] reported the clinical outcomes of multilevel CSM treated by laminectomy and lateral mass plate fusion. Severe myelopathy, advanced age, and myelomalacia on preoperative magnetic resonance imaging had no prognostic value for improvement of myelopathy.[56]

Many authors have attempted to compare various procedures for the surgical treatment of cervical myelopathy. González-Feria et al.[62] compared clinical outcomes among anterior decompression and fusion, laminectomy, and laminectomy and fusion. Laminectomy and fusion showed greater recovery than with the other two procedures. Yoon et al.[63] recently performed a systematic review comparing outcomes after laminectomy and fusion versus laminoplasty in cases with cervical myelopathy, and concluded that there is low-quality evidence that laminectomy and fusion and laminoplasty procedures are similarly effective in treating CSM. A few studies have compared the outcomes of laminectomy versus laminectomy and fusion. Both treatment strategies showed similar clinical improvements.[64,65]

## REFERENCES


1. Epstein JA, Epstein NE. The surgical management of cervical spinal stenosis, spondylosis, and myeloradiculopathy by means of the posterior approach. In: Clark CR (Ed). The Cervical Spine Research Society Editorial Committee. The Cervical Spine, 2nd edition. Philadelphia: JB Lippincott; 1989. pp. 625-43.
2. Wong AS, Massicotte EM, Fehlings MG. Surgical treatment of cervical myeloradiculopathy associated with movement disorders: indications, technique, and clinical outcome. J Spinal Disord Tech. 2005;18(Suppl):S107-14.
3. Epstein NE. Laminectomy for cervical myelopathy. Spinal Cord. 2003;41:317-27.
4. An HS, Ahn NU. Posterior decompressive procedures for the cervical spine. Instr Course Lect. 2003;52:471-7.
5. Epstein N. Posterior approaches in the management of cervical spondylosis and ossification of the posterior longitudinal ligament. Surg Neurol. 2002;58(3-4): 194-207; discussion 207-8.
6. Benzel EC, Lancon J, Kesterson L, et al. Cervical laminectomy and dentate ligament section for cervical spondylotic myelopathy. J Spinal Disord. 1991;4:286-95.
7. Epstein NE. Laminectomy with posterior wiring and fusion for cervical ossification of the posterior longitudinal ligament, spondylosis, ossification of the yellow ligament, stenosis, and instability: a study of 5 patients. J Spinal Disord. 1999;12: 461-6.
8. Heller JG, Edwards CC 2nd, Murakami H, et al. Laminoplasty versus laminectomy and fusion for multilevel cervical myelopathy: an independent matched cohort analysis. Spine. 2001;26:1330-36.
9. Yonenobu K, Fuji T, Ono K, et al. Choice of surgical treatment for multisegmental cervical spondylotic myelopathy. Spine. 1985;10:710-16.
10. Hamanishi C, Tanaka S. Bilateral multilevel laminectomy with or without posterolateral fusion for cervical spondylotic myelopathy: relationship to type of onset and time until operation. J Neurosurg. 1996;85:447-51.
11. Yamazaki A, Homma T, Uchiyama S, et al. Morphologic limitations of posterior decompression by midsagittal splitting method for myelopathy caused by ossification of the posterior longitudinal ligament in the cervical spine. Spine. 1999; 24: 32-4.
12. Komotar RJ, Mocco J, Kaiser MG. Surgical management of cervical myelopathy: indications and techniques for laminectomy and fusion. Spine J. 2006;6(6 Suppl): 252S-67S
13. Epstein N, Epstein JA. Treatment of cervical myelopathy: Part A. Laminectomy. In: TCSR Society (Ed). The Cervical Spine. Philadelphia: Lippincott Williams & Wilkins; 2005. pp. 1043-56.
14. Bell DF, Walker JL, O'Connor G, et al. Spinal deformity after multiple-level cervical laminectomy in children. Spine. 1994;19:406-11.
15. Deutsch H, Haid RW, Rodts GE, et al. Postlaminectomy cervical deformity. Neurosurg Focus. 2003;15:E5.

16. Yasuoka S, Peterson HA, Laws ER Jr, et al. Pathogenesis and prophylaxis of postlaminectomy deformity of the spine after multiple level laminectomy: difference between children and adults. Neurosurgery. 1981;9:145-52.
17. Yoshihara H, Yoneoka D. Trends in the treatment for traumatic central cord syndrome without bone injury in the United States from 2000 to 2009. J Trauma Acute Care Surg. 2013;75(3):453-8.
18. Horgan MA, Kellogg JX, Chesnut RM. Posterior cervical arthrodesis and stabilization: an early report using a novel lateral mass screw and rod technique. Neurosurgery. 1999;44:1267-71; discussion 1271-2
19. Errico T, Uhl R, Cooper P, Casar R, McHenry T: Pullout strength comparison of two methods of orienting screw insertion in the lateral masses of the bovine cervical spine. J Spinal Disord. 1992;5:459-63.
20. Heller JG, Carlson GD, Abitbol JJ, et al. Anatomic comparison of the Roy-Camille and Magerl techniques for screw placement in the lower cervical spine. Spine (Phila Pa 1976). 1991;(10 Suppl):S552-7.
21. Heller JG, Estes BT, Zaouali M, et al. Biomechanical study of screws in the lateral masses: variables affecting pull-out resistance. J Bone Joint Surg Am. 1996;78:1315-1321.
22. Merola AA, Castro BA, Alongi PR, et al. Anatomic consideration for standard and modified techniques of cervical lateral mass screw placement. Spine J. 2002;2: 430-35.
23. Seybold EA, Baker JA, Criscitiello AA, et al. Characteristics of unicortical and bicortical lateral mass screws in the cervical spine. Spine (Phila Pa 1976). 1999; 24:2397-2403.
24. Wellman BJ, Follett KA, Traynelis VC. Complications of posterior articular mass plate fixation of the subaxial cervical spine in 43 consecutive patients. Spine (Phila Pa 1976). 1998;23:193-200.
25. Heller JG, Silcox DH III, Sutterlin CE III. Complications of posterior cervical plating. Spine (Phila Pa 1976). 1995; 20:2442- 8.
26. Johnston TL, Karaikovic EE, Lautenschlager EP, et al. Cervical pedicle screws vs. lateral mass screws: uniplanar fatigue analysis and residual pullout strengths. Spine J. 2006;6:667-72.
27. Jones EL, Heller JG, Silcox DH, et al. Cervical pedicle screws versus lateral mass screws. Anatomic feasibility and biomechanical comparison. Spine (Phila Pa 1976). 1997; 22:977-82.
28. Abumi K, Shono Y, Ito M, et al. Complications of pedicle screw fixation in reconstructive surgery of the cervical spine. Spine (Phila Pa 1976). 2000;25:962-9.
29. Jeanneret B, Magerl F, Ward EH, et al. Posterior stabilization of the cervical spine with hook plates. Spine. 1991;16(3 Suppl):S56-63.
30. An HS, Gordin R, Renner K. Anatomic considerations for plate-screw fixation of the cervical spine. Spine. 1991;16(10 Suppl):S548-51.
31. Anderson PA, Henley MB, Grady MS, et al. Posterior cervical arthrodesis with AO reconstruction plates and bonegraft. Spine. 1991;16(3 Suppl):S72-9.
32. Abumi K, Kaneda K. Pedicle screw fixation for nontraumatic lesions of the cervical spine. Spine (Phila Pa 1976). 1997;22(16):1853-63.
33. Ludwig SC, Kowalski JM, Edwards CC 2nd, et al. Cervical pedicle screws: comparative accuracy of two insertion techniques. Spine. 2000;25:2675-81.
34. Ludwig SC, Kramer DL, Balderston RA, et al. Placement of pedicle screws in the human cadaveric cervical spine: comparative accuracy of three techniques. Spine. 2000; 25:1655-67
35. Richter M, Cakir B, Schmidt R. Cervical pedicle screws: conventional versus computer-assisted placement of cannulated screws. Spine (Phila Pa 1976). 2005; 30:2280-87.
36. Dai L, Ni B, Yuan W, et al. Radiculopathy after laminectomy for cervical compression myelopathy. J Bone Joint Surg (Br). 1998; 80: 846-9.
37. Kaptain GJ, Simmons NE, Replogle RE, et al. Incidence and outcome of kyphotic deformity following laminectomy for cervical spondylotic myelopathy. J Neurosurg (US). 2000;92(2 Suppl):199-204.
38. Kato Y, Iwasaki M, Fuji T, et al. Long-term follow- up results of laminectomy for cervical myelopathy caused by ossification of the posterior longitudinal ligament.J Neurosurg. 1998;89: 217-23.
39. Ryken TC, Heary RF, Matz PG, et al.; Joint Section on Disorders of the Spine and Peripheral Nerves of the American Association of Neurological Surgeons and Congress of Neurological Surgeons. Cervical laminectomy for the treatment of cervical degenerative myelopathy. J Neurosurg Spine. 2009;11(2):142-9.
40. Raynor RB, Pugh J, Shapiro I. Cervical facetectomy and its effect on spine strength. J Neurosurg. 1985;63:278-82.
41. Zdeblick TA, Zou D, Warden KE, et al. Cervical stability after foraminotomy: a biomechanical in vitro analysis. J Bone Joint Surg Am. 1992;74:22-7.
42. Yoshihara H, Passias PG, Errico TJ. Screw-related complications in the subaxial cervical spine with the use of lateral mass versus cervical pedicle screws: a systematic review. J Neurosurg Spine. 2013;19(5):614-23.
43. Kast E, Mohr K, Richter HP, et al. Complications of transpedicular screw fixation in the cervical spine. Eur Spine J. 2006;15:327-34.
44. Neo M, Sakamoto T, Fujibayashi S, et al. The clinical risk of vertebral artery injury from cervical pedicle screws inserted in degenerative vertebrae. Spine (Phila Pa 1976). 2005;30:2800-5.
45. Abumi K, Shono Y, Taneichi H, et al. Correction of cervical kyphosis using pedicle screw fixation systems. Spine (Phila Pa 1976). 1999;24:2389-96.
46. Yukawa Y, Kato F, Ito K, et al. Placement and complications of cervical pedicle screws in 144 cervical trauma patients using pedicle axis view techniques by fluoroscope. Eur Spine J. 2009;18:1293-9.
47. Nakashima H, Yukawa Y, Imagama S, et al. Complications of cervical pedicle screw fixation for nontraumatic lesions: a multicenter study of 84 patients. Clinical article. J Neurosurg Spine. 2012;16:238-47.

48. Yoshimoto H, Sato S, Hyakumachi T, et al. Clinical accuracy of cervical pedicle screw insertion using lateral fluoroscopy: a radiographic analysis of the learning curve. Eur Spine J. 2009;18:1326-34.
49. Yukawa Y, Kato F, Ito K, et al. Placement and complications of cervical pedicle screws in 144 cervical trauma patients using pedicle axis view techniques by fluoroscope. Eur Spine J. 2009;18:1293-9.
50. Snow RB, Weiner H. Cervical laminectomy and foraminotomy as surgical treatment of cervical spondylosis: a follow-up study with analysis of failures. J Spinal Disord. 1993;6:245-50; discussion 250-1.
51. Ebersold MJ, Pare MC, Quast LM. Surgical treatment for cervical spondylotic myelopathy. J Neurosurg. 1995;82: 745-51.
52. Adams CB, Logue V. Studies in cervical spondylotic myelopathy. 3. Some functional effects of operations for cervical spondylotic myelopathy. Brain. 1971;94: 587-94.
53. Smith-Hammond CA, New KC, Pietrobon R, et al. Prospective analysis of incidence and risk factors of dysphagia in spine surgery patients: comparison of anterior cervical, posterior cervical, and lumbar procedures. Spine. 2004;29: 1441-6.
54. An HS, Ahn NU. Posterior decompressive procedures for the cervical spine. Instr Course Lect. 2003;52:471-7.
55. Yonenobu K, Fuji T, Ono K, et al. Choice of surgical treatment for multisegmental cervical spondylotic myelopathy. Spine. 1985;10:710-16.
56. Huang RC, Girardi FP, Poynton AR, et al. Treatment of multilevel cervical spondylotic myeloradiculopathy with posterior decompression and fusion with lateral mass plate fixation and local bone graft. J Spinal Disord Tech. 2003; 16:123-9.
57. Lee SE, Chung CK, Jahng TA, et al. Long-term outcome of laminectomy for cervical ossification of the posterior longitudinal ligament. J Neurosurg Spine. 2013; 18(5):465-71.
58. Carol MP, Ducker TB. Cervical spondylotic myelopathies: surgical treatment. J Spinal Disord. 1988;1(1):59-65.
59. Anderson PA, Matz PG, Groff MW, et al.; Joint Section on Disorders of the Spine and Peripheral Nerves of the American Association of Neurological Surgeons and Congress of Neurological Surgeons. Laminectomy and fusion for the treatment of cervical degenerative myelopathy. J Neurosurg Spine. 2009;11(2):150-6.
60. Kumar VG, Rea GL, Mervis LJ, et al. Cervical spondylotic myelopathy: functional and radiographic long-term outcome after laminectomy and posterior fusion. Neurosurgery. 1999;44:771-7; discussion 777-8.
61. Morio Y, Yamamoto K, Teshima R, et al. Clinicoradiologic study of cervical laminoplasty with posterolateral fusion or bone graft. Spine. 2000;25:190-96.
62. González-Feria L, Peraita-Peraita P. Cervical spondylotic myelopathy: a cooperative study. Clin Neurol Neurosurg. 1975;78(1):19-33.
63. Yoon ST, Hashimoto RE, Raich A, et al. Outcomes after laminoplasty compared with laminectomy and fusion in patients with cervical myelopathy: a systematic review. Spine (Phila Pa 1976). 2013;38(22 Suppl 1):S183-94.
64. Hamanishi C, Tanaka S. Bilateral multilevel laminectomy with or without posterolateral fusion for cervical spondylotic myelopathy: relationship to type of onset and time until operation. J Neurosurg. 1996;85(3):447-51.
65. Perez-Lopez C, Isla A, Alvarez F, et al. [Efficacy of arthrodesis in the posterior approach of cervical myelopathy: comparative study of a series of 36 cases.] Neurocirugia (Astur). 2001;12:316-24.

Chapter 18

# Cervical Laminoplasty: Techniques and Outcomes

*John A Buza III, Themistocles S Protopsaltis*

## INTRODUCTION

Cervical laminoplasty is a posterior spinal procedure in which the laminae are repositioned or reshaped without intersegmental fusion in order to increase the volume of the spinal canal. Laminoplasty is used for the treatment of cervical spondylotic myelopathy, which is most commonly caused by cervical spondylosis or ossification of the posterior longitudinal ligament (OPLL), resulting in significant narrowing of the spinal canal. A number of techniques have traditionally been used to treat cervical spondylosis or OPLL leading to cervical spondylotic myelopathy, including anterior decompression with or without fusion, multilevel corpectomy, laminectomy with or without fusion, and laminoplasty.

Laminoplasty was developed in Japan in the 1970s to address many of the complications related to laminectomy alone. The earliest outcomes of the surgical treatment of cervical spondylosis with wide laminectomy and section of the dentate ligament were very poor.[1] In 1956, Clarke and Robinson described four different types of laminectomy: laminectomy alone, laminectomy with section of the dentate ligaments, laminectomy with removal of disk material, and laminectomy with opening of the dura for inspection and closure; none of them demonstrated satisfactory results.[2] Given the poor results with early outcomes of laminectomy, spinal surgeons were forced to search for alternatives. In the United States, Smith and Robinson developed an anterior approach to the cervical spine, which was believed to have less morbidity than laminectomy and safer removal of the degenerated disk without violating the spinal cord.[3,4] Early studies of the anterior approach in the 1970s demonstrated favorable outcomes, and the anterior approach was adopted as the first line option throughout the United States and Europe.[5]

While these advancements were encouraging, Japanese surgeons found that the primary cause of cervical myelopathy in their patient population was OPLL, thereby limiting the utility of the anterior approach. This forced Japanese surgeons to continue to refine the posterior approach. Perhaps the biggest advancement in this regard was the development of the high-speed drill in Japan, allowing safer and more precise decompression of the cervical spine. Laminoplasty was first described by Oyama and Hattori in 1972, and was primarily designed to prevent the formation of the post-laminectomy membrane.[6] In this technique, the spinous processes were first removed, and then a significant amount of the dorsal cortical bone including the medial one-third of the pedicle was removed. A Z-shape was incised in the thinned lamina, the laminae were lifted as a unit, and silk sutures were placed to maintain their position (Fig. 18.1). This technique did not become popular due to its technical complexity. In 1977, Hirabayashi et al. developed the simpler technique of expansive "open-door" laminoplasty, in which a unilateral laminar hinge is created and maintained to expand the canal.[7] Itoh et al. further modified this technique by using a bone block to stabilize the lifted

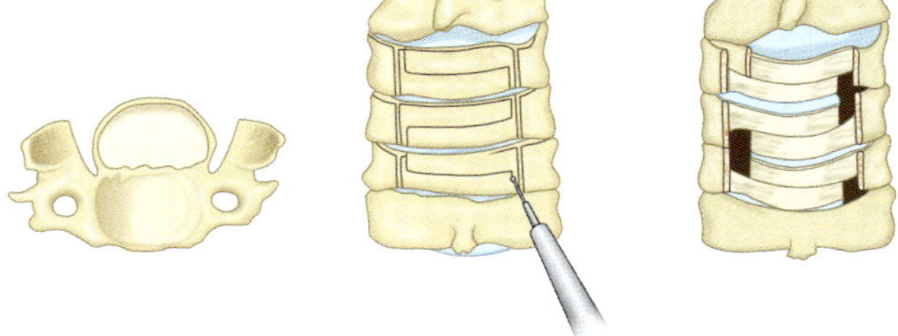

**Fig. 18.1:** Hattori's method. The spinous processes are first removed, and then a significant amount of the dorsal cortical bone including the medial one-third of the pedicle is removed. A Z-shape was incised in the thinned lamina, the lamina were lifted as a unit, and silk sutures were placed to maintain their position. *Source*: Redrawn from Kawai S, Sunago K, Doi K, Saika M, Taguchi T. Cervical laminoplasty (Hattori's method). Procedure and follow-up results. Spine. Nov 1988;13(11):1245-50.

lamina, which is referred to as "en bloc laminoplasty."[8] In 1980, Kurokawa et al. developed "double-door" laminoplasty, in which the spinous processes are split in the midline (similar to a French door) and maintained with suture or small bone grafts.[9] While there are numerous modifications of these techniques, the open-door and double-door laminoplasties are generally regarded as the two main types of procedures used today.

## CERVICAL SPONDYLOSIS

A thorough understanding of the anatomy, pathology, biomechanics, clinical presentation, and radiographic evaluation of cervical spondylosis is essential for the proper management of patients with this condition. While this was covered in depth in earlier chapters, a few key points are pertinent to review prior to discussion of cervical laminoplasty. Cervical spondylosis is the most common progressive disorder of the aging cervical spine, and is the result of degeneration of the intervertebral disks and facet joints of the cervical spine.[10-12] Spondylosis is therefore a natural process of aging; it occurs in 10% of individuals by the age of 25 years and 95% of individuals by the age of 65 years.[13] However, only a small portion of patients with spondylosis develop cervical myelopathy.[13]

In any patient with suspected cervical myelopathy, the diagnostic workup should include cervical radiographs, computed tomography (CT), and magnetic resonance imaging (MRI). Cervical X-rays should include anteroposterior (AP), lateral, oblique, and flexion-extension views; it is important to evaluate for kyphosis, subluxations, loss of disk height, foraminal osteophytes, or autofusions of adjacent segments.[10,12-14] On the lateral radiograph, local kyphosis exceeding 13° is a significant risk factor for poor postoperative prognosis.[15] If kyphosis >13° is detected, fusion should be considered.[15] One important parameter to calculate on the lateral radiograph is the Torg-Pavlov ratio, which is the size of the canal divided by the size of the vertebral body. This is measured by taking the distance between the posterior vertebral body line and the spinolaminar line, and dividing by the distance between the anterior vertebral body line and posterior body line (Fig. 18.2). The normal value is >1.0, and stenosis is typically defined by a ratio ≤0.82. Flexion-extension lateral radiographs are also obtained to assess for any significant instability. After obtaining radiographs, CT scan can help to better define the size and shape of the spinal canal, facet, uncovertebral joints, and transverse foramina. Computed tomography scan is arguably the best imaging modality to assess bone quality.[13] Magnetic resonance imaging is most useful in evaluating the spinal cord, spinal canal diameter, intervertebral disks, and vertebral ligaments.[10,12-14,16-18] Abnormal signal within the spinal cord on preoperative MRI is associated with poor postoperative outcome scores.[19] Several MRI measurements also have prognostic importance. The transverse area of the spinal cord at the maximal level of compression has been shown to relate to postoperative outcomes. Yamazaki et al. found that areas of 42 mm² correlated with excellent outcomes and areas of 31 mm² correlated with good outcomes using the Japanese Orthopedic Association score system.[20] The compression ratio should also be measured, defined as the smallest sagittal cord diameter divided by the largest transverse cord diameter, is associated with a poor prognosis when the value is <0.4. In addition to imaging studies, other studies including electromyography, nerve conduction studies, and somatosensory evoked potentials may also help delineate the nature and severity of the radiculopathy or myelopathy.

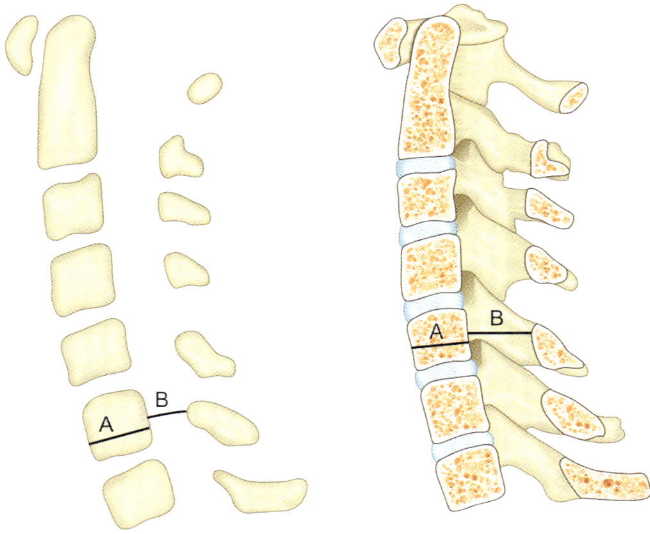


**Fig. 18.2:** The Torg-Pavlov ratio is the size of the canal divided by the size of the vertebral body. This is measured by taking the distance between the posterior vertebral body line and the spinolaminar line, and dividing by the distance between the anterior vertebral body line and posterior body line.
*Source*: Redrawn from Boxell CM, et al. Cervical laminoplasty: indications and techniques. In: Quinones-Hinojosa A (Ed). Schmidek and Sweet's Operative Neurosurgical Techniques. Philadelphia: Elsevier; 2012.

The pathogenesis of cervical spondylosis has implications for its treatment and the use of laminoplasty. The

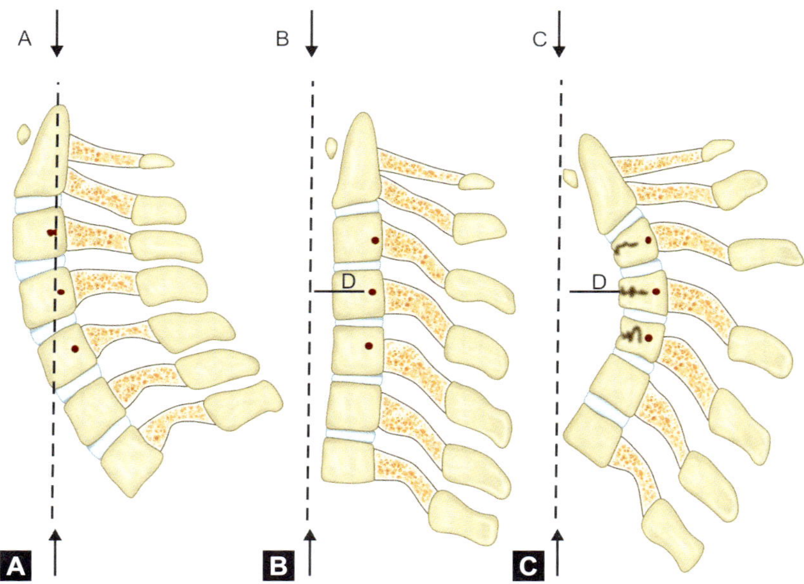


**Figs. 18.3A to C:** (A) Normal cervical lordosis; the dorsal vertebral body height is less than the ventral vertebral body height. (B) Loss of lordosis caused by loss of ventral disk interspace height, which occurs with the natural degenerative process. (C) Cervical kyphosis; further exaggeration of this deformity leads to ventral vertebral body compression.
*Source*: Redrawn from Benzel EC. Biomechanics of Spine Stabilization. Rolling Meadows, IL: American Association of Neurological Surgeons Publications; 2001.

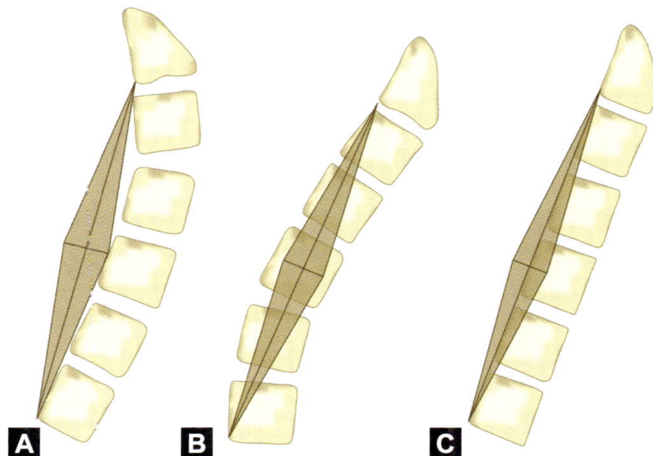

**Figs. 18.4A to C:** A line is drawn from the dorsocaudal aspect of the vertebral body of C2 to the dorsocaudal aspect of the vertebral body of C7. (A) Midsagittal section of the cervical spine demonstrating lordotic posture. (B) Midsagittal section in effective cervical kyphosis. (C) A "straightened" cervical spine.
*Source*: Redrawn from Benzel EC. Biomechanics of Spine Stabilization. Rolling Meadows, IL: American Association of Neurological Surgeons Publications; 2001.

reduction in sagittal spinal canal diameter that leads to cervical spondylosis begins with cervical disk desiccation.[12] As the nucleus pulposus begins to lose elasticity and becomes more fibrous, the annulus fibrosus takes more of the responsibility for weight bearing and may bulge into the spinal canal.[12,21-24] Importantly, this loss of disk height occurs ventrally and leads to a gradual loss of cervical lordosis until a kyphotic deformity exists (Figs. 18.3A to C).[21] Narrowing of the spinal canal may then be the result of a number of pathologic changes, including bulging or herniated nucleated disks, thickened laminae, thickened or buckling ligamentum flavum, thickened posterior longitudinal ligament, degenerative and hypertrophied facet joints, and degenerative uncovertebral joints.[12,23,25-27] One important aspect of this pathologic process is that the spinal cord may become tethered in both the sagittal and coronal planes. In the sagittal plane, an "effective kyphosis" may lead to both elongation and distortion of the spinal cord as it is tethered over the kyphosis (sagittal bowstring effect).[12,17,21,28] To help determine the configuration of the cervical spine, a line may be drawn from the dorsocaudal aspect of the vertebral body of C2 to the dorsocaudal aspect of the vertebral body of C7 (Figs. 18.4A to C). An "effective kyphosis" is identified when no part of the dorsal aspect of any of the vertebral bodies from C3 to C7 crosses this line. The spinal cord may also be tethered in the coronal plane by the dentate ligaments or nerve roots, known as the coronal bowstring effect (Figs. 18.5A to C).

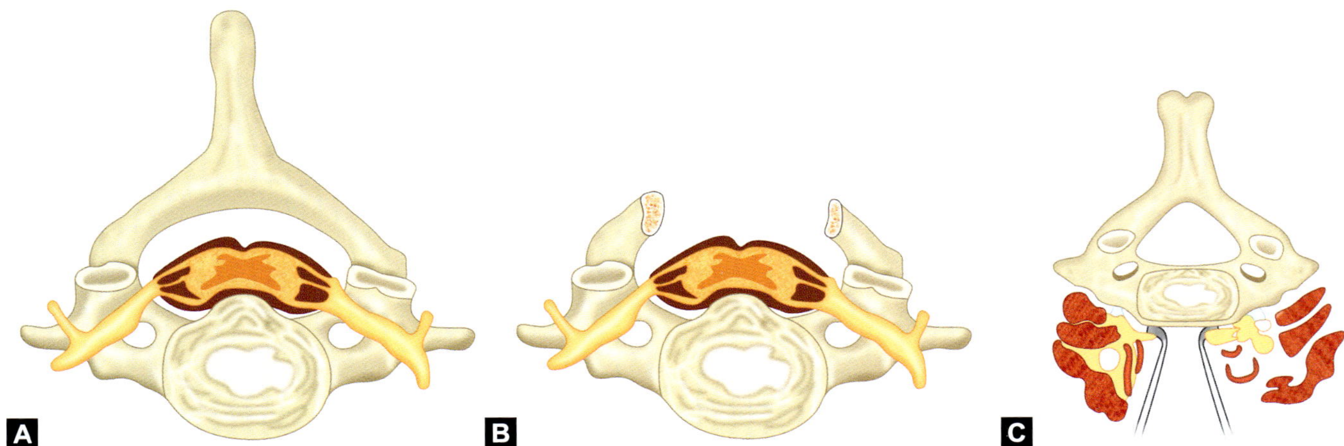


**Figs. 18.5A to C:** (A) Coronal plane tethering occurs when either the nerve roots or the dentate ligaments tether the spinal cord in the coronal plane. (B) Laminectomy does not help to relieve the distortion. (C) Ventral decompression helps to relieve this distortion. *Source*: Redrawn from Benzel EC. Biomechanics of Spine Stabilization. Rolling Meadows, IL: American Association of Neurological Surgeons Publications; 2001.

Both the sagittal and coronal bowstring effects are critical when considering surgical options for cervical spondylotic myelopathy, as dorsal decompression procedures (i.e. laminectomy) may worsen the deformity. This bowstring effect also has important implications for the use of laminoplasty, which theoretically works by allowing the spinal cord to shift posteriorly into the augmented space.

## INDICATIONS AND CONTRAINDICATIONS

The surgical options for decompression of the cervical spine in cervical spondylotic myelopathy include anterior decompression and fusion, laminectomy with or without posterior fusion, and cervical laminoplasty. The procedure of choice depends on a number of factors, including the number of vertebral segments involved, the source and location of compression, cervical alignment, and surgeon experience with the procedure. The first decision is typically whether to perform an anterior or posterior procedure. An anterior procedure is generally used in the presence of anterior compressive factors that are limited to one or two vertebral levels. Anterior decompression allows direct removal of the anterior compressive abnormality and fusion with the use of bone graft with or without instrumentation. Studies have reported up to 92% good to excellent results with this approach.[29] However, there are disadvantages to this approach as well, including adjacent segment degeneration, fusion rates, graft healing, and approach-related complications including dysphagia, recurrent laryngeal nerve injury, carotid sheath injury, or esophageal injury.[30-34] As reported by Hilibrand et al., the long-term risk of adjacent level disease following anterior fusion surgery may be as high as 25%.[32] The rate of pseudarthrosis increases with each segmental level added to an anterior decompression and fusion.[35] For this reason, most surgeons prefer to perform an anterior decompression when only one or two levels are involved, and there is a high rate of neurological improvement and predictable solid fusion.

Historically, laminectomy without fusion was used to decompress cervical stenosis when multiple levels were involved. The major complication of this technique was the development of postlaminectomy kyphosis secondary to iatrogenic destabilization of the cervical spine. Biomechanical studies of the cervical spine have demonstrated that up to 64% of load transmission occurs through the posterior column, including the facet joints and articular processes.[36] Loss of this posterior arch can result in significant instability, which may result in an anterior shift of the weight-bearing axis.[37] The kyphosis that results from this shift causes most weight to be borne by the anterior vertebral bodies and disks, which leads to worsening degeneration and spondylosis.[38,39] Instability may be prevented by posterior cervical fusion with instrumentation, but complications including failure of fusion, loss of fixation, and adjacent segment degeneration have all been reported despite this modification.[39]

The problem of postoperative kyphosis following laminectomy prompted the development of laminoplasty, which attempts to maintain postoperative stability by retaining the bulk of the posterior elements. The primary goals of laminoplasty are to expand the spinal canal, prevent the formation of the post-laminectomy membrane, and preserve the posterior structure of the cervical spine to attain stability. The two main indications for laminoplasty include OPLL and multilevel cervical spondylosis involving three or more motion segments. Relative indications include patients with recurrent myelopathy following prior ACDF procedure, and patients with increased risk for nonunion, including smokers and those with metabolic bone disease. Contraindications include a significant kyphotic deformity and one- or two-level disease. This is due to the fact that the procedure relies on the free migration of the spinal cord away from the ventral compressive structures, which has been demonstrated using postoperative CT scan.[40,41] The presence of a neutral or lordotic alignment is not a prerequisite for performing laminoplasty, however. Suda et al. recommended that patients with cervical kyphosis up to 13° may still benefit from laminoplasty so long as there are no cord signal changes on T2 MRI.[15] If there are cord changes on T2 MRI, then the upper limit of acceptable kyphosis is <5°.[15] Relative contraindications to perform laminoplasty include epidural fibrosis, large OPLL lesions occupying >50–60% of the AP canal diameter, and axial neck pain as the patient's chief complaint.

## LAMINOPLASTY TECHNIQUES

A variety of laminoplasty techniques have been described in the literature. All techniques are similar in that they expand the cervical canal and preserve some or all of the posterior elements. While there are many modifications, all techniques can be grouped into one of two main types of procedures. The first is the Hirabayashi or "open-door" laminoplasty, in which one side of the lamina, along with the spinous process and ligamentum flavum, is hinged open. The second is the Kurokawa or "double-door" laminoplasty, in which a midline opening is created and the left and right hemi-laminae hinge open bilaterally. There are modifications of these two major techniques, which will be discussed further below. A third technique, known as "en bloc" laminoplasty, involves complete removal of the lamina followed by reconstruction of the lamina. This will be discussed below as well.

## PATIENT POSITIONING AND PREPARATION

The patient is placed in the supine position with the neck minimally extended for endotracheal intubation. In patients with severe spinal cord compression, awake fiberoptic intubation may be performed to decrease the risk of spinal cord injury. Many surgeons use neurophysiological monitoring such as somatosensory evoked potentials and motor evoked potentials, although there is still some debate as to whether or not this information actually improves safety and patient outcomes. Prepositioning baseline neuromonitoring signals can be obtained; however, in many cases of advanced myelopathy, these signals are absent or unreliable. In these cases, the surgeon may also choose to perform a wake-up test after positioning in the prone position, especially if neuromonitoring signals are absent at baseline. Use of a Mayfield three-pin head vise aids in control of the head and neck in positioning and is optimal for maintaining cervical alignment in a neutral position. The Mayfield vise allows the surgeon to easily control the degree of flexion or extension, and has the added benefit of reducing pressure on the patient's eyes. The Jackson cradle or an Amsco table with chest rolls can be utilized to lower venous pressure by elevating the thoracic cage and decompressing the abdomen, which diminishes operative blood loss. The superolateral aspects of both shoulders are taped to the caudal aspect of the operating table to assist with radiographic visualization of the lower cervical levels intraoperatively. Of note, untaping the shoulders at the end of the procedure facilitates closure. After prepping and draping the surgical site in usual sterile fashion, the midline may be infiltrated with 1% lidocaine with epinephrine to minimize skin bleeding.

## SURGICAL APPROACH

A standard midline incision is used, dissecting down to the fascia using either monopolar or bipolar electrocautery to control bleeding. The fascia is incised with monopolar cautery. At this point, the surgeon may choose to either perform a standard bilateral subperiosteal dissection or a posterior element sparing approach. In the standard approach, the subperiosteal dissection is used to reflect the soft tissue structures off of the spinous processes, lamina, and medial aspects of the facets bilaterally. Great care should be taken during this aspect of the procedure to avoid damaging the facet capsules bilaterally. The dissection should be limited to the lamina that needs to be included in the laminoplasty. When possible, a laminoplasty limited to the C4-C6 levels should be performed as some studies show that this better maintains the muscular attachments to C2 and C7, which helps to minimize neck pain and maintain cervical alignment. The caudal one-third of the lamina above the highest level of the laminoplasty can be excised in a "dome laminectomy." The spinous processes of each level of the laminoplasty are cut approximately 5 mm from the base of the lamina. The spinous processes of C7 and C6 (when substantial enough) can be utilized as structural autograft for the reconstructed lamina. The remaining smaller spinous processes are morselized for subsequent autografting in the hinges of the lamina.

## OPEN-DOOR LAMINOPLASTY

Creation of an open-door laminoplasty involves making bone cuts at the junction of the lamina and facet complex bilaterally. On one side, a bicortical cut is performed along each lamina. This side will act as the "door" that can swing open. The bicortical cut is performed using a high-speed air drill; drilling proceeds through both the outer and inner cortical margin at the lamina facet junction, aiming medially toward the dura and away from the facet joints. On the contralateral side to the bicortical or "door" side, the "hinge" is created through which the door will swing open. The surgeon chooses which side will be the "open" side and which will be the "hinge" side, but as a rule of thumb, the side with the most compression or the most clinically symptomatic side should be the "open" side. If a foraminotomy is necessary, this is best performed on the open-door side.

Creation of the hinge is a crucial step in open-door laminoplasty. A high-speed air drill with a small burr should be used to drill through the outer cortex and cancellous bone at the lamina-facet junction, leaving the inner cortex intact. Care must be taken not to thin the inner cortex to the point where it fractures. Proper thinning of the laminar bone should create a spring-like resistance to deformation. However, if too little bone is drilled, this can lead to fracture if the hinge is forced open prematurely. If the contralateral bicortical "open" door is created first, the surgeon may test the hinge with gentle finger pressure. The inner cortex should be carefully thinned until gentle finger pressure opens the laminoplasty segment. In order to "open the door," the ligamentum flavum must be removed along the length of the open door (usually with a Kerrison punch). Two small curettes are advanced into the gap and the door is slowly opened, resulting in a green-stick "fracture" through the hinged side. The lamina should be moved as one unit in order to preserve the intraspinous ligaments and midline ligamentum flavum, both of which act as dorsal stabilizing structures. The AP diameter of the canal should be increased by approximately 4 mm, and then can be held open with a variety of techniques, including sutures, allograft spacers, and instrumentation with the use of specialized open-door laminoplasty plates.

## DOUBLE-DOOR OR "FRENCH DOOR" LAMINOPLASTY

Creation of a double-door laminoplasty involves making bilateral hinges at the junction of the lamina and facet complex bilaterally. A high-speed air drill with a matchstick neuro-soft-touch tip is utilized to create a midline trough through the lamina. The combination of the soft-touch burr tip and brisk progress with the burr minimizes risk to the dura. The caudal portion of the lamina is protected by the ligamentum flavum, so caution should be applied at the cephalad portion of the lamina. A craniotome with a footplate can also be utilized for the midline lamina cut as an alternative. The soft-touch burr is utilized along the outer cortical margin at the lamina facet junction, aiming medially toward the dura and away from the facet joints on both sides and leaving the inner cortex intact. Care must be taken not to thin the inner cortex to the point where it fractures. Proper thinning of the laminar bone should create a spring-like resistance to deformation. However, if too little bone is drilled, this can lead to fracture if the hinge is forced open prematurely. The inner cortex should be carefully thinned until gentle finger pressure opens the laminoplasty segment. In order to open the double door, the ligamentum flavum must be removed caudal and cephalad to the laminoplasty with a Kerrison punch. Two small curettes are advanced into the gap and the door is slowly opened, resulting in a green-stick "fracture" on each side of the lamina. The lamina should be moved as one unit in order to preserve the intraspinous ligaments and midline ligamentum flavum, both of which act as dorsal stabilizing structures. The AP diameter of the canal should be increased by approximately 4 mm, and then can be held open with autograft and allograft spacers that can be sutured to the lamina with drill holes using 5-0 ethibond suture or specialized open-door laminoplasty plates. If a foraminotomy is necessary, it should be performed prior to creation of the hinges. Laminoplasty plates are recommended wherever a foraminotomy is performed since the size of the hinged lamina will be small.

## OUTCOMES

The results of cervical laminoplasty have proven to be similar to anterior discectomy and fusion, laminectomy, and laminectomy with fusion in patient functional outcome measures.[27,42-46] No single laminoplasty technique has proven to be superior to any other.[47-49] The Japanese Orthopaedic Association score is the most common scoring system used to compare preoperative and postoperative outcomes for cervical laminoplasty, and most authors use this scoring system to calculate a mean recovery rate.[50] A literature review found that a mean recovery rate of roughly 55% (ranging anywhere from 20% to 80%) can be expected following cervical laminoplasty, and that roughly 80% of patients will see improvement of scores following cervical laminoplasty.[51] Again, there does not appear to be a significant difference in recovery rate when comparing open-door and double-door laminoplasty techniques.[52]

In addition to recovery rate, postoperative cervical alignment and range of motion are frequently reported outcome measures. It has been reported that worsening spinal alignment occurs in 22% to 53% of patients after undergoing laminoplasty.[6,19,45,53-57] Unfortunately, no specific technique can prevent the development of some degree of kyphosis after laminoplasty. Additionally, the laminoplasty technique will not restore lordosis in an already kyphotic spine. There is evidence to suggest that modern instrumentation techniques may lead to improved preservation of lordosis.[58] In addition to worsening spinal alignment, laminoplasty is associated with an aggregate loss of approximately 50% range of motion as reported in the literature.[52] This loss of range of motion may not be clinically relevant, however, as several authors have noted that it is in fact beneficial. One theory is that a loss of range of motion will limit dynamic factors that are thought to contribute to myelopathy.[54] Other authors have advocated for the importance of maintaining postoperative range of motion, arguing that it will decrease axial neck pain after laminoplasty and prevent adjacent segment cervical disease.[59]

## COMPLICATIONS

Complications after laminoplasty are similar to those after laminectomy and include wound complications, postoperative axial neck pain, reduced range of motion, canal restenosis, motor nerve root palsy, and the loss of cervical lordosis. Two complications that are particularly common after laminoplasty are C5 nerve root palsies and axial neck pain. The mean rate of clinically evident C5 nerve root palsy has been estimated to be approximately 8% after laminoplasty and does not vary with the laminoplasty technique.[51] Although the mechanism of C5 palsy is controversial, it is presumably due to a tethering effect on the nerve root near the apex of the lordosis that is induced by excessive posterior cord shift after decompression.[60] While many cases of C5 nerve palsy resolve spontaneously, a subset of patients have continued radiculopathy at long-term follow-up.[51,61]

Axial neck pain is a common patient complaint after laminoplasty but is not consistently reported in the literature. An estimated incidence varies from 6% to 60% and may vary based on surgical technique, the time at which neck pain is reported after surgery, or the surgeon's personal assessment of what constitutes neck pain.[52] Axial neck pain following laminoplasty may be due to surgical dissection around the facet joints. While axial neck pain begins shortly after surgery, it usually resolves after 1 year. Nonsteroidal anti-inflammatory medications and cervical stretching have been suggested to help alleviate this pain, although they have never been proven.[52]

## CONCLUSION

Cervical laminoplasty is a posterior spinal procedure in which the laminae are repositioned or reshaped without intersegmental fusion in order to increase the volume of the spinal canal. Laminoplasty is used for the treatment of cervical spondylotic myelopathy, which is most commonly caused by cervical spondylosis or OPLL. A thorough understanding of these disease processes is essential for the proper management of patients with this condition. A variety of laminoplasty techniques have been described in the literature, but all of them can be grouped into one of two main types of procedures. The first is the Hirabayashi or "open-door" laminoplasty, in which one side of the lamina, along with the spinous process and ligamentum flavum, is hinged open. The second is the Kurokawa or "double-door" laminoplasty, in which a midline opening is created and the left and right hemilaminae hinge open bilaterally. A mean recovery rate of roughly 55% can be expected following cervical laminoplasty, and roughly 80% of patients will see improvement of outcome scores following cervical laminoplasty. While complications are similar to those following laminectomy, C5 nerve root palsy and axial neck pain are particularly common after laminoplasty and must be discussed with the patient prior to surgery.

## REFERENCES


1. Yuhl ET, Hanna D, Rasmussen T, et al. Diagnosis and surgical therapy of chronic midline cervical disk protrusions. Neurology. 1955;5(7):494-509.
2. Clarke E, Robinson PK. Cervical myelopathy: a complication of cervical spondylosis. Brain. 1956;79(3):483-510.
3. Robinson RA, Smith G. Anterolateral cervical disc removal and interbody fusion for cervical disc syndrome. Bull Johns Hopkins Med J. 1955;96:223-4.
4. Smith GW, Robinson RA. The treatment of certain cervical-spine disorders by anterior removal of the intervertebral disc and interbody fusion. J Bone Joint Surg Am. 1958;40-A(3):607-24.
5. Bohlman H. Cervical spondylosis with moderate to severe myelopathy: a report of seventeen cases treated by Robinson anterior cervical discectomy and fusion. Spine. 1977;2:151.
6. Kawai S, Sunago K, Doi K, et al. Cervical laminoplasty (Hattori's method). Procedure and follow-up results. Spine. 1988;13(11):1245-50.
7. Hirabayashi K, Watanabe K, Wakano K, et al. Expansive open-door laminoplasty for cervical spinal stenotic myelopathy. Spine. 1983;8(7):693-9.
8. Itoh T, Tsuji H. Technical improvements and results of laminoplasty for compressive myelopathy in the cervical spine. Spine. 1985;10(8):729-36.
9. Kurokawa T, Tsuyama N, Tanaka H, et al. Enlargement of the spinal canal by the sagittal splitting of the spinous process. (In Japanese). Bessatsu Seikeigeka. 1982;2:234-40.
10. Crandall PH, Batzdorf U. Cervical spondylotic myelopathy. J Neurosurg. 1966;25 (1):57-66.
11. Ebersold MJ, Pare MC, Quast LM. Surgical treatment for cervical spondylitic myelopathy. J Neurosurg. 1995; 82 (5):745-51.
12. Ferguson RJ, Caplan LR. Cervical spondylitic myelopathy. Neurol Clin. 1985;3 (2):373-82.
13. Garfin SR. Cervical degenerative disorders: etiology, presentation, and imaging studies. Instr Course Lect. 2000; 49:335-8.
14. Alker G. Neuroradiology of cervical spondylotic myelopathy. Spine. 1988;13(7): 850-53.
15. Suda K, Abumi K, Ito M, et al. Local kyphosis reduces surgical outcomes of expansive open-door laminoplasty for cervical spondylotic myelopathy. Spine. 2003; 28(12):1258-62.
16. Arnasson O, Carlsson CA, Pellettieri L. Surgical and conservative treatment of cervical spondylotic radiculopathy and myelopathy. Acta Neurochirurgica. 1987;84(1-2):48-53.
17. Fager CA. Results of adequate posterior decompression in the relief of spondylotic cervical myelopathy. J Neurosurg. 1973;38(6):684-92.
18. McCormick WE, Steinmetz MP, Benzel EC. Cervical spondylotic myelopathy: make the difficult diagnosis, then refer for surgery. Cleveland Clinic J Med. 2003;70(10): 899-904.
19. Mochida J, Nomura T, Chiba M, et al. Modified expansive open-door laminoplasty in cervical myelopathy. J Spinal Disord. 1999;12(5):386-91.
20. Yamazaki T, Yanaka K, Sato H, et al. Cervical spondylotic myelopathy: surgical results and factors affecting outcome with special reference to age differences. Neurosurgery. 2003;52(1):122-26; discussion 126.
21. Benzel EC. Biomechanics of Spine Stabilization. Rolling Meadows, IL: American Association of Neurological Surgeons Publications; 2001.
22. Emery SE. Cervical spondylotic myelopathy: diagnosis and treatment. J Amer Acad Orthop Surg. 2001;9(6):376-88.
23. Saunders RL, Wilson DH. The surgery of cervical disk disease: new perspectives. Clin Orthop Rel Res. 1980(146):119-27.
24. Verbiest H. The management of cervical spondylosis. Clin Neurosurg. 1973;20: 262-94.
25. Epstein JA, Epstein BS, Lavine LS, et al. Cervical myeloradiculopathy caused by arthrotic hypertrophy of the posterior facets and laminae. J Neurosurg. 1978;49 (3):387-92.
26. Hirabayashi K, Bohlman HH. Multilevel cervical spondylosis. Laminoplasty versus anterior decompression. Spine. 1995;20(15):1732-34.
27. White AA, 3rd, Panjabi MM. Biomechanical considerations in the surgical management of cervical spondylotic myelopathy. Spine. 1988;13(7):856-60.
28. Fager CA. Reversal of cervical myelopathy by adequate posterior decompression. Lahey Clinic Found Bull. 1969;18 (3):99-108.
29. Herkowitz HN. A comparison of anterior cervical fusion, cervical laminectomy, and cervical laminoplasty for the surgical management of multiple level spondylotic radiculopathy. Spine. 1988;13(7):774-80.
30. Emery SE, Bohlman HH, Bolesta MJ, et al. Anterior cervical decompression and arthrodesis for the treatment of cervical spondylotic myelopathy. Two to seventeen-year follow-up. J Bone Joint Surg. 1998;80(7):941-51.
31. Mayr MT, Subach BR, Comey CH, et al. Cervical spinal stenosis: outcome after anterior corpectomy, allograft reconstruction, and instrumentation. J Neurosurg. 2002;96 (1 Suppl):10-6.
32. Hilibrand AS, Carlson GD, Palumbo MA, et al. Radiculopathy and myelopathy at segments adjacent to the site of a previous anterior cervical arthrodesis. J Bone Joint Surg. 1999;81(4):519-28.
33. Flynn TB. Neurologic complications of anterior cervical interbody fusion. Spine. 1982;7(6):536-39.
34. Riew KD, Sethi NS, Devney J, et al. Complications of buttress plate stabilization of cervical corpectomy. Spine. 1999;24(22):2404-10.
35. Farey ID, McAfee PC, Davis RF, et al. Pseudarthrosis of the cervical spine after anterior arthrodesis. Treatment by posterior nerve-root decompression, stabilization, and arthrodesis. J Bone Joint Surg. 1990;72(8):1171-77.
36. Pal GP, Sherk HH. The vertical stability of the cervical spine. Spine. 1988;13(5):447-49.
37. Raynor RB, Moskovich R, Zidel P, et al. Alterations in primary and coupled neck motions after facetectomy. Neurosurgery. 1987;21(5):681-87.
38. Albert TJ, Vacarro A. Postlaminectomy kyphosis. Spine. 1998;23(24):2738-45.

39. Houten JK, Cooper PR. Laminectomy and posterior cervical plating for multilevel cervical spondylotic myelopathy and ossification of the posterior longitudinal ligament: effects on cervical alignment, spinal cord compression, and neurological outcome. Neurosurgery. 2003;52(5):1081-87; discussion 1087-88.
40. Aita I, Hayashi K, Wadano Y, et al. Posterior movement and enlargement of the spinal cord after cervical laminoplasty. J Bone Joint Surg. 1998;80(1):33-7.
41. Sodeyama T, Goto S, Mochizuki M, et al. Effect of decompression enlargement laminoplasty for posterior shifting of the spinal cord. Spine. 1999;24(15):1527-31; discussion 1531-2.
42. Mummaneni PV, Kaiser MG, Matz PG, et al. Cervical surgical techniques for the treatment of cervical spondylotic myelopathy. J Neurosurg Spine. 2009;11(2):130-41.
43. Nakano N, Nakano T, Nakano K. Comparison of the results of laminectomy and open-door laminoplasty for cervical spondylotic myeloradiculopathy and ossification of the posterior longitudinal ligament. Spine. 1988;13(7):792-94.
44. Hasegawa K, Homma T, Chiba Y, et al. Effects of surgical treatment for cervical spondylotic myelopathy in patients > or = 70 years of age: a retrospective comparative study. J Spin Disor Tech. 2002;15(6):458-60.
45. Wada E, Suzuki S, Kanazawa A, et al. Subtotal corpectomy versus laminoplasty for multilevel cervical spondylotic myelopathy: a long-term follow-up study over 10 years. Spine. 2001;26(13):1443-47; discussion 1448.
46. Yoshida M, Tamaki T, Kawakami M, et al. Indication and clinical results of laminoplasty for cervical myelopathy caused by disc herniation with developmental canal stenosis. Spine. 1998;23(22):2391-97.
47. Edwards CC, 2nd, Heller JG, Murakami H. Corpectomy versus laminoplasty for multilevel cervical myelopathy: an independent matched-cohort analysis. Spine. 2002;27(11): 1168-75.
48. Iwasaki M, Ebara S, Miyamoto S, et al. Expansive laminoplasty for cervical radiculomyelopathy due to soft disc herniation. Spine. 1996;21(1):32-8.
49. Kawakami M, Tamaki T, Iwasaki H, et al. A comparative study of surgical approaches for cervical compressive myelopathy. Clin Orthop Rel Res. 2000(381):129-36.
50. Satomi K, Nishu Y, Kohno T, et al. Long-term follow-up studies of open-door expansive laminoplasty for cervical stenotic myelopathy. Spine. 1994;19(5):507-10.
51. Ratliff JK, Cooper PR. Cervical laminoplasty: a critical review. J Neurosurg. 2003;98(3 Suppl):230-38.
52. Steinmetz MP, Resnick DK. Cervical laminoplasty. Spine J. 2006;6(6 Suppl):274S-81S.
53. Edwards CC, 2nd, Heller JG, Silcox DH, 3rd. T-Saw laminoplasty for the management of cervical spondylotic myelopathy: clinical and radiographic outcome. Spine. 2000;25(14):1788-94.
54. Kimura I, Shingu H, Nasu Y. Long-term follow-up of cervical spondylotic myelopathy treated by canal-expansive laminoplasty. J Bone Joint Surg. 1995;77(6): 956-61.
55. Lee TT, Manzano GR, Green BA. Modified open-door cervical expansive laminoplasty for spondylotic myelopathy: operative technique, outcome, and predictors for gait improvement. J Neurosurg. 1997;86(1):64-8.
56. Yonenobu K, Hosono N, Iwasaki M, et al. Laminoplasty versus subtotal corpectomy. A comparative study of results in multisegmental cervical spondylotic myelopathy. Spine. 1992;17(11):1281-84.
57. Matsunaga S, Sakou T, Nakanisi K. Analysis of the cervical spine alignment following laminoplasty and laminectomy. Spinal Cord. 1999;37(1):20-4.
58. O'Brien MF, Peterson D, Casey AT, et al. A novel technique for laminoplasty augmentation of spinal canal area using titanium miniplate stabilization. A computerized morphometric analysis. Spine. 1996;21(4):474-83; discussion 484.
59. Shaffrey CI, Wiggins GC, Piccirilli CB, et al. Modified open-door laminoplasty for treatment of neurological deficits in younger patients with congenital spinal stenosis: analysis of clinical and radiographic data. J Neurosurg. 1999;90(2 Suppl):170-77.
60. Tsuzuki N, Abe R, Saiki K, et al. Extradural tethering effect as one mechanism of radiculopathy complicating posterior decompression of the cervical spinal cord. Spine. 1996;21(2):203-11.
61. Kawaguchi Y, Kanamori M, Ishihara H, et al. Minimum 10-year follow-up after en bloc cervical laminoplasty. Clin Orthop Rel Res. 2003(411):129-39.

Chapter 19

# Instrumentation Techniques of the Occiput, Upper Cervical Spine, and Subaxial Spine

*Afshin E Razi, Yong Kim, Ahmed Saleh*

## INTRODUCTION

Cervical spine pathology is often multifaceted and complex. Cervical spine pathologies necessitating surgical intervention may be secondary to a wide variety of causes, including trauma, degenerative disease, inflammatory arthritidies, congenital anomalies, tumors, and infections. As with many surgical ailments, the anatomy will often dictate the patient presentation, symptoms, treatments, and operative approach.

## ANATOMY

### Surgical Anatomy

The anatomy of the cervical spine is intricate and complex. A thorough understanding of the normal anatomy of the occiput and cervical spine is of paramount importance for the surgeon to understand cervical pathology, as well as to navigate and successfully instrument the cervical spine. An understanding of the soft tissue, bony, ligamentous, vascular, and muscular anatomy will benefit the surgeon in accessing the spine in a safe manner, while addressing the pathology at hand.

#### *Occiput*

The external bony landmarks on the occiput and their muscular attachment will dictate the location, safety, strength, and effectiveness of occipital hardware. There are four bony landmarks on the occiput that are visible at the time of surgery: the posterior edge of the foramen magnum, the superior nuchal line, the inferior nuchal line, and the external occipital protuberance. The superior nuchal line provides the attachment of the sternocleidomastoid muscle and trapezius. The insertion of the rectus capitus posterior major and minor occurs at the inferior nuchal line. The attachment of the semispinalis capitus and the oblique capitus superior occurs between the superior and inferior nuchal lines. The external occipital protuberance provides the attachment site of ligamentum nuchae.[1]

Of equal importance to the surgeon is the internal bony anatomy of the occiput due to its proximity to sensitive intracranial structures. The internal bony anatomy is in large part dictated by the anatomy of the human brain. The cerebral fossae and the cerebellar fossae create a central bony point called the internal occipital protuberance, and the dura creates the venous sinus.[2] The transverse venous sinus runs in the right and left transverse sulci and merges at the level of the external occipital protuberance to form the confluence of sinuses, which extends vertically and superiorly to form the superior sagittal sulcus.[1] The confluence of sinuses is also referred to as the trocula.

Several anatomic studies have been performed to help determine the safest and most effective way to insert screws for a screw-and-rod or a screw-and-plate construct for an occipital-cervical fusion. Studies have revealed that the thickest bone in the occiput is found at the level of the external occipital protuberance, which ranges from 11.5 to 15.1 mm in males and from 9.7 to 12.0 mm in females.[3] These studies confirmed that there is a great deal of variation in the location of the sinuses, and that there is no specific anatomic landmark on the outer table that definitively predicts the safety of a bicortical screw.[4]

#### *Atlas (C1)*

The first cervical vertebra (C1) is referred to as the atlas, for its ability to support the skull. This vertebra contains no vertebral body; it is composed of an anterior arch, posterior arch, and two lateral masses. The anterior arch articulates with the axis, via a ligamentous complex and plays an integral role in the cervical spine rotation and stability. The posterior arch completes the ring of the atlas to provide spinal foramen in which the spinal cord is housed and protected by the bony anatomy. The lateral masses are composed of a large, concave, superior articulating facet bilaterally, which articulates with the base of the skull and provides a significant portion of flexion and extension of the skull.[5] Laterally located in each lateral mass is a transverse foramen, which the vertebral artery traverses through before turning posteriorly and entering foramen magnum. Medial to the transverse foramen and lateral to the spinal foramen is a large lateral mass in which hardware can be effectively and safely placed.

### *Axis (C2)*

The second cervical vertebra (C2) is referred to as the axis, for its role as a pivot point in which the atlas and the skull rotate about. Arising from the vertebral body is the odontoid process, which provides the pivot point for rotation. The odontoid process articulates anteriorly with the anterior arch of the atlas and posteriorly with the transverse ligament, which is part of the ligamentous complex imparting stability to the segment. The axis has a strong lamina and pedicles that form the spinal foramen.[5] The transverse foramen provides a passage for the vertebral artery laterally. Posteriorly the spinous process of the axis is large, bifid in structure, and serves as the insertion site of many of the posterior cervical muscles.

### *Subaxial Cervical Spine (C3-C7)*

The subaxial cervical vertebrae all have an anterior body, which is usually wider in the medial to lateral dimension than it is in the anterior to posterior dimension. Each of these vertebrae also contains a bifid spinous process up to C6, which serves as a muscular attachment site. The spinous process of the seventh cervical vertebra is not bifid, but longer and more prominent, and therefore, C7 is referred to as the vertebral prominence. Also at each level, there is a transverse foramen in which the vertebral artery traverses. At the level of C7, however, the artery usually does not pass through the foramen, but anterior to it. Posteriorly the spinal canal is protected by a long and narrow lamina. Laterally, there are the lateral masses and pedicles, which are of great importance and interest in hardware placement. The subaxial cervical pedicles are short and narrow. The lateral masses, which support the superior and inferior articulating processes, are broad and strong, with the anterior border of the lateral mass being the transverse foramen.[5]

### *Ligamentous Anatomy*

The ligamentous anatomy of the cervical spine plays an important role in the stability of the spine. The cervical vertebral bodies are connected anteriorly via the anterior longitudinal ligament and posteriorly via posterior longitudinal ligament. These ligaments are broad and thin in the anterior-to-posterior dimension. The ligamentum flavum connect the lamina of the spine to one another, attaching from the undersurface of one lamina, to the top of the other .[5,6] All of the spinous processes are connected through a ligamentous complex that includes the supraspinous ligament and the interspinous ligament.

The atlantoaxial joint also has a unique and important ligamentous complex. The largest and strongest of these ligaments is the transverse ligament, whose primary role is to hold the odontoid up against the anterior arch of the atlas. The ligament originates from one side of the atlantal arch and inserts on the contralateral side. The alar ligaments originate from the odontoid process and attach onto the occipital condyles. The primary role of the alar ligaments is to prevent excessive axial rotation.[7] The apical ligament attaches from the tip of the odontoid process onto the anterior wall of foramen magnum, and its role appears to be a restraint to the occiput in both axial tension and anterior shear.[8]

### *Vascular Anatomy*

The path of the vertebral artery is of great interest and importance when contemplating surgical intervention of the cervical spine. The vertebral artery arises from the subclavian artery and enters the transverse foramen at the level of C6. Although there is a transverse foramen at C7, the artery usually travels anterior to the foramen at this level. After entering the transverse foramen at the level of C6, the artery traverses through each of the transverse foramen from C6 to C1. After traversing through the transverse foramen at C1, the artery courses posteriorly, medially, and superiorly where it enters the foramen magnum and anastomoses with the contralateral vertebral artery, forming the basilar artery.[9,10] In both anterior and posterior cervical spinal surgery, it is of utmost importance to appreciate and respect the anatomy of the vertebral artery and to be prepared to deal with aberrant anatomy, which may complicate the case.

## FIXATION TECHNIQUES

### Occipitocervical Fixation

Occipitocervical fusion has many diverse clinical indications, including tumors, subluxation secondary to longstanding rheumatoid arthritis, traumatic occipitocervical dislocation, ankylosing spondylitis causing severe deformity, degenerative arthritis, and cervical osteomyelitis.[11,12] Occipitocervical fusions are technically demanding procedures that require a thorough understanding of the anatomy, hardware, and biomechanics to be successfully completed. Simply stated, there are two segments to a successful occipital fixation construct. First, there must be adequate and strong fixation in the occiput; secondly, the occiput must be anchored to the cervical spine.

Prior to the advent and popularization of the current screw and rod or plate systems, occipital cervical fusions were achieved using either fibular or iliac crest strut grafting. These constructs were fixated with a wire construct, weaving the wires through the occiput, spinous process, or lamina of the atlas.[11,12] These constructs often required supplement external fixation in the form of a halo traction or Minerva casting, until a solid fusion had occurred. With advances in hardware and surgical techniques, this need for supplemental external immobilization has been obviated. These advances in hardware technology have demonstrated the biomechanical superiority of screw constructs. In a biomechanical study testing six methods of occipitocervical fixation, using a screw-and-rod construct or a screw-and-plate construct proved to be biomechanically superior when compared to a sublaminar wire and bone grafting technique. Screw constructs have also decreased the number of fusion levels required to achieve stable fixation. With sublaminar wire constructs, fusion usually extended down to C3, whereas with the current screw constructs, the fusion can be stopped at C2. This study showed that a screw construct using screws can decrease the number of fusion levels required, while remaining biomechanically superior.[13] Another biomechanical study examining the difference between various screw constructs versus wiring techniques also revealed the inferiority of wiring in flexion, extension, and torsion.[14]

As previously stated, occipital fixation is most dependent on the safety and efficacy of screw placement. The anatomic study by Ebraheim et al. revealed that the thickest bone in the occiput is at the level of the external occipital protuberance, where it ranged from 11.5 to 15.1 mm in males and from 9.7 to 12.0 mm in females.[3] The study also revealed that the thickness of the bone thinned considerably as the occiput curved laterally. This anatomic study revealed that 2 cm lateral at the level of the external occipital protuberance there was still a minimum of 8 mm of bone. The dural sinuses are contained directly beneath the thickest portions of the occiput, and the conclusion of this study was that screw fixation in the form of an 8 mm unicortical screw can be safely inserted at the level of the superior nuchal line extending 2 cm from the midline, 1 cm from the midline, 1 cm inferior to the external occipital protuberance, 0.5 cm from the midline, and 2 cm inferior to the external occipital protuberance.[3] Other anatomic studies looking at how the inner, middle, and outer table of the occiput contribute to the thickness of the bone revealed that the middle and outer tables contribute the most to the thickness of the occiput while the inner table contributes the least, averaging approximately only 2 mm in both males and females.[4]

Another anatomic study by Nadim et al. investigated the proximity of the venous sinuses from the center of the external occipital protuberance. This study used an inside-out technique to mark the sinuses and the trocula, then measure the distance of upper and lower borders of these structures from the external occipital protuberance. The upper border of the trocula was on average 12.6 mm above the external occipital protuberance, while the lower border was approximately 4.7 mm away. The study also showed that 1 cm lateral to the external occipital protuberance, the upper border of the transverse sinus was 7.3 mm away and the lower border 6.5 mm away. The authors concluded that screws inserted at the level of the external occipital protuberance or 1 cm below it will cause an injury to the sinuses, and therefore recommended screw placement a minimum of 2 cm below the superior nuchal line.[15]

Given the proximity of the screws to the sinuses, Haher et al. performed a biomechanical study to determine the differences in pullout strength between a bicortical screw, a unicortical screw, and wire fixation. They found that although there was a significant difference in the pullout strength between a unicortical screw and a bicortical screw, this difference only existed in the thickest bone at the external occipital protuberance. However, as the screws were placed further away from this point, the difference in pullout strength between the unicortical screw and bicortical screw decreased.[16] Thus, they concluded that unicortical fixation approached the pullout strength of bicortical fixation in the occiput. They hypothesized that this similarity in pullout strength was due to the larger thickness of the outer table of the occiput and minimal inner table thickness, as shown in the study by Zipnick et al.

With the advent of neuronavigational technology available to spine surgeons in the operating room, newer techniques for occipital fixation are being developed. One technique that has recently been explored is the placement of an occipital condylar screw. For the fixation to adequately support occipitocervical fusion, a bicortical screw must be used in the occipital condyle. This technique is highly challenging due to the close proximity of the sensitive structures such as the vertebral artery, emissary vein, and hypoglossal nerve.[17,18] Occipital condylar screw fixation can be considered in cases where a salvage procedure may be necessary, such as in the case of an occipitocervical pseudoarthrosis, or in a patient who had a prior posterior craniotomy.

The technique for the placement of an occipital condylar screw involves the standard midline posterior incision and exposure of posterior arch of C1 and lateral masses of C2. Once the medial border of the occipital condyle is identified, dissection is continued in a subperiosteal fashion to avoid injury to the neurovascular structures. The entry point for the occipital condylar screw was determined to be 4–5 mm lateral to the posterior medial edge of the condyle at the junction with the occipital bone at the condylar fossa.[18] A radiographic study examining the optimal screw trajectory revealed that a middle or lateral starting point in the condyle had the highest success rate of placement. They defined the middle entry point as the midpoint between the lateral and medial borders of the condyle. The medial and lateral entry points were defined as being 3 mm medial or lateral to the middle point. This study also revealed that it was difficult to identify a specific amount of medial angulation required to place the screw within the long axis of the condyle, and therefore they recommended that the angulation should be determined by studying the patient's preoperative computed tomography (CT) scan.[19] A biomechanical study comparing occipital condylar screw fixation to standard occipital plating, both with a C1 lateral mass, and C2 par screw anchors revealed that the constructs were biomechanically equivalent in terms of stiffness, range of motion in flexion-extension, lateral bending, and axial rotation flexibility tests of a physiologic magnitude.[20]

Another technique that has been described for occipital cervical fusion is an inside-out technique. This procedure requires a standard midline posterior approach, extended approximately 2–3 cm superior to the external occipital protuberance. Standard C1-C2 lateral mass screws or transarticular screws are placed. A plate is then contoured to the occiput and a burr hole is made that will allow for clearance of the head of the screw; then a keyway is created, guiding the screw to the desired position. The screw is then secured to the plate with a nut. In this technique, either an iliac crest or rib bone graft is then secured to the plate to form a solid arthrodesis.[21,22]

The position of occipital fusion is also of importance to the surgeon. The goal is to fuse the occiput in the position of maximal function for the patient. It is considered that occipitocervical neutral is the most functional position for fusion. In a radiographic study, Phillip et al. determined that a neutral position of the cranium occurs at an occipitocervical angle of 44°. The occipitocervical angle is defined as the junction between a line drawn from the basion to opisthion and the superior endplate of C3. This is an important radiographic assessment that can be used intraoperatively to ensure an adequate and functional position of occipital cervical fusion.[23]

## Atlantoaxial Fixation

### *Brooks and Jenkins Technique*

There are many causes of atlantoaxial instability. Some congenital disorders that contribute to instability are odontoid aplasia or hypoplasia and os odontoideum. Trauma, inflammatory disorders, and neoplastic disease may also present with atlantoaxial instability. Historically, rheumatoid arthritis was one of the leading causes of atlantoaxial instability requiring surgical stabilization. However, with the advent of effective disease-modifying agents such as adalimumab and etanercept, the number of patients requiring surgical stabilization for atlantoaxial instability has significantly decreased.

One of the earliest techniques described for treating this disorder was the Gallie technique, which called for bone graft to be secured with a wire passing beneath the arch of C1 and wrapped under and around the C2 spinous process. In 1978, Brooks and Jenkins modified and refined this technique by using sublaminar wires at both C1 and C2 and called it the wedge compression method. Of their original case series, 11 out of 15 patients had a solid C1-C2 fusion at the time of follow-up, one patient had spontaneously fused from C1-C3, one patient required a fusion extended to the occiput due to a fracture of the posterior arch of C1, and one patient died spontaneously 2 months postoperatively from an unknown cause.[24]

In the technique described by Brooks and Jenkins, the patient is placed in the prone position with standard cranial pin fixation for the head. Intraoperative fluoroscopy is then used to ensure that the neck is placed in a position to reduce the atlantoaxial joint. The incision is then made from the occiput and extended down to C4 or C5. The posterior arch of the atlas is exposed using a subperiosteal dissection, and this dissection is extended laterally. The spinous process and lamina of the axis are exposed, taking care not to disturb the C2-C3 articulation. The surfaces of the atlas and axis that will be in contact with the bone graft are then curreted. Next, using an aneurysm needle, a Mersilene suture is passed underneath the arch of the atlas, and then passed under the lamina of the axis on each side. The suture is then used as a guide to pass 20-gauge wire under the arch of C1 and lamina of C2 bilaterally. Bone graft is then harvested from the iliac crest and two grafts measuring 1.25 cm × 3.5 cm are obtained. The grafts are then beveled to fit in the interval between the arch of the atlas and lamina of the axis, and held in position by tightening and twisting the 20-gauge wire.

There are, however, several limitations to the use of the Brooks and Jenkins technique. This technique is contraindicated in patients with a fracture of the arch of the atlas as this arch is one of the anchor points of the bone graft. Jenkins and Brooks recommended in their original article that in patients where a defect of the arch exists, the fusion should be extended to the occiput.[24] Today, however, options such as transarticular screw fixation or the Harms technique can be used to treat atlantoaxial instability as well as allow for preservation of occipitocervical motion in these patients. Also, this technique required postoperative immobilization to protect the cervical spine until bony union occurred. The authors used either a Minerva cast or a Sternal-occipital-mandibular brace for postoperative immobilization.

### *Transarticular Screw Fixation of the Atlantoaxial Joint*

The transarticular screw technique was first introduced in 1986 by Magerl and Seeman as a method of fixation in patients suffering from atlantoaxial instability.[25] This technique has been shown to be effective in many causes of atlantoaxial instability, including rheumatoid arthritis, trauma, and congenital disorders.[26,27] The technique uses two screws that traverse four cortices each through the C1-C2 articulation to afford atlantoaxial stability. Advantages of this technique include strong fixation obviating the need for halo immobilization after surgery, low implant cost, a high fusion rate, and the ability to perform the procedure even if a defect of the posterior elements of C1 exists. Disadvantages of transarticular screw fixation include a technically demanding procedure, difficulty in achieving an adequate reduction in cases with substantial deformity, and anatomic restraints eliminating some patients as candidates for this procedure.[25, 28]

It is important to obtain a preoperative CT scan in order to plan screw trajectory and lengths as well as to assess the patient's anatomy, which may preclude transarticular screw fixation.[28,29] In a radiographic study examining the C1-C2 anatomy on CT scans, it was determined that 20% of subjects had anatomic anomalies that would preclude placing a transarticular screw on at least one side. The most common anomaly that was found preventing screw placement was a high-riding transverse foramen that would place the vertebral artery at risk. Only 3% of the patients had anatomic restraints preventing transarticular screw placement bilaterally.[29] In another radiographic CT study defining unacceptable risk of transarticular screw placement as <3.5 mm of space available for the screw and "risky" as between 3.5 and 4.5 mm of space available for the screw, 23.4% of patients fell into one of these two categories.[30] More recently, these numbers have been challenged by an magnetic resonance imaging study examining vertebral artery location in 30 patients with atlantoaxial instability, which revealed that 40% of these patients had vertebral artery anatomy precluding transarticular screw placement on at least one side. The authors noted that in this study, the patients' anatomy was distorted secondary to the deformity caused by the atlantoaxial instability.[31]

*Techniques*[28]

1. Place the patient in the prone position with standard cranial pin fixation for the head, and place the head slightly flexed, which may aid in screw trajectory. Placing the patient in the reverse Trendelenburg position may help decrease venous bleeding during the procedure.

2. Ensure adequate reduction and optimize the image on the intraoperative fluoroscopy. Test under fluoroscopy if the trajectory required for the transarticular screw can be achieved given the patient's anatomy and positioning.
3. Incision is made from the external occipital protuberance to C3, and a subperiosteal technique is used to expose the posterior elements of the occiput, atlas, axis, and C3.
4. The entry point for the screw is 2–3 mm lateral to the medial border of the pars of C2 and 2–3 mm superior to the C2-C3 articulation. The optimal entry point and trajectory should be determined through careful preoperative planning of the patient's CT scan.
5. The C1-C2 can be curetted or burred and bone graft can be placed in the joint to promote a bony union.
6. Use fluoroscopy to determine the optimal screw trajectory. The drill bit may be inserted percutaneously and a drill guide used if the length of the incision does not allow for the optimal angle.
7. A starting hole may be started with an awl, and the drill passed in the desired direction under direct fluoroscopic guidance.
8. Tap the entire length of the drill hole.
9. Insert the desired screw. A polyaxial screw may be used if the surgeon is anticipating extension of fusion to the occiput or subaxial spine.
10. In patients where only one transarticular screw can be safely placed, the fixation can be augmented with autograft via cable fixation. [28,32]

In addition to this most commonly used posterior approach to the C1-C2 transarticular screw, anterior and anterolateral approaches have also been described.[33]

As previously stated, transarticular screw fixation is a technically demanding procedure, in which lack of accuracy can have severe and detrimental effects on the patient. In a retrospective study examining postoperative CT scans of 112 transarticular screws placed via a standard technique, 95.5% of the screws were in adequate position, two screws were placed too medial, two screws were placed too lateral, and one screw was placed too inferiorly. Of all the screws, 69.4% perforated the anterior cortex.[34] There were no neurological deficits that were identified in this study; however, anterior perforation may cause injury to the hypoglossal nerve or internal carotid artery.[33]

Due to the sensitive anatomy of the region, complications associated with transarticular screw fixation may be catastrophic. It is imperative that the surgeon be prepared to deal with an intraoperative injury to the vertebral artery. It is recommended that if brisk bleeding is expressed from the drill hole, a vertebral artery injury should be assumed and the screw should be placed to gain fixation and stop the bleeding. Screw placement should not be attempted on the contralateral side, and the patient should receive a postoperative CT angiogram to assess the vertebral arteries.[28]

### *Harms Technique*

As previously stated, transarticular screw fixation is not anatomically feasible in up to 23% of patients. For this reason, Harms devised a novel technique in 2001 using a C1 lateral mass screw and C2 pedicle screw connected with a rod construct to achieve stability and fusion of the atlantoaxial joint. He believed that this technique minimized the risk of injury to the vertebral artery and allowed for improved reduction of the atlantoaxial joint. In his original article, he retrospectively reviewed 37 patients in which the polyaxial screw and rod construct had been performed, all of whom went on to a solid fusion, and none of whom had a vertebral artery or dural injury.[35]

*Techniques*[35]

1. Place the patient in the prone position with standard cranial pin fixation for the head.
2. Ensure adequate C1-C2 visualization using intraoperative fluoroscopy.
3. Incision is made from the occiput to C3, and a subperiosteal technique is used to expose the posterior elements of the occiput, atlas, axis, and C3. The dissection must be taken to the lateral border of the C1-C2 articulation.
4. Identify the C2 nerve root and retract it caudally to expose the entry point of the C1 screw. The entry point of the C1 screw is in the middle of the junction of the C1 posterior arch and the midpoint of the posterior inferior part of the C1 lateral mass. The trajectory of the screw should be placed in 5–10° of convergence in the axial plane, and should remain parallel to the inferior arch of C1 in the sagittal plane.[36]
5. A pilot hole is drilled at the entry point using a high-speed burr. The hole is tapped and a polyaxial screw of the appropriate length is placed into the lateral mass of C1. Verify the position of the screw using intraoperative fluoroscopy.
6. Identify the medial border of the pars of C2 and identify the entry point of the C2 screw. The entry

point of the C2 pedicle screw is defined as being in the superomedial quadrant formed by the intersection of a line that bisects the C2 pars vertically, and the other that bisects the lamina horizontally.[36] Make the entry point of the C2 pedicle screw with a high-speed burr. Using a 2 mm drill bit, a pilot hole is drilled approximately 20–30° medially and superiorly. The hole is then tapped and a polyaxial screw of the appropriate length is placed. Verify the position of the screw using intraoperative fluoroscopy.

7. Fix the rods to the polyaxial screws bilaterally.
8. Decorticate C1-C2 posteriorly and the C1-C2 articulation. Bone may be acquired from the iliac crest if additional bone graft is desired.

Several studies have compared the fusion rates and biomechanical strength of the three C1-C2 fusion techniques described. In one study comparing the fusion rate of the modified Gallie technique with the transarticular screw technique, the inferiority of the Gallie technique was exposed. The Gallie technique went on to achieve a bony fusion in only 58% of patients with a 6.9-year average follow-up, while the transarticular screw technique achieved arthrodesis in 100% of the patients.[37] One patient in this series did, however, have an injury to the vertebral artery with transarticular screw fixation.

A meta-analysis reviewing the literature comparing transarticular screw fixation with screw-and-rod constructs like the Harms technique revealed fusion rates of 94.6% for transarticular screws and 97.5% for screw-and-rod constructs. However, there was more variability in the technique and graft material used with the screw-and-rod constructs.[38] Both, however, were determined to have a very reliable fusion rate when compared to the previously studied fusion rate of the Gallie technique.

Another meta-analysis comparing the vertebral artery injuries of transarticular screws with screw-and-rod constructs revealed that vertebral artery injuries with transarticular screw placement occurred in 26 of 3,627 or 0.72% of the implanted transarticular screws compared with 10 out of 2,979 or 0.34% of C2 pedicle screws. It was determined that two deaths were directly attributable to these injuries in patients undergoing transarticular screw placement. In one patient, a unilateral vertebral artery injury resulted in a brainstem stroke; in another, bilateral vertebral artery occlusion was the cause of death.[39] Due to this uncommon but highly devastating complication that may occur during the placement of transarticular screws, most spinal surgeons now prefer utilizing the Harms technique over transarticular screw techniques whenever it is feasible.

## Subaxial Cervical Spine

### *Lateral Mass Screw Fixation*

Historically, the fixation of the subaxial cervical spine was limited to the use of laminar hooks and sublaminar or interspinous wires. These constructs often required cortical bone graft to aid in construct stability as well as postoperative immobilization with a halo. Lateral mass screws have been safely used in the cervical spine for over 20 years. They were originally developed when screw-and-plate constructs were being used for cervical spine arthrodesis. Even though the use of screw-and-plate constructs is decreasing in favor of screw-and-rod constructs, the techniques and insertions of these lateral mass screws has not changed drastically. Lateral mass screws in the United States are widely used by both orthopedic surgeons and neurosurgeons under "physician-directed use." There, however, remains no official classification regarding the usage of these implants by the Food and Drug Administration (FDA). Several organizations such as the American Academy of Orthopaedics, the Cervical Spine Research Society, and the North American Spine Society have advocated for the FDA to classify lateral mass screws as a Class 2 medical device.

The technique was originally described by Roy-Camille, and several other surgeons have made modifications, most notably Magerl, Louis, Anderson, and An. Although the concept of placing a screw into the lateral mass is the same in each, the entry point and screw trajectory differ. The goals of lateral mass screw placement are to contact the most bone providing the most structural support, while avoiding the structures at risk, the vertebral arteries and the cervical nerve roots. Depending on the screw technique used, lateral angulation of the screw is meant to avoid injury to the vertebral arties, while cephalad angulation is meant to decrease the risk of injury to the nerve root.

The original technique by Roy-Camille calls for the lateral mass screw entry point to be directly in the center of the lateral mass. A 2.0 mm drill bit is then used and directed to 0° of cephalad angulation of the screw and approximately 10° of lateral angulation. A 3.5 mm tap is then used, and a 3.5 mm screw is inserted.[40]

The technique described by Louis called for a screw entry point that intersected a vertical line 5 mm from the lateral edge of the facet joint, and a horizontal line drawn 3 mm inferior to the superior articulating facet. He used a 2.8 mm drill bit directed to 0° of cephalad angulation and 0° of lateral angulation. According to his study, the screw length using this technique was between 8 mm and 12 mm on average.[41]

The technique by Magerl was somewhat less detailed; however, the screw trajectory was significantly different than that of Roy-Camille. He described his screw entry point as slightly medial and cranial to the center of the articular mass. He directed the screw parallel to the direction of the adjacent facet joint, which resulted in approximately 25° of cephalad angulation and 25° of lateral angulation. He stated that this technique would most effectively prevent injury to the sensitive neurological structures while maximizing the screw lengths. However, his technique did not specify the size of the drill bit used or whether he would tap the hole prior to screw insertion. He would use a 2.7 mm screw or a 3.5 mm screw, depending on the size of the articulating process.[42]

Anderson's technique called for an entry point that was similar to that of Roy-Camille's. His entry point was 1 mm medial to the center point of the lateral mass. He used a 2 mm Kirshner wire as a drill bit, and the drill bit was directed to 30–40° of cephalad angulation and 10° of lateral angulation. He then tapped the dorsal cortex of the drill hole with a 3.5 mm tap and placed a 3.5 mm screw. His average screw length using this technique was 16–18 mm.[43]

The modification by An, which he determined via a cadaveric study, described the entry point for the lateral mass screw as 1 mm medial to the center of the lateral mass. The screw trajectory that he determined to be the safest was approximately 15–18° in the cephalad direction and 30–33° in the lateral direction. The average screw length of this technique was between 10 mm and 11 mm.[44]

Several studies have been performed comparing these different lateral mass screw techniques. Most studies compare the two most popular lateral mass screws, the Roy-Camille technique and the Magerl technique. An early cadaveric study revealed that a safe screw length was 14–15 mm in the Roy-Camille technique and 15–16 mm in the Magerl technique at the C3-C6 levels.[45] A CT scan study analyzing the anatomy of the lateral mass revealed that there was significant difference in the size of the lateral masses depending on gender and spinal level. Comparing the screw lengths that can be placed in the lateral masses of C3-C7, the study revealed that the screws placed in C4-C6 were consistently the longest screws, while the lateral mass screw of C7 was the shortest.[46] The study also revealed that on average the screw length placed via the Magerl technique was 2.6 mm longer at C3-C6 levels, and approximately 1.3 mm longer at the C7 level. The mean screw length of the C3-C6 levels using the Roy-Camille technique was 11.7–12.9 mm in males and 11.0–11.5 mm in females. The mean screw length of the C3-C6 levels using the Magerl technique was 14.0–15.6 mm in males and 13.2–14.0 mm in females. The mean screw length at C7 was 9.8 mm in males and 8.5 mm in females using the Roy-Camille technique, and 11.4 mm in males and 9.6 mm in females using the Magerl technique.[46]

Several studies have also been performed investigating the safety of these lateral mass screw techniques with regard to the nerve root. A cadaveric study in which surgeons placed lateral mass screws using both the Roy-Camille technique and the Magerl technique revealed that nerve root injury occurred in 0.8% of the Roy-Camille screws and 7.3% of the Magerl screws. The study, however, also revealed that the screws placed later on in the study were less likely to cause nerve root injury, suggesting that the Roy-Camille screws had a longer learning curve to successful placement.[47] In another cadaveric study, the Magerl, Anderson, and An techniques were used to place 20 mm screws in all specimens, intentionally overpenetrating the ventral cortex to determine which technique would cause the greatest rate of nerve root violation. This study revealed the An technique had the lowest rate of nerve root violation at 60%, compared to 95% for the Magerl technique and 90% for the Anderson technique.[48]

### *Cervical Pedicle Screw Fixation*

Similarly to lateral mass screw fixation of the cervical spine, cervical pedicle screws have been used by surgeons for approximately 20 years; however, there still remains no FDA approval of pedicle screws in the cervical spine. The advantage of pedicle screws is that they provide three-column support, making them biomechanically superior to lateral mass screws.

The insertion of cervical pedicle screws is technically demanding due to the sensitive surrounding neurovascular structures. The structures at risk include the spinal cord, nerve roots, and the vertebral artery. Anatomic studies have revealed the distance between the pedicle and the inferior nerve root to range 1.0–2.5 mm, while there is no distance at all between the pedicle and the superior nerve root. This study also revealed that the distance between the medial pedicle and the dura ranged 2.4–3.1 mm in all specimens.[49] The size of the pedicle is also small and can be variable; a cadaveric anatomic study revealed that the average C3 pedicle width was 4.9 mm with a range of 3.7–5.4 mm, and the average C7 pedicle with was 6.9 mm with a range of 5.1–6.5 mm. This study revealed that the pedicle size did get progressively larger from C3-C7 and that the pedicle size in females was smaller than that of males.[49] In an anatomic study using a CT reconstruction model, it was found that the distance of the vertebral artery from the lateral border of the pedicle was only approximately 1.1 mm at C2, 2 mm at C6, and 6.5 mm at C7. The large difference between the C7 and the other cervical levels was due to 80% of the patients in the study having a vertebral artery that was lateral to the transverse foramen at that level.[50] With all of these anatomic restraints, the insertion of pedicle screws is a high-risk procedure; some surgeons have opted to use CT-guided methods for the insertion of these screws.[51]

The first surgeon to describe subaxial cervical pedicle screw fixation was Abumi in 1994. His technique for the insertion of these pedicle screws called for a subperiosteal dissection lateral enough to expose the lateral margins of the facet joints. The entry point for the screw was described as slightly lateral to the center of the articular mass and close to the posterior margin of the superior articular surface, taking into consideration the anatomy. A high-speed burr was used to penetrate the posterior cortex and widened until the entrance of the pedicle was visible. A probe was then used to confirm both the medial and lateral borders of the pedicle, and a lateral fluoroscopic image was obtained to confirm trajectory and screw length. He described the trajectory of his screw as 30–40° medial to the midline in the transverse plane and parallel to the upper end plate in the sagittal plane. Abumi's original technique called for the insertion of a 4.5 mm screw.[52] In his updated technique, he began to tap the screw pilot hole that was created and used screw diameters varying from 3.5 mm to 4.5 mm, with screw lengths varying between 20–28 mm.[53] The optimal transverse and sagittal trajectory was examined by CT reconstruction techniques and revealed that the angle differs according to each spinal level. The highest transverse angle was seen at C3 at a mean angle of 46°, while the lowest was seen at C7 with a mean angle of 28°. The sagittal angle also differed, with the optimal trajectory being 7° superior at C3, neutral at C5, and 2° inferior at C2.[54]

The complications of cervical pedicle screw insertion were explored retrospectively by Abumi as well. In his series of 180 patients, 712 cervical pedicle screws were placed and 669 of the screws were imaged postoperatively via CT scan. Of the 180 patients, 7 patients declined a postoperative CT scan, and 4 patients died in the early postoperative period. Of the remaining 169 patients, after excluding the patients who were fused due to a tumor, he achieved a fusion rated of 99.4%. In this series, he reported one vertebral artery injury and two cervical radiculopathies secondary to screw impingement on the nerve root, one of which improved with nonsurgical management; the other improved with screw removal. This study also looked at the rate of screw perforation at each of the vertebral levels regardless of their clinical significance. A total of 6.7% of the screws placed perforated the pedicle, with the highest rate being at the C4 pedicle at 10.6% and the lowest at the C2 pedicle at 4.1%.[55]

Given the highly sensitive neurovascular structures and the technically demanding procedure, the benefits of cervical pedicle screw fixation must outweigh the risks. Cervical pedicle screws provide a point of fixation across all three spinal columns. The first biomechanical study comparing the pullout strength between cervical pedicle screws and lateral mass screws was conducted by Jones et al. In their cadaveric study, they used 56 cervical vertebrae (C2-C7) in which the right and left sides were randomized to either a cervical pedicle screw or a lateral mass screw placed using the An technique. The study confirmed the superiority of cervical pedicle screws. The mean load-to-failure of the cervicle pedicle screws were 677 N compared to 355 N for the lateral mass screws.[56]

### *Transarticular Screw Fixation of the Subaxial Cervical Spine*

Transarticular screw fixation may also be used in the subaxial cervical spine. Although less popular than inserting lateral mass screws in the subaxial cervical spine, transarticular screws can be inserted as the primary mode of fixation, to supplement anterior fusion constructs, or in posterior cervical spine revision cases. There are, however, limitations to the use of these screws. Transfacet screw fixation is contraindicated in cases in which the lateral masses are comminuted and in cases of deformity requiring correction.[57]

This screw technique was first described by Roy-Camille in 1972 but has since been refined by several surgeons, including Takayasu and DalCanto. In Takayasu's technique, a superiosteal dissection is performed exposing the facet joints bilaterally. The facet joints are then curetted to remove the articular cartilage and bone graft is placed into the facet joints. The entry point of the screw is midway between the lateral border of the lamina and the lateral bone margin of the articular pillar in the mediolateral position, and midway to the caudal third of the articular pillar between the superior and inferior facets joints in the rostrocaudal position. After using an awl for the starting point, a drill is used under fluoroscopic guidance to drill through four cortices at an angle of 60–80° inferior and 0° medial to lateral. A 10 to 18 mm screw is then inserted. In his series of 81 screws in 25 patients, he identified no vertebral artery or nerve root injuries.[58] DalCanto modified the technique slightly by aiming the screws approximately 20° laterally, which he determined through his cadaveric study was a safer trajectory in order to avoid vertebral artery injury. DalCanto also demonstrated that there were no significant differences in range of motion and load-to failure between transarticular facet screw constructs and lateral mass screw-and-plate fixation.[59]

## REFERENCES


1. Roberts DA, Doherty BJ, Heggeness MH. Quantitative anatomy of the occiput and the biomechanics of screw fixation. Spine. 1998;23(10):1100-1108.
2. Henry G. Gray's Anatomy: The Classic Collector's Edition. New York, NY: Crown; 1977.
3. Ebraheim NA, Lu J, Biyani A, et al. An anatomic study of the thickness of the occipital bone: implications for occipitocervical instrumentation. Spine. 1996;21 (15):1725-9.
4. Zipnick RI, Merola AA, Gorup J, et al. Occipital morphology: an anatomic guide to internal fixation. Spine. 1996; 21(15):1719-24.
5. Southwick WO, Keggi K. The normal cervical spine. J Bone Joint Surg Am.. 1964; 46(8):1767-77.
6. Panjabi MM, Oxland TR, Parks EH. Quantitative anatomy of cervical spine ligaments. Part II. Middle and lower cervical spine. J Spinal Disord. 1991;4(3):277-83.
7. Dvorak J, Panjabi MM. Functional anatomy of the alar ligaments. Spine. 1987; 12(2):183-9.
8. Panjabi MM, Oxland TR, Parks EH. Quantitative anatomy of cervical spine ligaments. Part I. Upper cervical spine. J Spinal Disord. 1991;4(3):270-6.
9. Heary RF, Albert TJ, Ludwig SC, et al. Surgical anatomy of the vertebral arteries. Spine. 1996;21:2074-80.
10. Eskander MS, Drew JM, Aubin ME, et al. Vertebral artery anatomy: a review of two hundred and fifty MRI scans. Spine. 2010;35:2035-40.
11. Wertheim SB, Bohlman HH. Occipitocervical fusion. Indications, technique, and long-term results in thirteen patients. J Bone Joint Surg Am. 1987;69(6):833-6.
12. Stock GH, Vaccaro A, Brown AK, et al. Contemporary Posterior Occipital Fixation. J Bone Joint Surg Am. 2006; 88(7):1642-9.
13. Hurlbert RJ, Crawford NR, Choi WG, et al. A biomechanical evaluation of occipitocervical instrumentation: screw compared with wire fixation. J Neurosurg. 1999;90(1):84-90.
14. Sutterlin CE, Bianchi JR, Kunz DN, et al. Biomechanical evaluation of occipitocervical fixation devices. J Spinal Disord. 2001;14(3):185-92.
15. Nadim Y, Lu J, Sabry FF, et al. Occipital screws in occipitocervical fusion and their relation to the venous sinuses: an anatomic and radiographic study. Orthopedics. 2000; 23(7):717-9.
16. Haher TR, Yeung AW, Caruso SA, et al. Occipital screw pullout strength: a biomechanical investigation of occipital morphology. Spine. 1999;24(1):5-9.
17. Marca FL, Zubay G, Morrison T, et al. Cadaveric study for placement of occipital condyle screw: technique and effects on surrounding anatomic structures. J Neurosurg Spine. 2008;9:347-53.
18. Uribe JS, Ramos E, Vale F. Feasibility of occipital condyle screw placement for occipitocervical fixation: a cadaveric study and description of a novel technique. J Spinal Disorder Tech. 2008;21:540-6.
19. Lee JO, Buchowski JM, Lee KM, et al. Optimal trajectory for the occipital condylar screw. Spine. 2012;37(5):385-92.
20. Uribe JS, Ramos E, Youssef AS, et al. Craniocervical fixation with occipital condyle screws: biomechanical analysis of a novel technique. Spine. 2010;35(9):931-8.
21. Pait TG, Al-Mefty O, Boop FA, et al. Inside-outside technique for posterior occipitocervical spine instrumentation and stabilization: preliminary results. J Neurosurg. 1999;90:1-7.
22. Sandhu FA, Pait TG, Benzel E, et al. Occipitocervical fusion for rheumatoid arthritis using the inside-outside stabilization technique. Spine. 2003;28(4):414-9.
23. Phillips FM, Phillips CS, Wetzel FT, et al. Occipitocervical neutral position possible surgical implications. Spine. 1999; 24(8):775-8.
24. Brooks AL, Jenkins EB. Atlanto-axial arthrodesis by the Wedge compression method. J Bone Joint Surg Am. 1978; 60-A(3):279-84.
25. Magerl F, Seeman P. Stable posterior fusion of the atlas and axis by transarticular screw fixation. Cervical Spine. 1986;322-7.
26. Grob D. Transarticular screw fixation for atlanto-occipital dislocation. Spine. 2001;26:703-7.
27. Nagaria J, Kelleher MO, McEvoy L, et al. C1-C2 Transarticular screw fixation for atlantoaxial instability due to rheumatoid arthritis: a seven-year analysis of outcome. Spine. 2009; 34:2880-5.
28. Finn MA, Apfelbaum RI. Atlantoaxial transarticular screw fixation: update on technique and outcomes in 269 patients. Neurosurgery. 2010;66(3):A184-92.

29. Paramore CG, Dickman CA, Sonntag VK. The anatomical suitability of the C1-2 complex for transarticular screw fixation. J Neurosurg. 1996; 85:221-4.
30. Jun BY. Anatomic study for ideal and safe posterior C1-C2 transarticular screw fixation. Spine. 1998;23(15):1703-7.
31. Lau SW, Sun LK, Lai R, et al. Study of the anatomical variations of vertebral artery in C2 vertebra with magnetic resonance imaging and its application in the C1-C2 transarticular screw fixation. Spine. 2010;35(11):1136-43.
32. Bransford RJ, Lee MJ, Reis A. Posterior fixation of the upper cervical spine: contemporary techniques. J Am Acad Orthop Surg. 2011;19:63-71.
33. Cavalcanti DD, Agrawal A, Garcia-Gonzalez U, et al. Anterolateral C1-C2 transarticular fixation for atlantoaxial arthrodesis: landmarks, working area, and angles of approach. Neurosurgery. 2010;67:38-42.
34. Fujii T, Oda T, Kato Y, et al. Accuracy of atlantoaxial transarticular screw insertion. Spine. 2000;25:1760-4.
35. Harms J, Melcher RP. Posterior C1-C2 fusion with polyaxial screw and rod fixation. Spine. 2001;26(22):2467-71.
36. Schulz R, Macchiavello N, Fernandez E, et al. Harms C1-C2 instrumentation technique. Spine. 2011;36:945-50.
37. Farey ID, Smith N. Modified Gallie technique versus transarticular screw fixation in C1-C2 fusion. Clin Orthop Relat Res. 1999;359:126-36.
38. Elliot RE, Tanweer O, Boah A, et al. Outcome comparison of atlantoaxial fusion with transarticular screws and screw-rod constructs: meta-analysis and review of the literature. J Spinal Disorder Tech. 2014;27:11-28.
39. Elliot RE, Tanweer O, Boah A, et al. Comparison of screw malposition and vertebral artery injury of C2 pedicle and transarticular screws: meta-analysis and review of the literature. J Spinal Disord Tech. 2014;27(6):305-15.
40. Roy-Camille R, Saillant G, Mazel C. Internal fixation of the unstable cervical spine by a posterior osteosynthesis with plates and screws. In: Cervical Spine Research Society (Ed), The Cervical Spine. New York, NY: JB Lippincott; 1989. pp. 390-403.
41. Nazarian SM, Louis RP. Posterior internal fixation with screw plates in traumatic lesions of the cervical spine. Spine. 1991;16(3):S64-71.
42. Jeanneret B, Magerl F, Ward H, et al. Posterior stabilization of the cervical spine with hook plates. Spine. 1991;16(3):S56-63.
43. Anderson PA, Henley MB, Grady MS, et al. Posterior cervical arthrodesis with AO reconstruction plates and bone graft. Spine. 1991;16(3):S72-9.
44. An HS, Gordin R, Renner K. Anatomic considerations for plate-screw fixation of the cervical spine. Spine. 1991; 16(10):S548-51.
45. Ebraheim NA, Klausner T, Xu R, et al. Safe lateral-mass screw lengths in the Roy-Camille and Magerl techniques: an anatomic study. Spine. 1998;23:1739-42.
46. Stemper BD, Marawar SV, Yoganandan N, et al. Quantitative anatomy of subaxial cervical lateral mass. An analysis of safe screw lengths for Roy-Camille and Magerl techniques. Spine. 2008;33:893-7.
47. Heller JG, Carlson GD, Abitbol JJ, et al. Anatomic comparison of the Roy-Camille and Magerl techniques for screw placement in the lower cervical spine. Spine. 1991;16:S552-7.
48. Xu R, Haman SP, Ebraheim NA, Yeasting RA. The anatomic relation of lateral mass screws to the spinal nerves: a comparison of the Magerl, Anderson, and An techniques. Spine (Phila Pa 1976). 1999;24(19):2057-61.
49. Ugur HC, Attar A, Uz A, et al. Surgical anatomic evaluation of the cervical pedicle and adjacent neural structures. Neurosurgery. 2000;47(5):1162-9.
50. Tomasino A, Parikh K, Koller H, et al. The vertebral artery and the cervical pedicle: morphometric analysis of a critical neighborhood. J Neurosurg Spine. 2010; 13: 52-60.
51. Ludwig S, Kramer D, Vaccaro A, et al. Transpedicle screw fixation of the cervical spine. Clin Orthop Relat Res. 1999;359:77-88.
52. Abumi K, Itoh H, Taneichi H, et al. Transpedicular screw fixation for traumatic lesions of the middle and lower cervical spine: description of the techniques and preliminary report. J Spinal Disord. 1994;7(1):19-28.
53. Abumi K, Kaneda K. Pedicle screw fixation for nontraumatic lesions of the cervical spine. Spine. 1997;22(16):1853-61.
54. Lee D, Lee S, Kang S, et al. Optimal entry points and trajectories for cervical placement into subaxial cervical vertebrae. Eur Spine J. 2001;20:905-11.
55. Abumi K , Shono Y, Ito M, et al. Complications of pedicle screw fixation in reconstructive surgery of the cervical spine. Spine. 2000;8:962-9.
56. Jones E, Heller J, Silcox D, et al. Cervical pedicle screws versus lateral mass screws: anatomic feasibility and biomechanical comparison. Spine. 1997;22(9):977-82.
57. Aydogan M, Enercan M, Hamzaoglu A, et al. Reconstruction of the subaxial cervical spine using lateral mass and facet screw instrumentation. Spine. 2012; 37(5):E335-41.
58. Takayasu M, Hara M, Yamauchi K, et al. Transarticular screw fixation in the middle and lower cervical spine. J Neurosurg. 2003;99:132-6.
59. DalCanto R, Lieberman I, Inceoglu S, et al. biomechanical comparison of transarticular facet screws to lateral mass plates in two-level instrumentations of the cervical spine. Spine. 2005;30(8):897-902.

Chapter 20

# Neurological and Vascular Complications after Surgery for Cervical Myelopathy

*Hideki Sudo*

## C5 PALSY AS A NEUROLOGICAL COMPLICATION

### Epidemiology

Both anterior cervical decompression and fusion and posterior decompressive surgery, such as laminoplasty with or without instrumentation, are widely used procedures to treat cervical myelopathy. However, C5 palsy remains a serious complication that affects the surgical outcome. Postoperative C5 palsy is defined as new paresis of the deltoid muscle and/or the biceps brachii muscle after surgery without any deterioration of myelopathic symptoms.[1] About half of affected patients complain of sensory deficits and/or intractable pain in the shoulder region as well as muscle weakness, whereas the other half manifest only motor weakness in the C5 area.[1,2] Reportedly, 92% of C5 palsies occur unilaterally and the remaining 8% affect muscles bilaterally.[2] Most cases of C5 palsy occur within a week after surgery. The incidence of C5 palsy after anterior surgery was 1.6–12.1%[3,4] and after cervical posterior decompression surgery was 0–30%.[2,4] Gandhoke et al.[5] found no difference in the rate of C5 palsy (6.5%) between anterior cervical corpectomy and fusion ($n$ = 31) and laminoplasty ($n$ = 31) to treat cervical myelopathy. Nassr et al.[4] reviewed 630 North American patients and reported that the incidence of C5 palsy was highest for laminectomy and fusion (9.5%), followed by corpectomy with posterior fusion (8.4%), corpectomy (5.1%), and laminoplasty (4.8%); however, these differences did not reach statistical significance. The total incidence was 6.7% irrespective of the surgical procedure, and there was a significantly higher incidence in males (8.6%) than in females (4.5%).

### Causes of C5 Palsy

*Local Nerve Root Trauma During Surgery*

A number of causes of C5 palsy have been suggested: iatrogenic (related to the surgical procedure), nerve root impairment, and pathology of the spinal cord.[6-9] Using the transverse processes of fresh porcine lumbar spines, Hosono et al.[10] suggested that tissues around the drilled bone, especially nerve roots, could be damaged by the heat generated from the tip of a high-speed drill, leading to nerve root palsy; in this case, nerve root impairment would be classified as an iatrogenic injury. However, their hypothesis cannot explain why, in certain cases, C5 palsy develops several days after the surgery.

*Root Impairment and Tethering of the Nerve Root*

The superior articular process of C5 protrudes in a more anterior direction than that of other cervical vertebrae, and the rootlets of the C5 segment are shorter than those of other segments.[5] Furthermore, the C5 segment is usually the point at which the extent of posterior shift of the cord is greatest.[5] Tsuzuki et al.[11] conducted an anatomical study using human cadavers and concluded that the exertion of traction forces on extradural portions of anterior and posterior roots by the posteriorly expanded dura might have a major role in the occurrence of paralysis after posterior decompression of the spinal cord. Katsumi et al.[12] reported that the C4-C5 foramen was significantly narrower on T2-weighted magnetic resonance imaging (MRI) in the C5 palsy group (9/141 cases) than in the nonpalsy group. They suggested that the main etiology of C5 palsy was C5 nerve root impairment induced by pre-existing C4-C5 foraminal stenosis.[12] Imagama et al.[9] reviewed 1,858 patients who had undergone cervical laminoplasty and identified 43 patients (2.3%) who had developed C5 palsy. Computed tomographic (CT) scanning of the C5 palsy group revealed significant narrowing of the C4-C5 foramen and a larger superior articular process compared to those in the nonpalsy group.[9] In addition, on MRI, the posterior shift of the spinal cord at C4-C5 was significantly greater in the C5 palsy group than in the nonpalsy group, which indicated tethering of the nerve root (Figs. 20.1A and B).[9] They also found that 80% of cases in which nerve

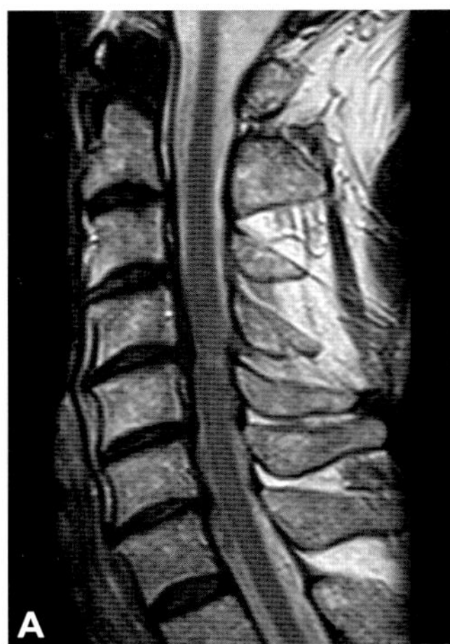

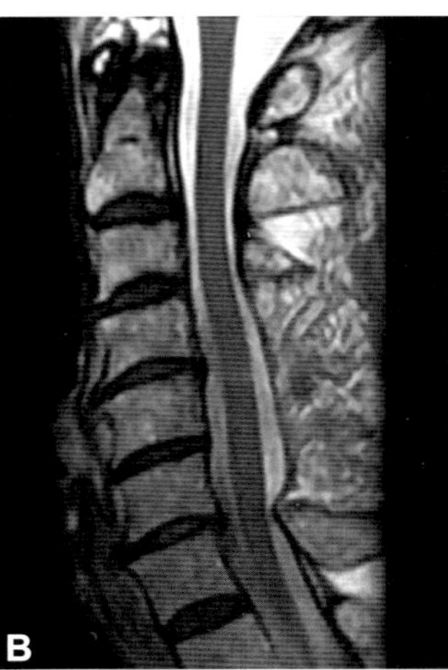


**Figs. 20.1A and B:** A 72-year-old man with cervical spondylotic myelopathy had disturbances of gait and fine finger movement control. (A) A preoperative T2-weighted sagittal magnetic resonance imaging (MRI) image of the cervical spine is shown. He underwent open-door laminoplasty. However, muscle weakness of the left deltoid [Manual Muscle Test (MMT) score of 2] and biceps brachii (MMT score of 2) started 2 days after the operation. (B) A postoperative T2-weighted sagittal MRI is shown. There were no obvious findings of C4-5 foraminal stenosis, but posterior shift of the spinal cord was observed. C5 palsy completely recovered spontaneously within 1 month. Tethering of the nerve root is thought to be due to the posterior shift of the spinal cord.

root impairment was suspected clinically were cases of C5 palsy accompanied by pain in the distribution of the C5 root, thereby suggesting that C5 palsy is more likely to be caused by C5 impairment than by spinal cord pathology.[9]

### *Reperfusion Injury*

Chiba et al.[6] analyzed 15 patients in whom postoperative segmental motor paralysis developed after expansive open-door laminoplasty; they found that mechanical injuries of the nerve root alone could not fully explain the cause of this paralysis for the following reasons: (1) The incidence of paralysis was not affected by the cervical alignment or the cause of spinal cord compression; (2) more than half of the paralyzed patients experienced multisegmental paralysis and bilateral involvements; and (3) no sensory disturbance was present in the concomitant segment in most of the patients. They reported that the delayed onset of paralysis, dysesthesia of the upper extremities, and the presence of T2 high-signal-intensity zones on MRI suggested that a certain impairment in the gray matter of the spinal cord may have an important role in the development of postoperative segmental motor paralysis.[6] T2 high-signal-intensity zones might represent changes in the microcirculatory spinal cord kinetics caused by congestion from rapid reperfusion of the blood flow after decompression.[6] In the central nervous system, rapid reperfusion of the blood flow after ischemia causes further damage to hypoxic tissues.[6,13] A rapid rise in $pO_2$ induces a risk for oxidative cell injury caused by the formation of free radicals and other toxic products of oxidative reactions.[6,14] Although there has not been direct evidence to support the reperfusion theory, the etiology of segmental motor paralysis may be multifactorial; in addition to nerve root pathology, the impairment of spinal cord autoregulation may be a factor in the development of segmental paralysis in some cases.[6] Ikegami et al.[15] reported that the existence of preoperative T2 high-signal-intensity zones was not a significant risk for the occurrence of postoperative segmental motor paralysis, but the intensity change significantly influenced the severity of the paralysis, which suggested that preoperative spinal cord damage has some additive effects on the severity of segmental motor paralysis.

## Prognosis

C5 palsy often resolves spontaneously, and previous studies have reported good prognosis for neurological and functional recovery.[2,16,17] Sakaura et al.[2] reported that differences in the overall rates of recovery between cases of severe [Manual Muscle Test (MMT) score of 1–2] and mild (MMT score of 3–4) deltoid paresis were not significant, and patients with postoperative C5 palsy generally had a good prognosis for functional recovery; however, cases of severe paralysis required significantly longer recovery times than did the mild cases. Conversely, irreversible cases of C5 palsy have also been reported.[3,9,18] For patients severely paralyzed at onset (MMT score of 0–2), conservative treatment may not be indicated.[9] C5 palsy adds significant burdens to patients' quality of life and to healthcare system costs.[19]

## Preventing C5 Palsy

There is no reliable way of completely preventing C5 palsy, but several approaches have been suggested to decrease its occurrence. Symmetric decompression achieved by open-door laminoplasty might introduce imbalanced rotational movement of the spinal cord and result in C5 palsy.[20] Double-door laminoplasty is recommended to minimize C5 palsy, particularly if the patient has ossification of the posterior longitudinal ligament.[20] Eskander et al.[21] reviewed 176 patients who underwent anterior decompression or corpectomy at the C4–C6 levels and suggested that spinal cord rotation was a strong and significant predictor of C5 palsy. In their study, patients were classified into three types: type 1 represented mild rotation (0°–5°), type 2 represented moderate rotation (6°–10°), and type 3 represented severe rotation (≥11°). C5 palsy occurred in none of the 159 patients with type 1 rotation, 8 of 13 with type 2 rotation, and 4 of 4 with type 3 rotation.[21] These results indicate that patients with greater degrees of spinal cord rotation and subsequent cord displacement were also at greater risk of C5 palsy in anterior surgery.[21] Odate et al.[22] stated that surgeons should consider restricting decompression width to <15 mm and avoid asymmetric decompression to reduce the incidence of C5 palsy in the anterior approach.

Prophylactic C4-C5 foraminotomy reduces the risk of C5 palsy.[1,9,23] If a patient has a stenotic C4-C5 foramen and a prominent articular process, palsy may be avoided by performing a concomitant foraminotomy.[9] Komagata et al.[24] reported that bilateral C4-C5 foraminotomy with open-door laminoplasty decreased the incidence of C5 palsy to 0.6%. Their partial foraminotomy decompresses nerve roots from branch point to entry point of the foramen. The foraminotomy is reported to be useful for treating even postoperative C5 palsy.[23] Excessive expansion by laminoplasty also should be avoided to prevent the C5 nerve root from becoming tethered by a posterior shift of the spinal cord.[9]

C5 palsy after posterior fusion with instrumentation also has been reported.[23,25-27] The incidence of C5 palsy was significantly higher for spinal instrumented fusion combined with laminoplasty than for laminoplasty alone.[26] Correction using posterior instrumentation of kyphosis and spondylolisthesis is a risk factor for iatrogenic foraminal stenosis leading to C5 palsy.[26] Kyphosis correction at C4-C5 is achieved by the posterior shift of the C4 vertebra and shortening of the disk height at C4-C5, which eventually causes foraminal stenosis at C4-C5 (Figs. 20.2A and B).[25] Wu et al.[27] recommended the use of an appropriate distraction maneuver between spinal segments during placement of the rod to prevent iatrogenic foraminal stenosis. To avoid significant posterior shift of the spinal cord, excessive kyphosis correction should not be performed.[23,25] Hojo et al.[25] recommended avoiding excessive correction of cervical kyphosis exceeding 9.7° per segment and kyphosis correction mainly at C4-C5 because

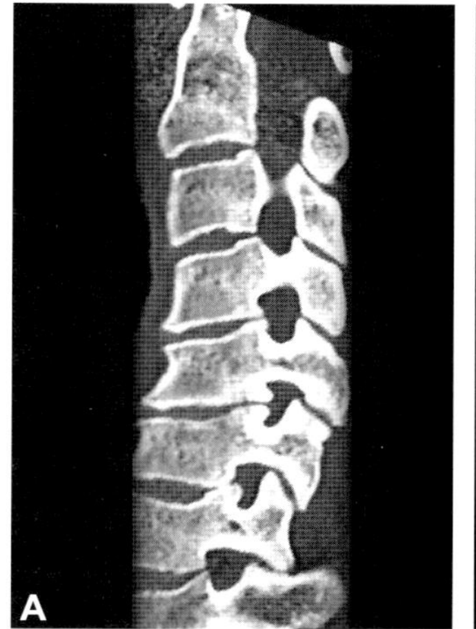


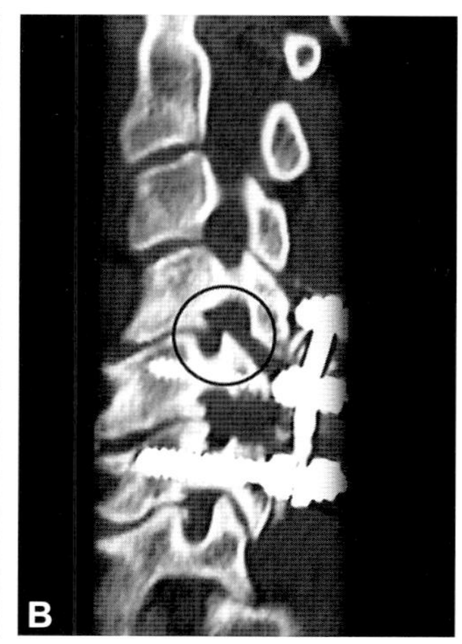


**Figs. 20.2A and B:** Postoperative iatrogenic foraminal stenosis. A 41-year-old-man had undergone laminoplasty combined with C4-C6 posterior instrumentation with pedicle screws for cervical myelopathy with segmental instability. Left C5-6 foraminotomy was also performed because foraminal stenosis was observed on preoperative sagittal reconstructed computed tomography (CT) imaging (A). Seven days after the surgery, muscle weakness of the left deltoid [Manual Muscle Test (MMT) score of 2] and biceps brachii (MMT score of 3) was observed. Postoperative CT showed that the C4 vertebra translated posteriorly, which indicated that the nerve root was impinged between the bony spar of the C4 vertebra and the superior articular process of C5 (B; circle). He underwent additional bilateral C4-5 foraminotomy. The next day, there were clearly signs of recovery, and his muscle weakness returned to normal in 3 months.

it may cause both foraminal stenosis at C4-C5 foramen and the most dramatic posterior shift of the spinal cord at C4-C5 segment.

Another choice for kyphosis correction is the anterior surgery. It is easy to apply a distraction force between vertebral bodies, which widens the disk space to create cervical lordosis.[25] Herman et al.[28] reported that the average kyphosis correction angle was 21°, and Ferch et al.[29] reported that it was 11°. Neither study reported any postoperative late neurological complications. The reasons for this were thought to be that the correction angle achieved by anterior surgery was smaller than that achieved by posterior surgery and that intervertebral graft could enlarge the intervertebral foramina.[25]

The use of intraoperative neurophysiological monitoring in surgical decompression surgery for cervical myelopathy may assist the surgeon in taking corrective measures to reduce or prevent permanent neurological deficits.[30,31] Clark et al.[31] found a correlation between decreased intraoperative transcranial motor-evoked potentials (MEPs) and postoperative new neurological deficits

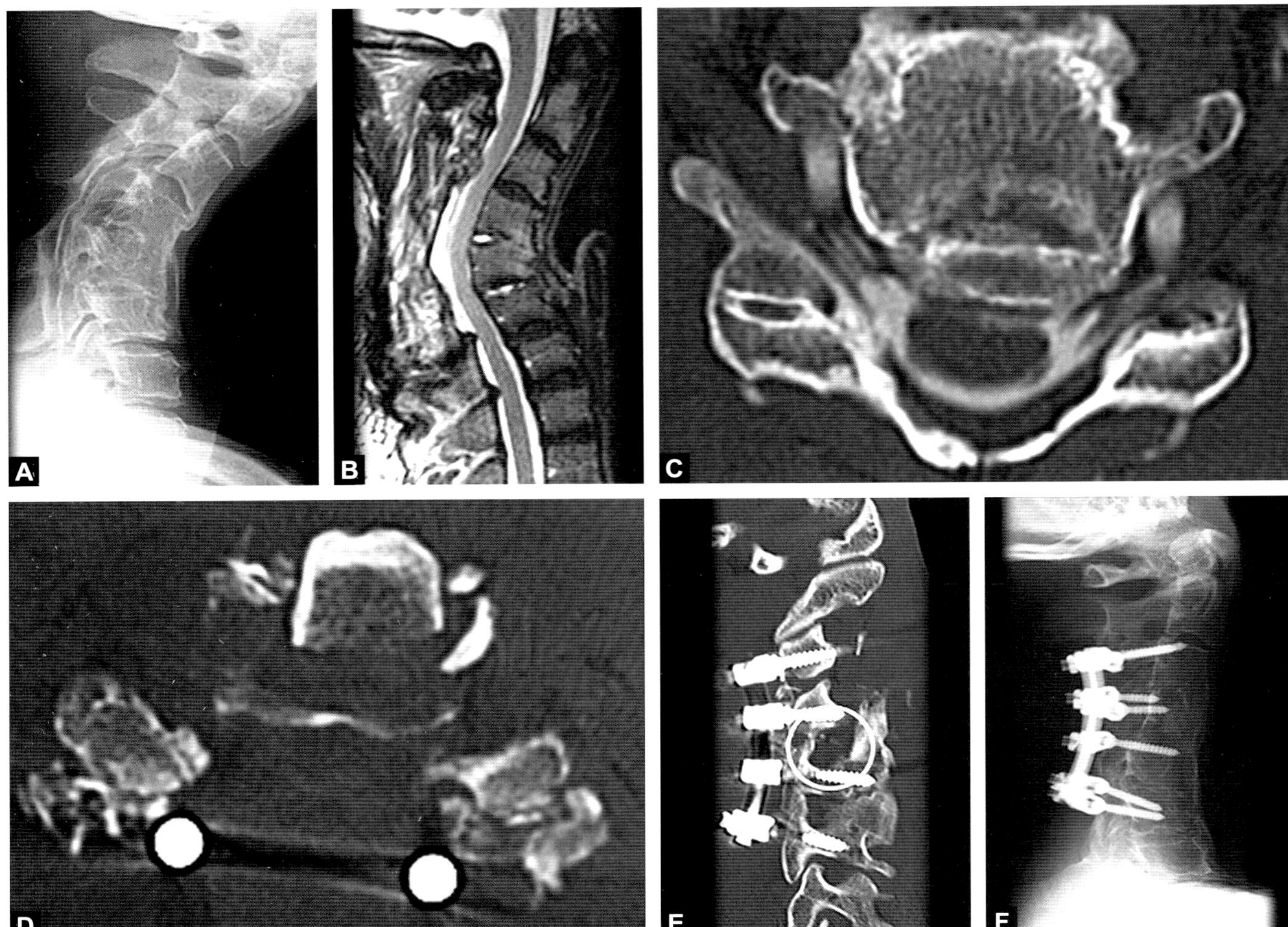

**Figs. 20.3A to F:** A 48-year-old man was unable maintain a horizontal gaze in addition to neck pain. The etiology of his cervical kyphosis was unknown. (A) Lateral cervical spine radiography showed cervical kyphosis. (B) Sagittal magnetic resonance imaging showed that the spinal cord was draped over the vertebral body. (C) Computed tomography (CT) angiogram at C4-5 showed a bone spur located in front of the bilateral vertebral artery. He underwent combined anterior and posterior surgeries with iliac bone graft. These included corpectomy of C4, uncinectomy of bilateral C4 and C5, laminectomy of C3-C6, and foraminotomy of C3-C4 and C4-C5. Intraoperative transcranial motor-evoked potentials showed no abnormal signs. However, 4 days after surgery, muscle weakness of the left deltoid [Manual Muscle Test (MMT) score of 2] and biceps brachii (MMT score of 4) were observed. Postoperative CT showed no obvious foraminal stenosis at C4-5 (D; axial image at C4-5 level, E; sagittal reformatted CT image showing the C4-5 foramen; circle). C5 palsy recovered spontaneously within 4 months. The posterior shift of the spinal cord after surgery may have caused the late neurological deficits after correction of cervical kyphosis.

in patients with cervical myelopathy. Sensitivity varied depending on the patient's comorbidities, age, and preoperative neurological function. However, the sensitivity increased to 100% in elderly patients and in patients with preoperative motor deficits. The sensitivity and positive predictive values of the deltoid and biceps MEP changes in predicting C5 palsy were 67% and 67%, respectively.[31] Bhalodia et al.[32] reported that the sensitivity and specificity of MEPs monitoring for identifying acute-onset deltoid weakness were 100% and 99%, respectively, and for spontaneous electromyography monitoring were only 20% and 92%, respectively. They concluded that MEPs monitoring is a highly sensitive and specific technique for detecting C5 palsy that manifests immediately upon waking from anesthesia. However, delayed-onset C5 palsy cannot be predicted by intraoperative neuromonitoring via either modality (Figs. 20.3A to F).[32]

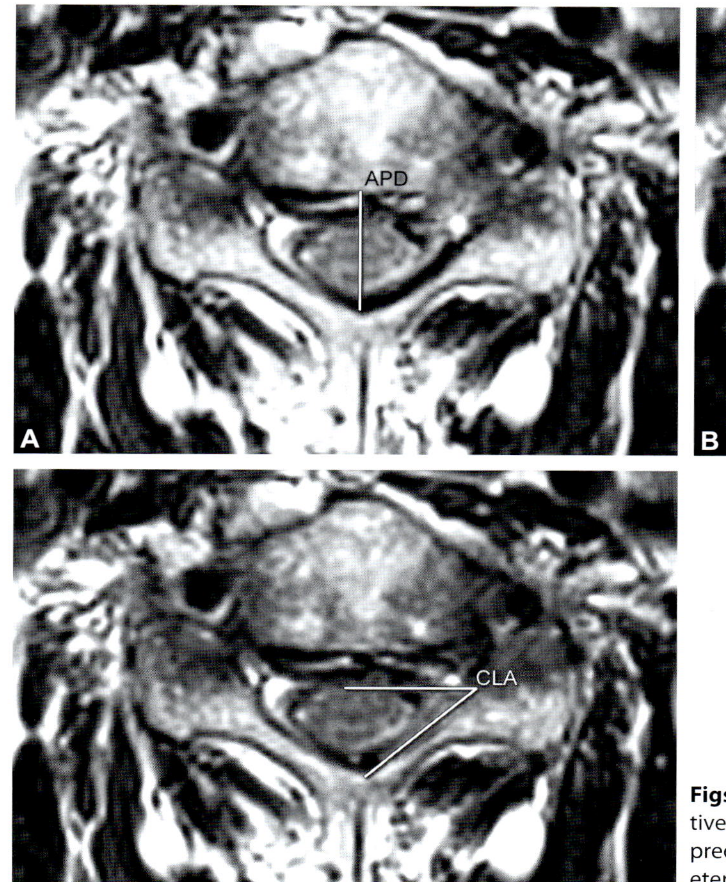


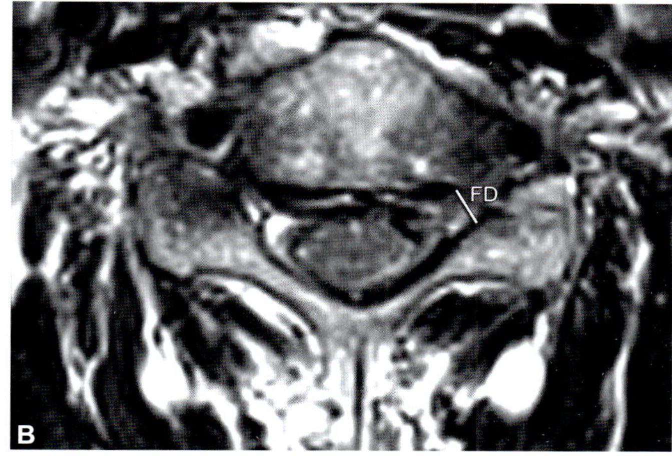


**Figs. 20.4A to C:** A formula predicts development of postoperative C5 palsy for patients with cervical myelopathy by measuring preoperative anteroposterior diameter (A; APD), foraminal diameter (B; FD), and cord-lamina angle (C; CLA) on T2-weighted magnetic resonance imaging.

Recently, Lubelski et al.[33] established a formula to predict the development of postoperative C5 palsy after decompression surgery for patients with cervical myelopathy by measuring preoperative anteroposterior diameter (APD), foraminal diameter (FD), and cord-lamina angle (CLA) on MRI (Figs. 20.4A to C). Using the three variables in a predictive model, they found that the odds ratios of having palsy for APD, FD, and CLA were 0.3, 0.02, and 1.4, respectively. For every 1 mm increase in APD and FD, the odds of developing palsy decreased 69% and 98%, respectively. In contrast, for every 1° increase in CLA, the odds of developing palsy increased by 43%. The associated equation for the fitted logistic regression model was as follows:

$$\log (p/1 - p) = -0.81 - [1.16 \bullet (\text{APD})] - [4.00 \times (\text{FD})] + [0.35 \times (\text{CLA})]$$

This prediction formula may enable better patient selection as well as preparation of patients who have an increased probability of developing C5 palsy.[33]

## VERTEBRAL ARTERY INJURY AS A VASCULAR COMPLICATION

### Epidemiology

Iatrogenic vertebral artery (VA) injury is a rare complication of cervical spinal surgery, but it can result in catastrophic complications, such as arteriovenous fistulae, late-onset hemorrhage, pseudoaneurysm and thrombosis with embolic incidents, cerebral ischemia, stroke, and even death.[34] The vascular complications might occur days to years later. Ischemia occurring immediately after surgery could be the result of complete occlusion of the vessels, whereas those occurring much later could be the result of emboli from a partially occluded VA.[34]

Vertebral artery injury can occur during both anterior cervical decompression and fusion and posterior instrumentation surgery. The incidence in anterior cervical decompression and fusion is 0.18–0.5%[35,36] and that in posterior atlantoaxial transarticular screw fixation is

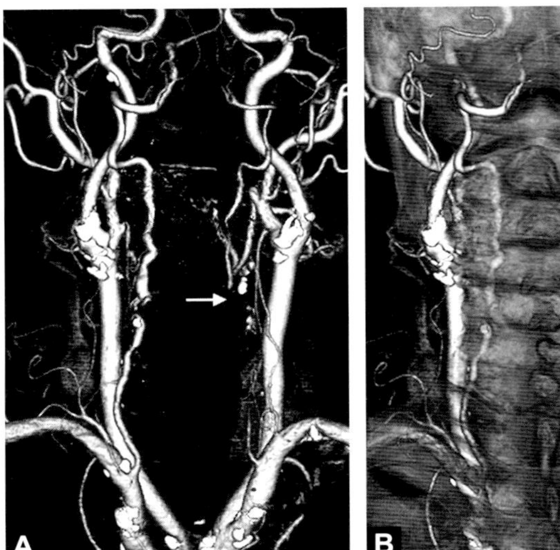
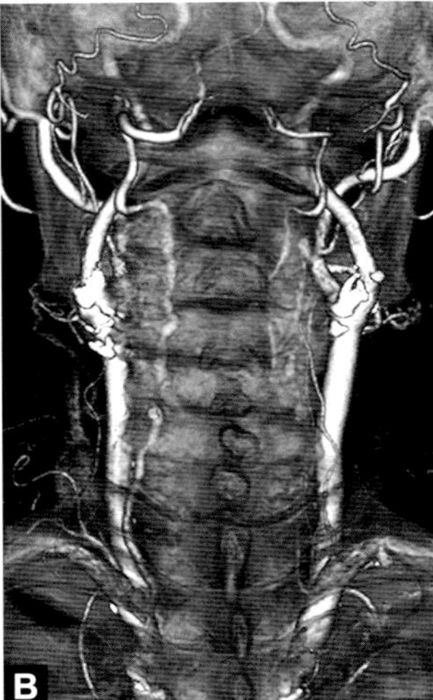

**Figs. 20.5A and B:** Preoperative three-dimensional computed tomographic angiogram showing the disrupted right vertebral artery (A; arrow). (B) An integrated image of the vascular and cervical spine is shown.

1.3–8.2%.[35,37] In a systematic literature review, Coe et al.[38] reported that no cases of VA injury were identified in 758 patients who underwent lateral mass screw fixation in the cervical spine. Similarly, in a systematic review, Yoshihara et al.[39] stated that VA injuries were extremely rare following the use of both lateral mass screws and cervical pedicle screws in the subaxial cervical spine, although they were significantly more common when using cervical pedicle screws.

## Anomalies in the VAs and Circle of Willis

During posterior instrumentation surgery, there is a risk bleeding or cerebral infarction from injury to a VA because of the penetration of a screw into the transverse foramen.[40] However, VA occlusion is rarely symptomatic because there is usually sufficient collateral blood supply from the contralateral side and the circle of Willis.[41,42] In patients with occlusion of both VAs, both the posterior communicating artery and the first segment of the posterior cerebral artery (P1), which constitute the posterior part of the circle of Willis, are essential collateral vessels for the basilar artery;[42,43] these collaterals can respond quickly to low perfusion pressure by a simple reversal of flow.[42] Therefore, their size and patency may be a risk factor for cerebral infarction in patients whose VAs have been occluded or rendered stenotic by cervical instrumentation (Figs. 20.5A and B).[42]

Sano et al.[43] measured the diameters of VA, P1, and basilar artery, and they determined the rate of formation of an anomalous VA and the variation in the posterior portions of the circle of Willis. They showed that a hypoplastic VA (<2.2 mm in diameter), a hypoplastic P1 (<1 mm in diameter), and a hypoplastic P1 (<1 mm in diameter) were present in 11%, 81%, and 13% of patients, respectively.[43] Nagahama et al.[42] used three-dimensional CT angiography (3D-CTA) to investigate the incidence of anomalies in VAs and circle of Willis in 55 consecutive patients who had undergone instrumented posterior fusion of the cervical spine. The frequencies of abnormal VA blood flow and VA dominance were 58.2% and 40%, respectively. The posterior communicating artery was occluded on one side in 41.8% of the patients and bilaterally in 38.2%. Variations in VAs and the circle of Willis were not significantly related to the presence or absence of the posterior communicating arteries. Importantly, 18.2% of the patients showed characteristic variations in the circle of Willis with unilateral VA stenosis or a dominant VA, which indicated that a high rate of anatomical variations led to lethal complications among these patients (Fig. 20.6).[42]

## Surgical Planning Algorithm for Posterior Instrumentation Surgery

Preoperative 3D-CTA can simultaneously show both VAs and the surrounding bony structures. Preoperative assessment of VAs and circle of Willis is essential if a posterior spinal fusion with instrumentation is to be performed safely. Flowchart 20.1 shows a 3D-CTA-based surgical planning algorithm for the different types of vascular anomalies.[42]

## Management of VA Injury

Management of VA injury includes direct tamponade, microsurgical repair, and surgical ligation. Direct hemostatic tamponade with hemostatic agents is often effective in managing acute bleeding. However, several cases of hemorrhage and fistula formation have been reported.[44] The simplest and most effective technique is screw placement, but screw insertion could lead to VA erosion with recurrent hemorrhage, distal embolization, or late infarction.[45] Microvascular repair preserves blood flow and minimizes the risk of ischemic complications.[34] Surgical ligation of VA can achieve hemostasis, but significant morbidity and mortality have been reported following

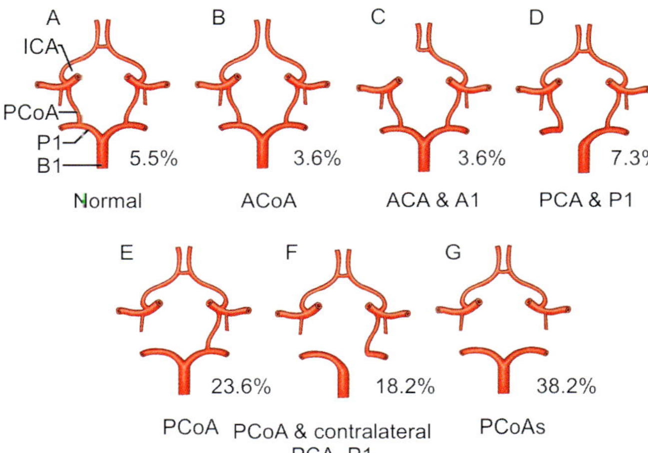


**Fig. 20.6:** Anatomical variations of the circle of Willis. In each case, the absence of an artery (depicted only on one side, but it can also be absent on the other side) and its frequency were investigated.

(ICA: Internal carotid artery; PCoA: Posterior communicating artery; P1: First segment of the posterior cerebral artery; BA: Basilar artery; ACoA: Anterior communicating artery; ACA: Anterior cerebral artery; A1: First segment of the anterior cerebral artery; PCA: Posterior cerebral artery).

*Source*: Reproduced with permission and copyright of the British Editorial Society of Bone and Joint Surgery. Nagahama K, Sudo H, Abumi K, et al. Anomalous vertebral and posterior communicating arteries as a risk factor in cervical instrumentation surgery. Bone Joint J. 2014;96-B:535-40.

**Flowchart 20.1:** A three-dimensional computed tomographic angiography-based surgical planning algorithm in the presence of the different types of vascular anomalies.

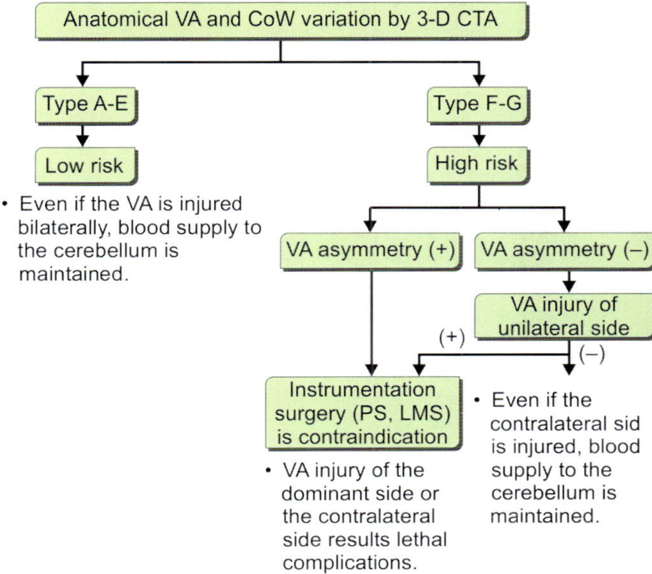


(VA: Vertebral artery; CoW: Circle of Willis; PS: Pedicle screw; LMS: Lateral mass screw).

*Source*: Reproduced with permission and copyright of the British Editorial Society of Bone and Joint Surgery. Nagahama K, Sudo H, Abumi K, et al. Anomalous vertebral and posterior communicating arteries as a risk factor in cervical instrumentation surgery. Bone Joint J. 2014;96-B:535-40.

this procedure.[46] Thus, ligation should only be considered when adequate collateral blood supply is confirmed by intraoperative angiography. Peng et al.[34] recommended performing immediate angiography even if an injury is managed with tamponade only or direct repair to detect vascular complications, confirming adequate collateral circulation, and determining the patency of a surgically repaired vessel or to detect any stenosis. In case of a patent contralateral VA or sufficient collateral posterior circulation, an alternative intervention for an injured VA can be total occlusion with coil embolization to prevent further complications.[34] Irrespective of the choice of intervention, follow-up evaluation of the vessel situation is necessary by MRI or CTA.

## CONCLUSION

Both C5 palsy and VA injury are rare but can occur during surgical management of cervical myelopathy. Careful preoperative evaluation using imaging techniques and careful and appropriate surgical procedures can reduce the risk of neurovascular complications.

## REFERENCES

1. Katsumi K, Yamazaki A, Watanabe K, et al. Can prophylactic bilateral C4/C5 foraminotomy prevent postoperative C5 palsy after open-door laminoplasty?: a prospective study. Spine (Phila Pa 1976). 2012;37:748-54.
2. Sakaura H, Hosono N, Mukai Y, et al. C5 palsy after decompression surgery for cervical myelopathy: review of the literature. Spine (Phila Pa 1976). 2003;28:2447-51.
3. Hashimoto M, Mochizuki M, Aiba A, et al. C5 palsy following anterior decompression and spinal fusion for cervical degenerative diseases. Eur Spine J. 2010;19:1702-10.
4. Nassr A, Eck JC, Ponnappan RK, et al. The incidence of C5 palsy after multilevel cervical decompression procedures: a review of 750 consecutive cases. Spine (Phila Pa 1976). 2012;37:174-8.
5. Gandhoke G, Wu JC, Rowland NC, et al. Anterior corpectomy versus posterior laminoplasty: is the risk of postoperative C-5 palsy different? Neurosurg Focus. 2011;31:E12.
6. Chiba K, Toyama Y, Matsumoto M, et al. Segmental motor paralysis after expansive open-door laminoplasty. Spine (Phila Pa 1976). 2002;27:2108-15.
7. Fan D, Schwartz DM, Vaccaro AR, et al. Intraoperative neurophysiologic detection of iatrogenic C5 nerve root injury

during laminectomy for cervical compression myelopathy. Spine (Phila Pa 1976). 2002;27:2499-502.
8. Hasegawa K, Homma T, Chiba Y. Upper extremity palsy following cervical decompression surgery results from a transient spinal cord lesion. Spine (Phila Pa 1976). 2007;32:E197-202.
9. Imagama S, Matsuyama Y, Yukawa Y, et al. C5 palsy after cervical laminoplasty: a multicentre study. J Bone Joint Surg Br. 2010;92:393-400.
10. Hosono N, Miwa T, Mukai Y, et al. Potential risk of thermal damage to cervical nerve roots by a high-speed drill. J Bone Joint Surg Br. 2009;91:1541-4.
11. Tsuzuki N, Zhogshi L, Abe R, et al. Paralysis of the arm after posterior decompression of the cervical spinal cord. I. Anatomical investigation of the mechanism of paralysis. Eur Spine J. 1993;2:191-6.
12. Katsumi K, Yamazaki A, Watanabe K, et al. Analysis of C5 palsy after cervical open-door laminoplasty: relationship between C5 palsy and foraminal stenosis. J Spinal Disord Tech. 2013;26:177-82.
13. Zhao M, Zhang Y, Liu L, et al. Somatosensory- and motor-evoked potentials in a rabbit model of spinal cord ischemia and reperfusion injury. Spine (Phila Pa 1976). 1997;22:1013-7.
14. Kim-Lee MH, Stokes BT, Yates AJ. Reperfusion paradox: a novel mode of glial cell injury. Glia. 1992;5:56-64.
15. Ikegami S, Tsutsumimoto T, Ohta H, et al. Preoperative spinal cord damage affects the characteristics and prognosis of segmental motor paralysis after cervical decompression surgery. Spine (Phila Pa 1976). 2014;39:463-8.
16. Satomi K, Nishu Y, Kohno T, et al. Long-term follow-up studies of open-door expansive laminoplasty for cervical stenotic myelopathy. Spine (Phila Pa 1976). 1994;19:507-10.
17. Uematsu Y, Tokuhashi Y, Matsuzaki H. Radiculopathy after laminoplasty of the cervical spine. Spine (Phila Pa 1976). 1998;23:2057-62.
18. Ikenaga M, Shikata J, Tanaka C. Radiculopathy of C-5 after anterior decompression for cervical myelopathy. J Neurosurg Spine. 2005;3:210-7.
19. Miller JA, Lubelski D, Alvin MD, et al. C5 Palsy following posterior cervical decompression and fusion: cost and quality of life implications. Spine J. 2014;14 (12):2854-60.
20. Kaneyama S, Sumi M, Kanatani T, et al. Prospective study and multivariate analysis of the incidence of C5 palsy after cervical laminoplasty. Spine (Phila Pa 1976). 2010;35:E1553-8.
21. Eskander MS, Balsis SM, Balinger C, et al. The association between preoperative spinal cord rotation and postoperative C5 nerve palsy. J Bone Joint Surg Am. 2012;94:1605-9.
22. Odate S, Shikata J, Yamamura S, et al. Extremely wide and asymmetric anterior decompression causes postoperative C5 palsy: an analysis of 32 patients with postoperative C5 palsy after anterior cervical decompression and fusion. Spine (Phila Pa 1976). 2013;38:2184-9.
23. Nakashima H, Imagama S, Yukawa Y, et al. Multivariate analysis of C-5 palsy incidence after cervical posterior fusion with instrumentation. J Neurosurg Spine. 2012;17:103-10.
24. Komagata M, Nishiyama M, Endo K, et al. Prophylaxis of C5 palsy after cervical expansive laminoplasty by bilateral partial foraminotomy. Spine J. 2004;4:650-5.
25. Hojo Y, Ito M, Abumi K, et al. A late neurological complication following posterior correction surgery of severe cervical kyphosis. Eur Spine J. 2011;20:890-8.
26. Yamanaka K, Tachibana T, Moriyama T, et al. C-5 palsy after cervical laminoplasty with instrumented posterior fusion. J Neurosurg Spine. 2014;20:1-4.
27. Wu FL, Sun Y, Pan SF, et al. Risk factors associated with upper extremity palsy after expansive open-door laminoplasty for cervical myelopathy. Spine J. 2014; 14:909-15.
28. Herman JM, Sonntag VK. Cervical corpectomy and plate fixation for postlaminectomy kyphosis. J Neurosurg. 1994;80 (6):963-70.
29. Ferch RD, Shad A, Cadoux-Hudson TA, et al. Anterior correction of cervical kyphotic deformity: effects on myelopathy, neck pain, and sagittal alignment. J Neurosurg. 2004;100 (1 Suppl Spine):13-9.
30. Currier BL. Neurological complications of cervical spine surgery: C5 palsy and intraoperative monitoring. Spine (Phila Pa 1976). 2012;37:E328-34.
31. Clark AJ, Ziewacz JE, Safaee M, et al. Intraoperative neuromonitoring with MEPs and prediction of postoperative neurological deficits in patients undergoing surgery for cervical and cervicothoracic myelopathy. Neurosurg Focus. 2013; 35:E7.
32. Bhalodia VM, Schwartz DM, Sestokas AK, et al. Efficacy of intraoperative monitoring of transcranial electrical stimulation-induced motor evoked potentials and spontaneous electromyography activity to identify acute-versus delayed-onset C-5 nerve root palsy during cervical spine surgery: clinical article. J Neurosurg Spine. 2013;19:395-402.
33. Lubelski D, Derakhshan A, Nowacki AS, et al. Predicting C5 palsy via the use of preoperative anatomic measurements. Spine J. 2014;14(9):1895-901.
34. Peng CW, Chou BT, Bendo JA, et al. Vertebral artery injury in cervical spine surgery: anatomical considerations, management, and preventive measures. Spine J. 2009;9:70-6.
35. Neo M, Fujibayashi S, Miyata M, et al. Vertebral artery injury during cervical spine surgery: a survey of more than 5600 operations. Spine (Phila Pa 1976). 2008;33:779-85.
36. Burke JP, Gerszten PC, Welch WC. Iatrogenic vertebral artery injury during anterior cervical spine surgery. Spine J. 2005;5:508-14.
37. Wright NM, Lauryssen C. Vertebral artery injury in C1-2 transarticular screw fixation: results of a survey of the AANS/CNS section on disorders of the spine and peripheral nerves. American Association of Neurological Surgeons/ Congress of Neurological Surgeons. J Neurosurg. 1998;88: 634-40.
38. Coe JD, Vaccaro AR, Dailey AT, et al. Lateral mass screw fixation in the cervical spine: a systematic literature review. J Bone Joint Surg Am. 2013;95:2136-43.
39. Yoshihara H, Passias PG, Errico TJ. Screw-related complications in the subaxial cervical spine with the use of lateral mass versus cervical pedicle screws: a systematic review. J Neurosurg Spine. 2013;19:614-23.
40. Abumi K, Ito M, Sudo H. Reconstruction of the subaxial cervical spine using pedicle screw instrumentation. Spine (Phila Pa 1976). 2012;37:E349-56.

41. Taneichi H, Suda K, Kajino T, et al. Traumatically induced vertebral artery occlusion associated with cervical spine injuries: prospective study using magnetic resonance angiography. Spine (Phila Pa 1976). 2005;30:1955-62.
42. Nagahama K, Sudo H, Abumi K, et al. Anomalous vertebral and posterior communicating arteries as a risk factor in cervical instrumentation surgery. Bone Joint J. 2014;96-B:535-40.
43. Sano A, Hirano T, Watanabe K, et al. Preoperative evaluation of the vertebral arteries and posterior portion of the circle of Willis for cervical spine surgery using 3-dimensional computed tomography angiography. Spine (Phila Pa 1976). 2013;38:E960-7.
44. Choi JW, Lee JK, Moon KS, et al. Endovascular embolization of iatrogenic vertebral artery injury during anterior cervical spine surgery: report of two cases and review of the literature. Spine (Phila Pa 1976). 2006;31:E891-4.
45. Maughan PH, Ducruet AF, Elhadi AM, et al. Multimodality management of vertebral artery injury sustained during cervical or craniocervical surgery. Neurosurgery. 2013;73(2 Suppl Operative):271-81.
46. Shintani A, Zervas NT. Consequence of ligation of the vertebral artery. J Neurosurg. 1972;36:447-50.

# Section 5

# Cervical Myelopathy in the Setting of Cervical Deformities

Chapter 21

# Cervical Myelopathy in the Setting of Cervical Deformities

*Shaleen Vira, Matthew A Spiegel, Virginie Lafage, Frank Schwab*

## INTRODUCTION

Rather than being a distinct clinical entity, cervical alignment plays an important role in the evaluation of any patient with cervical spine pathology. Alignment considerations permeate many of the distinct clinical entities that cause myelopathy but are particularly evident in cervical spondylotic myelopathy (CSM). Furthermore, there is a two-way association between alignment and myelopathy pathophysiology. Not only does the alignment affect the clinical course and response to intervention in myelopathic patients, but also the pathogenesis of myelopathy itself leads to derangements in cervical alignment. This chapter formulates these concepts into a cohesive framework for clinical application.

## WHAT IS CONSIDERED A CERVICAL DEFORMITY?

The function of the cervical spine in the setting of sagittal alignment is to maintain horizontal gaze.[1] There is a wide range of normal alignment as described in the preceding chapters, and there is a wide range of what is considered a deformity. Global, regional, and focal considerations contribute toward making a diagnosis of cervical deformity. Furthermore, depending on the particular deformity, either static or dynamic factors may play a larger role in the contribution of deformity to symptomatic myelopathy.

### Static Alignment

#### *Pathophysiology*

The pathophysiology of CSM can be summarized as symptomatic compression of the spinal column by spondylotic changes. The insult to the column can occur by direct compression from an offending structure or by indirect compression via vascular supply damage that then leads to cord dysfunction. Both static and dynamic pathophysiologic mechanisms are involved in this compressive etiology. Additionally, the alignment of the spine is intimately related to the pathophysiology of the disease. Accordingly, this section focuses on the static alignment factors that drive myelopathy.

Spondylosis is defined as the degenerative changes of the vertebrae, intervertebral disks, facets, and associated ligaments. Spondylotic degeneration is age-related, and not all patients experience myelopathic or radiculopathic symptoms. Imaging studies of asymptomatic individuals over age 60 show that spondylosis exists in the cervical spine, at one or more levels, in up to 95% of men and 89% of women.[2,3] Furthermore, in a consecutive autopsy series of 200 adults, spondylosis was demonstrated in 53.5% of specimens, with only 7.5% having had documented clinical evidence of myelopathy.[4] These findings imply that the development of CSM cannot be solely attributed to anatomical degeneration. This realization has encouraged clinicians to further investigate how alignment factors link degenerative changes to myelopathy.

#### *Kyphosis*

In 2012, Le Huec et al. reported that over one-third of their asymptomatic normative cohort presented with kyphotic cervical spines, but without any complaints.[5] This is an analogous to findings of Boden, that spondylotic changes are seen in many asymptomatic individuals.[2] Indeed, neither kyphosis nor spondylosis necessitates myelopathy, as the relationship between imagining findings and pathology is complex.

Nevertheless, kyphosis is one scenario that is known to lead to cervical myelopathy. Its pathological mechanism is through the degeneration of cervical intervertebral disks, as an early event in the cascade toward spondylosis. While normally, anterior disk height is greater than posterior disk height, in spondylosis, Lestini et al. explain that the ventral portion of the disk preferentially loses height, such that the final result is a loss of normal cervical lordosis (CL).[6] This, in turn, leads to greater forces being placed on ventral aspects of the vertebral bodies, resulting in cervical kyphosis.[7] To make matters worse, as anterior and posterior borders of the cervical curvature compress and lateral margins expand, kyphosis progresses further, spiraling the cascade.[8]

Cervical kyphosis forces the spinal cord to abut against the vertebral bodies, leading to compression of the anterior cord. If the cord is tethered by ligaments (dentate ligament) and cervical nerve roots, this can increase longitudinal cord tension.[9] Intramedullary pressure can increase from this cord tethering, which can then lead to neuronal loss and demyelination.

Kyphosis also yields indirect damage to the spine, via vascular insults. In a model of small game fowls, Shimizu et al. found that the degree of kyphosis is related to the amount of cord flattening and decreasing vascular supply, as the small feeder blood vessels for the cord become flattened and lead to ischemia.[8] Using angiography, it is easy to demonstrate that vascular supply to the anterior cord is decreased in kyphosis. Again, progressive kyphosis over time can exacerbate these changes, especially anteriorly where the mechanical compression is direct. Specifically, the anterior horn and anterior fasciculus preferentially experience neuronal loss and atrophy. Shimizu et al. also found that with advanced progression, the lateral and posterior fasciculi deteriorate as well.[8] Finally, Naderi et al. conclude that the presence of abnormal cervical curvature predicts decreased postoperative neurologic improvement, and patients with greater kyphosis experience more neck pain.[10,11]

## Sagittal Malalignment

Sagittal malalignment (as further explained in Chapter 3) is defined as anterior deviation of the C7 plumb line >50 mm from the posterior superior corner of S1.[12,13] Similar to kyphosis, sagittal malalignment has also been implicated as a contributor of cord flattening and increased cord tension, a cascade that as mentioned above, ultimately results in neurologic derangement.[14] In a cadaveric model, induced thoracic kyphosis (TK) of 51° and above resulted in a significant increase of intramedullary pressure, further supporting the link between alignment and the development of myelopathy.[15]

Tang et al. explain that in the presence of positive cervical sagittal alignment, the cervical spine may adopt drastic changes in curvature, namely, hyperlordosis of C1-C2, as a compensatory mechanism.[10] This compensation is driven by Dubousset's conus of economy.[1] Moreover, with increasing age, patients with CSM have decreased range of motion (ROM), with stiff soft tissue, to maintain the head-neck complex in optimal position.[17] Therefore, patients may not realize their full ROM in flexion, because of habitually keeping a stiff neck.[18,19] These compensatory changes are adapted by the human body in order to maintain horizontal gaze, and are actually maladaptive from the perspective of CSM.

Akin to this lordotic maladaptive cascade for maintenance of horizontal gaze is the relation between TK and lumbar lordosis (LL). It is known that the TK and LL curves adapt to patients' pelvic incidence (PI). Continuing the chain, the amount of CL must then also be proportional to the lower curves. Thus, in addition to CL correlating with sagittal vertical axis (SVA), CL also responds to angulations of PI, pelvic tilt (PT), TK, LL, T1 slope (T1S), and thoracic inlet angle (TIA).

Alternative hypotheses exist to explain the relationship between the cervical spinal alignment and thoracolumbar sagittal alignment. Traditionally it was thought that patients who have anterior malalignment of the spine (positive SVA), secondary to decrease in LL and/or an increase in TK, recruit cervical spine compensatory mechanisms (increasing CL). However, recent studies on adult spinal deformity patients with varying levels of sagittal malalignment demonstrate similar chin brow vertical angle and C2C7 SVA. Craniocervical parameters are markers of intrinsic deformity as opposed to compensation to thoracolumbar malalignment.[20] Similarly, when comparing patients who have undergone deformity under-correction with those who have undergone overcorrection, there is no difference in CL but significant differences in recruitment of compensatory mechanisms in the pelvis and lower extremities.[21] This nascent area of research certainly is an apt area for further inquiry.

The diagnosis and management of cervical deformities requires utmost appreciation of sagittal malalignment. Glassman et al. established that positive SVA is associated with a deterioration in quality of life (QOL) in patients with adult spinal deformity.[22] Furthermore, Tang et al. discovered that even a C2 SVA >40 mm (where 40–50 mm is still considered "normal") is a cause of concern for cervical misalignment, as poor health-related QOL (HRQOL) scores begin to correlate with worse outcomes, as assessed by the neck disability index (NDI).[10]

Villavicencio et al. conducted a double-blinded, randomized, controlled trial (elucidating that improved cervical Cobb angles do not correlate significantly with clinical outcomes, but maintaining or improving segmental sagittal alignment does have significant implications for improvement in outcome scores.[23]

The C2-C7 SVA is also correlated with other HRQOLs, such as the modified Japanese Orthopaedic Association (mJOA), $r = -0.282$. In preoperative patients, with sagittal malalignment as measured by increased C2-C7 SVA, the mJOA associates with worse functionality.[24] Alternatively, the C2-C7 Cobb was not found to significantly correlate with mJOA scores. Protopsaltis et al. examined over 150 patients with CSM, and confirmed that high baseline cervical SVAs (cSVA) correlated with significantly worse disability scores from the mJOA. Interestingly, the mean cSVAs of the high cSVA cohort were 39.4 ± 7.4 mm, suggesting that 40 mm may be a potential threshold below which cervical sagittal malalignment should be corrected.[25]

In a study by Smith et al. on preoperative myelopathic patients, mJOA scores were found to have differing relationships with magnetic resonance imaging (MRI) cervical alignment findings.[24] For kyphotic patients, there was moderate negative correlation between normalized cord volumes and cross-sectional areas to mJOA scores. However, for lordotic patients, mJOA scores were found to be positively correlated with cord volumes, external cord areas, and mean cross sectional areas. This suggests that the role of cord volume and area in myelopathy is dependent on alignment. Smith et al. postulated that kyphosis-induced tension could occur only after a certain threshold of alignment values, at which point cord redundancy might be exceeded and cord elasticity is maximized. However, they did not specifically find a correlation between preoperative kyphosis and severity of myelopathy. Nevertheless, when present, they concluded that consideration should be given to correct cervical kyphosis and cervical sagittal imbalance (C2-C7 SVA).[26]

With respect to cervicothoracic junction (CTJ) parameters, T1S was found to be the greatest predictor of C2-C7 SVA.[27] Kim et al. investigated the relationship between preoperative T1S and postoperative cervical sagittal alignment in patients undergoing laminoplasty. They found that patients with high preoperative T1S (above the 50th percentile), were more likely to have greater postoperative kyphotic changes at the 2-year follow-up.[28]

The future direction of cervical deformity correction in myelopathic patients should take on a comprehensive approach in assessing global, regional, and focal relationships between the cervical spine and the other segments of the vertebral column. To optimize cervical deformity correction, it has been recommended to closely examine T1S and TIA, because they drive and relate to CL.[28,29] However, because these regional parameters do not characterize global relationships in the spine, a thorough approach entails incorporating pelvic parameters as well.[25] Indeed, spinal regions are not independent of one another, and CL depends on TK, LL, and PI. Thus, Protopsaltis et al. describe CL as an adaptive spine segment, relative to changes in other spinal regions, for the ultimate purpose of maintaining a "conus of economy," and preserving horizontal gaze.[25]

As Ames et al. describe, there is a clear need for future prospective studies to further isolate the effects of cervical alignment on outcome measures with elimination of confounding variables. Analysis of the cervical regional alignment with respect to overall spinal pelvic alignment is critical. Additionally, evaluation of inter- and intrarater reliability for the cervical parameters requires further academic study as well.[26]

## Dynamic Alignment

The contribution of dynamic alignment to myelopathy enjoys a significant history. It accounts for positional changes in the neck contributing to symptoms of cord compression, and its study dates back to at least the 1950s. In 1952, Brain et al. demonstrated with myelographic studies that a C5-C6 disk protrusion causes cord compression in extension and but not in flexion.[30] Years later, in 1971, Adams et al. demonstrated the association between canal diameter and motion within the canal, where unstable segments have narrow canals. This was an early finding—that there is a dynamic component contributing to CSM.[31,32] Over the past half century, the visualization and understanding of how dynamic alignment influences myelopathic pathology has matured alongside the technological advancements in imaging modalities and quantitative analytic techniques. The goals of recent efforts in dynamic alignment have been to define relevant cervical dynamic parameters, establish statistical correlations between these parameters and HRQOL scores, and elucidate how dynamic alignment can explain differences of severity in myelopathy patients with similar degenerative findings on static imaging.

Dynamic elements can magnify static components of canal deformation through ligamentous and osseous pathology.[33] During cervical motion, the spinal cord is injured by osteophytic bars and diskal protrusion. Stenosis compromises the venous drainage, and anterior impingement plays a role in compression of the anterior spinal artery.[34,35] An already compressed cord can sustain further damage when exposed to longitudinal cord tension through repetitive flexion or extension movements.[36-39] With flexion, the spinal cord is draped over the vertebral bodies and can be compressed against osteophytic spurs and protruding disks.[26,37,40] During extension, the ligamentum flavum (or laminae) bulges inward, pinching the cord posteriorly and against the posterior margin of the vertebral body, ultimately causing a posterior stenosis.[35,37,41,42] Over time, these repetitive actions may lead to irreversible changes in the spinal cord.[18,34,43] These findings may also explain why there are heterogeneous outcomes with surgical decompression.

Dynamic radiographic studies demonstrate cervical cord changes upon flexion-extension, which may contribute to possible mechanisms of cervical myelopathy. Muhle et al. measured the sagittal cord diameter in 40 healthy subjects and found that, upon flexion, the cord diameter is significantly reduced compared with the neutral position.[38] Yanase et al. measured the cervical cord volume in healthy patients and found that it varies with sex, age, height, and body weight.[44]

Magnetic resonance imaging has been used to examine dynamic alignment in myelopathy patients. Yu et al. investigated the relationship of high-intensity lesions on T2-weighted MRI and dynamic changes of the cervical spine in patients with CSM.[45] On a T2-weighted MRI, they discovered that segmental hyperextension and ROM were risk factors for high-intensity lesions. These results are similar to those of Zhang et al., who showed that the cervical cord is significantly longer in flexion than in the neutral or extension positions.[46] The cord available space was found to be largest in the neutral position and smallest in the extension position. Furthermore, patients were more likely to have cord impingement in extension rather than in flexion.[46]

Matsunaga et al. stated that static pathology is exacerbated by dynamic elements.[33] Flexion induces a compression against ventral spondylotic bars, whereas extension induces a compression against the bulking ligamentum flavum. Muhle et al. described a "pincer effect" of impingement, from anterior and posterior degenerative elements, that leads to cord compression. Using kinematic MRI, they demonstrated functional cord impingement at early stages of degenerative disease, and progressive spinal stenosis with cervical cord impingement at advanced stages of degenerative disease.[47]

These dynamic findings spark a cascade of events, beginning with degenerative disk disease and ultimately progressing to myelopathy. In patients with CSM, flexion may be a larger contributor to the etiology, as cord impingement is exacerbated. However, in patients with primary cervical malalignment, in which kyphosis is the predominant position of the spine, the myelopathy may be due to cord lengthening, flattening, and vascular compromise.[46] In summary, ligamentous laxity with instability can lead to a pincer phenomenon with subluxation in flexion and extension.

Another pathway in which dynamic factors lead to myelopathy is through reduction of cord space and microvascular compromise.[37,48] The accumulation of static and dynamic degenerative changes reduces canal diameter and the overall sagittal mobility of the spine, leading to myelopathic progression.[32] Even nondegenerative etiologies such as athetoid-dystonic conditions, cervical dystonia, achondroplasia, and rugby players with repeated forced flexion and extension positions, can experience accelerated spondylosis with dynamic motion-related development of CSM.[49-54] In summary, biomechanical and motion-related factors may transiently compress the spinal cord, nerve roots, and their vascular supply.[34,36,40,43]

Very recently, investigators have delved even further into how dynamic factors drive myelopathy by studying ROM of the cervical spine in these patients. Park et al. studied the ROM in the cervical spine after extensive fusion, using the methodology of the occipitocervical angle (made by the anterior cervical fusion mass and the McGregor line) and the cervicosternal angle (made by the anterior cervical fusion mass and the anterior border of the sternum), in flexion and extension.[55] Similarly, Fujimori et al. examined the ROM after laminoplasty by simply looking at the difference between C2-C7 lordosis in flexion and extension.[56]

Liu et al. found that on a regional level, increased CL in flexion correlated with a worse Nurick grade. However, in their population, there were no correlations between regional parameters and Nurick, or HRQOLs in patients with cervical spine aligned in extension at baseline.[57] Their findings were consistent with the concept summarized above, that with active flexion, the length of the canal increases, and the cord and dura are stretched beyond their normal tension, with an unequal distribution, and held against spondylotic protrusions,[18,34,43] while in extension, the cervical spinal cord is relaxed and flaccid.[34] They postulated that CSM patients may instinctively guard the cord against further longitudinal tension by maintaining slight extension while in flexion.[34] This study also found a correlation between decreased ROM and higher Nurick grades

Finally, the CTJ, or cervicothoracic hinge, has been implicated in driving myelopathy on a dynamic basis. As the location of where the mobile neck transitions to a more fixed thoracic barrel, the CTJ is a biomechanically complex area. Bony destruction due to neoplasm, trauma, or surgical decompression at this location can result in major concern for spinal instability.[18,58,59] A biomechanical cadaveric study by Stemper et al. demonstrated that lower cervical joints are subjected to greater motions and higher likelihoods of injury in rear-impact motor vehicle accidents, mainly because the inertial loading is transferred from the seat to the CTJ.[59] It is no wonder that this transition zone, where the lordotic cervical spine blends to the kyphotic curvature of the thoracic spine, is a structurally critical area that is susceptible to many kinds of insults.[60,61] Furthermore, Cho et al. found that lower cervical laminae are thinner and weaker compared with upper thoracic vertebrae, again demonstrating another anatomical point of inflection that can be exploited by traumatic or repetitive motion.[18,61]

## Focal Alignment

In addition to global and regional alignment factors, there has been recent interest in examining the role of focal alignment that contributes to myelopathy in the setting of cervical deformities. Three common strategies to quantify focal alignment are calculating axes of rotation, counting the vertebral levels affected by spondylosis, and measuring spondylolisthesis.

### *Axes of Rotation*

Early conceptual attempts at quantifying positional changes in the cervical spine can be traced back to the instantaneous axis of rotation (IAR).[62] Pearcy et al. described that when using any two images depicting a starting and ending position of the vertebrae, the center is termed the IAR. However, throughout a particular motion, not all phases will occur about the same axis, such that consecutive pair of images are needed to define an IAR unique to a specific phase of movement. Pearcy et al. coined the term "centrode of motion," describing the locus that captures the series of IARs throughout the entire movement to be studied.[62] Amevo et al. delineated a normal zone (within which the IAR could fall), circumscribed by an abnormal zone, thereby eliminating the anterior versus posterior comparison.[63] They found that subjects with neck pain are significantly more likely to fall into the abnormal zone.[63] These studies suggest that there is a difference in the center of rotation (COR) between pathological and nonpathological cervical motion populations.

Dvorak et al. performed extensive analysis of flexion and extension radiographs among patients with degenerative changes, radicular syndromes, whiplash trauma, and prior normative data.[19,64,65] They found a trend for a more anterior IARs for each vertebrae, throughout a series of several radiographs, in the patient cohorts compared with a healthy population.[19] Lee et al. found that patients with an unstable cervical spine also had a head-neck axis of rotation that was more anterior than a healthy population, using motion analysis equipment instead of radiographic data.[66]

Liu et al. correlated these parameters with HRQOLs.[57] A more posterior COR correlates with a worse SF-36 physical component summary (PCS).[57] The cardinal determinant of where this center falls is determined by the compression forces of the muscles and compression stiffness of the disks.[67] Increased posterior muscle force tends to displace the center backward.[67] If the anterior stiffness of the disk is reduced, the center would also shift posteriorly.[67] Hence, a more posteriorly located COR could indicate collective stiffness of the posterior soft tissues, as well as increased disk (s) stiffness in C2 to C7.

Liu et al. extended our understanding of focal alignment by applying Dubousset's concept of "cone of balance" to segmental areas of the spinal column. They wrote that to conceptualize and visualize the flexion and extension motions of the cervical spine and its contributions to clinical presentation, Dubousset's cone should be applied to the region of the spinal column. Liu et al. developed a "dynamic cone of kinesis" and demonstrated that a smaller cone of kinesis, the dynamic cone of the cervical spine (as measured by an angle and an area from a fixed C7), is correlated with a worse Nurick grade. Furthermore, smaller cones also correlate with increased age, which is consistent with prior data that CSM occurs more frequently in older individuals.[57,68,69] With this model in mind, Liu et al. proposed to visualize the dynamic cervical spine in patients with CSM through their lens, the cone of kinesis, for the purposes of examining the pathology in a kinetic fashion.[57]

### *Number of Vertebrae Involved*

The number of vertebral levels involved in CSM has been correlated with severity. Global and regional parameters often fail to capture individual segmental pathology. Cervical spondylotic myelopathy arises from single- or multi-level disease processes, particularly in older populations.[68,69] Shinomiya et al., in an experimental study using cats as myelopathy models, inducing spinal cord compression by anteriorly applied screws, demonstrated that spinal cord compression at multiple levels causes more severe deterioration functionally and histologically than single-level compression.[70] Liu et al. found that increased number of segments with focal kyphosis was found to be correlated with a worse Nurick and mJOA in flexion.[57] They found that focal kyphosis clearly and significantly correlated with clinically apparent and patient-experienced myelopathy severity, especially when multiple areas of focal kyphosis exist along the cervical spine.

### *Spondylolisthesis*

The third important strategy in quantifying focal alignment is spondylolisthesis. Liu et al. identified the role of focal deformity, specifically listhesis (most likely degenerative spondylolisthesis in their patient population) and focal kyphosis, during dynamic neck motion studies.[57] They found that sagittal slip increases the degree of narrowing in the cervical canal. This sagittal feature by itself is responsible for a static component in CSM. While listhesis and axial rotation are all part of motion of the cervical spine, sagittal slip at C7-T1 in both flexion and extension correlates with worse mJOA. These findings provide a focal understanding of the previously described concept, that motion, through specific areas of spondylotic changes, can lead to myelopathy.[64]

Regarding focal alignment, increased spondylolisthesis correlates with worse mJOA and Nurick grade, especially at higher cervical levels. Overall lordosis does not significantly correlate with HRQOL. However, multiple levels of segmental kyphosis have been shown to contribute to regional disability.[25] Similarly, Oshima et al. found that the existence of local slip was a prognostic factor for surgery in patients with mild CSM.[71] These studies give clinical support to the cadaveric findings made by Chavanne, that increased cSVA or kyphosis results in increased intramedullary pressure, which, in turn, can worsen myelopathy.[14]

Liu et al. established that sagittal slip at C4-C5 correlates with worse NDI and PCS in extension.[57] Not only is C4-C5 one of the most common places of cord compression in the cervical spine for patients with CSM, second only to C6-C7, but Morio et al. retrospectively noted restriction of the C4-C5 ROM after laminoplasty improved clinical myelopathy symptoms.[3,37,72,73] Morio et al. also unearthed a significant correlation between C4-C5 intervertebral ROM and mJOA at the final postoperative follow-up ($R = -0.305$, $p = 0.031$), highlighting the impact of stabilizing this focal area.[73]

An increased maximum sagittal slip at any cervical level, as well as an increased C2-C3 slip, correlates with a worse mJOA in extension.[57] Although the cord is more lax in extension than in flexion, the cord can still be compressed between a spondylotic ridge and laminae, or a buckled ligamentum flavum.[34,37] Myelopathy severity correlates with extreme sagittal plane translation, regardless of the cervical level, with an element of extension bringing out the compressive focal aspects of the disease. Taken together, these results on focal abnormalities suggest that spondylolisthesis at C2-C3 and C7-T1 are associated with myelopathy severity.

Studies of focal alignment have shed light on the possible link between the pathophysiology of cord lengthening and tension, described in prior sections, and myelopathy severity. Using the kinetic cone theory, Liu et al. postulated that patients with smaller cones may have a normative ROM for their age and gender, but are potentially guarding their cords from tension or compression. Also, in patients with particularly long symptomatic periods before presentation, they may have exercised active or reflexogenic muscular restraint for so long that they have developed subsequent soft tissue stiffening. Consequentially, moving outside this cone then requires recruitment of more muscles, which are either chronically over-contracted or underused.[16,19] Loss of cone size may be more an end result of neurological compression, and not necessarily the inability to move. This culminates in a cycle of intentional hypomobility and stiffness. In a sense, surgery attempts to achieve what the patients are already living out in the course of their disease: stabilizing sagittal movement of the cervical spine.[39]

In summary, focal alignment has provided a new lens through which to view CSM. Quantifying the axis of rotation enables investigators to analyze the contribution local motion plays on the degenerative cascade of myelopathy. Understanding the levels and studying each level on an individual basis, through spondylolisthesis studies, helps explain the symptomology of these complex patients.

## Surgical Planning

The previous sections discussed the relationship between cervical alignment and clinical disability measures.[26] Attempts to improve cervical alignment in CSM patients represent an opportunity for surgeons to reduce disability and maximize outcomes. Other chapters extensively discuss surgical options for CSM. Rather than provide an incomplete discussion on this topic, this section aims to provide an overview of how alignment plays a role in surgical planning.

A key initial step in surgical planning is obtaining preoperative 3-ft standing radiographs to provide adequate visualization, from the external auditory canal (center of mass of the head) to the femoral heads. Next, the radiographic parameters discussed above should be appropriately measured. There are several software planning tools that aid the surgeon in incorporating these radiographic parameters into surgical planning. One software program that has gained popularity is Surgimap (Nemaris Inc.). Akbar et al. succinctly demonstrated how to utilize Surgimap in calculating radiographic parameters and planning deformity correction.[74] The ease and speed of these technologies have provided clinicians useful tools to synthesize large amounts of quantitative information with which to provide rapid and effective patient care.

After measuring the appropriate radiographic parameters, the surgeon must determine what the goals are, in terms of restoring these parameters to normal levels. The normative data for cervical parameters presented above provide useful information; however, these data are incomplete with respect to cervicothoracic and occipitocervical parameters, as some of these have not been rigorously evaluated in asymptomatic individuals.

Moreover, there is a lack of clearly defined indications as to the optimal amount of correction suggested to be performed with surgery. Nevertheless, several authors have proposed some general guidelines in optimizing the radiographic parameters outlined above that can potentially maximize surgical outcomes. Currently, a general guideline is to correct cervical kyphosis to as close to neutral as possible.[75] Several authors report successful results with correction of kyphosis for myelopathic patients. For example, Watanabe reports a series of 12 young patients (aged 12–22) with cervical flexion myelopathy who improve after surgical correction of their kyphosis.[76] Studies have shown that patients who underwent one- or two-level corpectomies for CSM, in which CL was maintained, have positive long-term HRQOL (mJOA score) outcomes.[77]

Protopsaltis et al. state that cervical alignment parameters are critical during surgical planning for cervical deformity correction.[25] Chin brow vertical angle, T1S, C2 SVA, and regional CL should be considered in planning strategies. These findings are consistent with the commonly held belief to correct kyphosis to as neutral as possible. Kim et al. specifically investigated post-laminoplasty and recommended that the preoperative T1S be measured, as the likelihood of developing kyphotic changes at 2 years increases with a higher preoperative T1S.[28]

Despite these successful results, the precise relationship between correcting alignment and myelopathy severity is not fully understood. Uchida et al., based on their review of 476 CSM cases, recommend that correction of sagittal alignment in patients with kyphosis above 10° may maximize the chance of neurologic improvement. However, they did not find correlation between preoperative mJOA score and preoperative kyphosis angle. They attribute this lack of correlation to the many potential confounding factors, including duration of symptoms, age, segmental instability, and irreversible changes in the spinal cord.[78] To recapitulate, while there are no strict guidelines as to what parameters should be corrected or what values they should be corrected to, the above studies highlight the importance that alignment plays in surgical planning strategies.

Finally, after determining what parameters the clinician chooses to correct, consideration must be given to the surgical approach that is employed to achieve these goals. Selecting the surgical approach to decompress the spine for CSM patients is subject to controversy.[79] Two common themes in these debates are (1) that posterior approaches alone may be inadequate treatment for myelopathy, and (2) that restoring sagittal alignment is critical in maximizing outcomes.

First, posterior approaches alone may destabilize the spine and promote kyphosis, which may worsen or lead to postsurgical myelopathy. The posterior neural arch is responsible for the majority of the load transmission through the cervical spine, as the natural biomechanics of the spine rely on a lordotic curve to distribute most of the load posteriorly. Removing it causes a significant loss of stability. It has been hypothesized that by removing the posterior arch-facet complex in laminectomies, there is a shift in load bearing from the posterior column to the anterior column. This can lead to vertebral body wedging, and eventually cervical kyphosis can manifest as sagittal malalignment. This cascade may facilitate progression of CSM, and indeed, postlaminectomy kyphosis may worsen myelopathy. Some authors suggest that performing laminectomies alone may destabilize the spine, and posterior approaches alone may not be sufficient to correct cervical lordotic alignment in the subaxial spine. If posterior decompression alone is undertaken or the cervical spine is fused in a kyphotic position, future myelopathy may develop.[25] Other authors have suggested that decompression alone, even ventral decompression, which does not decrease cord tension induced by kyphosis, may not result in optimal outcomes.[8]

Second, restoring sagittal malalignment has been recommended in CSM patients. In patients with sagittal malalignment with CSM, restoring the SVA with instrumentation can be a useful adjunct in decompression surgery to maximize chances for neurologic recovery. In addition, cervical myelopathy correction in patients without sagittal malalignment may develop postlaminectomy kyphosis, the most common etiology of cervical spinal deformity.[9,80] Returning to the underlying pathophysiology, adequately correcting the alignment may explain the conundrum experienced by past investigators that surgical decompression may fail to relieve symptoms. However, this point has not been rigorously demonstrated, and it remains unclear whether alignment correction in the cervical spine, in addition to adequate decompression, may further improve myelopathy scores and disability.[81,78,82] In summary, minimizing kyphosis and improving sagittal alignment are well-recognized objectives of surgical planning. Future surgical techniques and planning methodologies should be evaluated for their ability to meet these recognized goals.

Third, consideration must be given as to what levels to include in surgical intervention. Based on the importance of the cervicothoracic hinge described above, fusions ending at C7 raise concern about instability and adjacent segment disease.[16,58] Liu et al. found that listhesis at the CTJ correlates with worse mJOA scores, suggesting that instability between C7 and T1 is related to myelopathy severity.[57] Some surgeons routinely select C3 to C7 and others from C2 to T1. Based on the spondylolisthesis study by Liu et al., surgeons should consider focal alignment regarding instability at C2-C3 and C7-T1 when determining posterior fusion levels for patients with CSM.[57] In summary, special attention must be paid to areas in the cervical spine that are prone to instability, such as the CTJ, in order to adequately treat CSM and avoid untoward side effects of surgical intervention.

## CONCLUSION

The development and progression of cervical myelopathy are intimately related with cervical alignment. This chapter presents the static and dynamic bases of how global, regional, and focal derangements can lead to myelopathy. Some general guidelines for surgical planning that take into consideration these alignment issues are offered, with a focus on developing a common framework to view current and future intervention strategies for this complex pathology.

## REFERENCES


1. Dubousset J. Three-dimensional analysis of the scoliotic deformity. In: Weinstein S (Ed.). The Pediatric Spine: Principles and Practices. New York: Raven Press; 1994. pp. 479–96.
2. Boden S, McCowin P, Davis D, et al. Abnormal magnetic-resonance scans of the cervical spine in asymptomatic subjects. A prospective investigation. J Bone Jt Surg Am. 1990;72:1178-84.
3. Matsumoto M, Okada E, Ichihara D, et al. Modic changes in the cervical spine: prospective 10-year follow-up study in asymptomatic subjects. J Bone Joint Surg Br. 2012;94:678-83.
4. Hughes JTT, Brownell B. Necropsy observations on the spinal cord in cervical spondylosis. Riv Patol Nerv Ment. 1965;86:196-204.
5. Huec JC Le, Demezon H, Aunoble S. L'équilibre sagittal du rachis cervical sur une population asymptomatique : Nouveaux paramètres et valeurs standards Sagittal parameters of cervical global balance . Normative values from a prospective cohort of asymptomatic volunteers. E-Mémoires l'Académie Natl Chir. 2013;12:18-24.
6. Lestini WF, Wiesel SW. The pathogenesis of cervical spondylosis. Clin Orthop Relat Res. 1989(239):69-93.
7. Shedid D, Benzel EC. Cervical spondylosis anatomy: pathophysiology and biomechanics. Neurosurgery. 2007;60:S7-13.
8. Shimizu K, Nakamura M, Nishikawa Y, et al. Spinal kyphosis causes demyelination and neuronal loss in the spinal cord: a new model of kyphotic deformity using juvenile Japanese small game fowls. Spine (Phila Pa 1976). 2005;30:2388-92.
9. Albert TJ, Vaccaro AR. Postlaminectomy kyphosis. Spine (Phila Pa 1976). 1998; 23:2738-45.
10. Tang JA, Scheer JK, Smith JS, et al. The impact of standing regional cervical sagittal alignment on outcomes in posterior cervical fusion surgery. Neurosurgery. 2012;71:662-9; discussion 669.
11. Naderi S, Ozgen S, Pamir MN, et al. Cervical spondylotic myelopathy: surgical results and factors affecting prognosis. Neurosurgery. 1998;43:43-9; discussion 49-50.

12. Smith JS, Shaffrey CI, Lafage V, et al. Spontaneous improvement of cervical alignment after correction of global sagittal balance following pedicle subtraction osteotomy. J Neurosurg Spine. 2012;17:300-7.
13. Glassman SD, Bridwell K, Dimar JR, et al. The impact of positive sagittal balance in adult spinal deformity. Spine (Phila Pa 1976). 2005;30:2024-9.
14. Chavanne A, Pettigrew DB, Holtz JR, et al. Spinal cord intramedullary pressure in cervical kyphotic deformity: a cadaveric study. Spine (Phila Pa 1976). 2011;36: 1619-26.
15. Farley CW, Curt BA, Pettigrew DB, et al. Spinal cord intramedullary pressure in thoracic kyphotic deformity: a cadaveric study. Spine (Phila Pa 1976). 2012; 37:E224-30.
16. Hart RA, Tatsumi RL, Hiratzka JR, et al. Perioperative complications of combined anterior and posterior cervical decompression and fusion crossing the cervico-thoracic junction. Spine (Phila Pa 1976). 2008;33:2887-91.
17. Yukawa Y, Kato F, Suda K, et al. Age-related changes in osseous anatomy, alignment, and range of motion of the cervical spine. Part I: Radiographic data from over 1,200 asymptomatic subjects. Eur Spine J. 2012;21:1492-8.
18. O'Connell J, Brain R, Ritchie R, et al. Cervical Spondylosis. Proc R Soc Med. 1956;49:197-208.
19. Dvorak J, Panjabi MM, Novotny JE, et al. Clinical validation of functional flexion/extension radiographs of the cervical spine. Spine (Phila Pa 1976). 1993;18:120-7.
20. Lafage VC, Ferrero E, Lafage R, et al. Maintaining chin brow vertical angle (CBVA) and horizontal gaze in lumbar fatback deformity: full body analysis of the chain of compensation from the cervical spine to the feet. 2014.
21. Challier V, Lafage R, Ferrero E, et al. Full body Eos analysis of the maintenance of functional CBVA and horizontal gaze among hypo-lordotic versus hyperlordotic patients. 42nd Annual Meeting of Cervical Spine Research Society (CSRS), December 3-6 2014, Orlando, FL.
22. Glassman SD, Berven S, Bridwell K, et al. Correlation of radiographic parameters and clinical symptoms in adult scoliosis. Spine (Phila Pa 1976). 2005;30:682-8.
23. Villavicencio AT, Babuska JM, Ashton A, et al. Prospective randomized double blinded clinical study evaluating the correlation of clinical outcomes and cervical sagittal alignment. Neurosurgery. 2011;68:1.
24. Smith JS, Lafage V, Ryan DJ, et al. Association of myelopathy scores with cervical sagittal balance and normalized spinal cord volume: analysis of 56 preoperative cases from the AOSpine North America Myelopathy study. Spine (Phila Pa 1976). 2013;38:S161-70.
25. Protopsaltis TS, Fehlings MG, Liu S, et al. Impact of regional and focal cervical alignment on myelopathy severity: report of 151 patients. International Meeting for the Advancement of Spinal Techniques (IMAST), July 16-19 2014, Valencia, Spain.
26. Ames CP, Blondel B, Scheer JK, et al. Cervical radiographical alignment: comprehensive assessment techniques and potential importance in cervical myelopathy. Spine (Phila Pa 1976). 2013;38:S149-60.
27. Knott PT, Mardjetko SM, Techy F. The use of the T1 sagittal angle in predicting overall sagittal balance of the spine. Spine J. 2010;10:994-8.
28. Kim T-H, Lee SY, Kim YC, et al. T1 slope as a predictor of kyphotic alignment change after laminoplasty in patients with cervical myelopathy. Spine (Phila Pa 1976). 2013; 38:E992-7.
29. Schwab FJ, Smith VA, Biserni M, et al. Adult scoliosis: a quantitative radiographic and clinical analysis. Spine (Phila Pa 1976). 2002;27:387-92.
30. Brain WR, Northfield D, Wilkinson M. The neurological manifestations of cervical spondylosis. Brain. 1952;75:187-225.
31. Adams CB, Logue V. Studies in cervical spondylotic myelopathy. II. The movement and contour of the spine in relation to the neural complications of cervical spondylosis. Brain. 1971;94:568-86.
32. Adams CB, Logue V. Studies in cervical spondylotic myelopathy. I. Movement of the cervical roots, dura and cord, and their relation to the course of the extrathecal roots. Brain. 1971;94:557-68.
33. Matsunaga S, Komiya S, Toyama Y. Risk factors for development of myelopathy in patients with cervical spondylotic cord compression. Eur Spine J. 2015;24 Suppl 2:142-9.
34. Breig A, Turnbull I, Hassler O. Effects of mechanical stresses on the spinal cord in cervical spondylosis. A study on fresh cadaver material. J Neurosurg. 1966;25: 45-56.
35. Henderson FC, Geddes JF, Vaccaro AR, et al. Stretch-associated injury in cervical spondylotic myelopathy: new concept and review. Neurosurgery. 2005;56:1101-13; discussion 1101-13.
36. Karadimas SK, Erwin WM, Ely CG, et al. Pathophysiology and natural history of cervical spondylotic myelopathy. Spine (Phila Pa 1976). 2013;38:S21-36.
37. Toledano M, Bartleson JD. Cervical spondylotic myelopathy. Neurol Clin. 2013; 31:287-305.
38. Muhle C, Wiskirchen J, Weinert D, et al. Biomechanical aspects of the subarachnoid space and cervical cord in healthy individuals examined with kinematic magnetic resonance imaging. Spine (Phila Pa 1976). 1998;23:556-67.
39. Gruninger W, Gruss P. Stenosis and movement of the cervical spine in cervical myelopathy. Paraplegia. 1982;20:121-30.
40. Scheer JK, Tang JA, Smith JS, et al. Cervical spine alignment, sagittal deformity, and clinical implications. J Neurosurg Spine. 2013;19:141-59.
41. Taylor A. The mechanism of injury to the spinal cord in the neck without damage to the vertebral column. J Bone Jt Surg. 1951;33-B:543-7.
42. Kawaida H, Sakou T, Morizono Y, Yoshikuni N. Magnetic resonance imaging of upper cervical disorders in rheumatoid arthritis. Spine (Phila PA 1976). 1989; 14(11):1144-8.
43. Smith GW. The treatment of certain cervical-spine disorders by anterior removal of the intervertebral disc and interbody fusion. J Neurol Neurosurg Psychiat. 1960;23:214-21.
44. Yanase M, Matsuyama Y, Hirose K, et al. Measurement of the cervical spinal cord volume on MRI. J Spinal Disord Tech. 2006;19:125-9.
45. Yu L, Zhang Z, Ding Q, et al. Relationship between signal changes on T2-weighted magnetic resonance images and cervical dynamics in cervical spondylotic myelopathy. J Spinal Disord Tech. 2015;28(6):E365-7.
46. Zhang L, Zeitoun D, Rangel A, et al. Preoperative evaluation of the cervical spondylotic myelopathy with flexion-extension magnetic resonance imaging: about a prospective study of fifty patients. Spine (Phila Pa 1976). 2011;36:E1134-9.
47. Muhle C, Metzner J, Weinert D, et al. Classification system based on kinematic MR imaging in cervical spondylitic myelopathy. AJNR Am J Neuroradiol. 1998; 19:1763-71.

48. Baron EM, Young WF. Cervical spondylotic myelopathy: a brief review of its pathophysiology, clinical course, and diagnosis. Neurosurgery. 2007;60:S35-41.
49. El-Mallakh R, Rao K, Barwick M. Cervical myelopathy secondary to movement disorders: case report. Neurosurgery. 1989;24:902-5.
50. Ebara S, Harada T, Yamazaki Y, et al. Unstable cervical spine in athetoid cerebral palsy. Spine (Phila Pa 1976). 1989; 14:1154-9.
51. Hagenah J, Vieregge A, Vieregge P. Radiculopathy and myelopathy in patients with primary cervical dystonia. Eur Neurol. 2001;45:236-40.
52. Yoshii J, Traynelis VC. Achondroplasia and cervical laminoplasty. J Neurosurg Spine. 2009;11:417-20.
53. Pyeritz R, Sach G, Udvarhelyi G. Surgical intervention in achondroplasia: cervical and lumbar laminectomy for spinal stenosis in achondroplasia. Johns Hopkins Med J. 1980; 146:203-6.
54. Berge J, Marque B, Vital J, et al. Age-related changes to the cervical spines of front-line rugby players. Am J Sport Med. 1999;27:422-9.
55. Park MS, Mesfin A, Stoker GE, et al. Sagittal range of motion after extensive cervical fusion. Spine J. 2014;14:338-43.
56. Fujimori T, Le H, Ziewacz JE, et al. Is there a difference in range of motion, neck pain, and outcomes in patients with ossification of posterior longitudinal ligament versus those with cervical spondylosis, treated with plated laminoplasty? Neurosurg Focus. 2013;35:E9.
57. Liu S, Lafage R, Smith JS, et al. The impact of dynamic alignment, motion, and center of rotation on myelopathy grade and regional disability in cervical spondylotic myelopathy. J Neurosurg Spine. 2015 Aug 28:1-11.
58. Kreshak JL, Kim DH, Lindsey DP, et al. Posterior stabilization at the cervicothoracic junction: a biomechanical study. Spine (Phila Pa 1976). 2002;27:2763-70.
59. Stemper BD, Yoganandan N, Pintar FA, et al. The relationship between lower neck shear force and facet joint kinematics during automotive rear impacts. Clin Anat. 2011;24:319-26.
60. Ramieri A, Domenicucci M, Ciappetta P, et al. Spine surgery in neurological lesions of the cervicothoracic junction: multicentric experience on 33 consecutive cases. Eur Spine J. 2011;20 Suppl 1:S13-9.
61. Cho W, Eid AS, Chang UK. The use of pedicle screw-rod system for the posterior fixation in cervico-thoracic junction. J Korean Neurosurg Soc. 2010;48:46-52.
62. Pearcy M, Bogduk N. Instantaneous axes of rotation of the lumbar intervertebral joints. Spine (Phila Pa 1976). 1988; 12:1033-41.
63. Amevo B, Aprill C, Bogduk N. Abnormal instantaneous axes of rotation in patients with neck pain. Spine (Phila Pa 1976). 1992;17:748-56.
64. Dvorak J, Panjabi MM, Novotny JE, et al. In vivo flexion/extension of the normal cervical spine. J Orthop Res. 1991; 9:828-34.
65. Dvorak J, Antinnes JA, Panjabi MM, et al. Age and gender related normal motion of the cervical spine. Spine (Phila Pa 1976). 1992;17:S393-S398.
66. Lee SW, Draper ER, Hughes SPF. Instantaneous center of rotation and instability of the cervical spine. Spine (Phila Pa 1976). 1997;22:641-8.
67. Bogduk N, Amevo B, Pearcy M. A biological basis for instantaneous centres of rotation of the vertebral column. Proc Inst Mech Eng H. 1995;209:177-83.
68. Matz PG, Anderson PA, Holly LT, et al. The natural history of cervical spondylotic myelopathy. J Neurosurg Spine. 2009; 11:104-11.
69. Behrbalk E, Salame K, Regev GJ, et al. Delayed diagnosis of cervical spondylotic myelopathy by primary care physicians. Neurosurg Focus. 2013;35:E1.
70. Shinomiya K, Mutoh N, Furuya K. Study of experimental cervical spondylotic myelopathy. Spine (Phila Pa 1976). 1992;17:S838-7.
71. Oshima Y, Seichi A, Takeshita K, et al. Natural course and prognostic factors in patients with mild cervical spondylotic myelopathy with increased signal intensity on T2-weighted magnetic resonance imaging. Spine (Phila Pa 1976). 2012;37:1909-13.
72. Gore DR, Sepic SB, Gardner GM. Roentgenographic findings of the cervical spine in asymptomatic people. Spine (Phila Pa 1976). n.d.;11:521-4.
73. Morio Y, Yamamoto K, Teshima R, et al. Clinicoradiologic study of cervical laminoplasty with posterolateral fusion or bone graft. Spine (Phila Pa 1976). 2000;25:190-6.
74. Akbar M, Terran J, Ames CP, et al. Use of Surgimap spine in sagittal plane analysis, osteotomy planning, and correction calculation. Neurosurg Clin N Am. 2013;24:163-72.
75. Steinmetz MP, Stewart TJ, Kager CD, et al. Cervical deformity correction. Neurosurgery. 2007;60:S90-7.
76. Watanabe K, Hasegawa K, Hirano T, et al. Anterior spinal decompression and fusion for cervical flexion myelopathy in young patients. J Neurosurg Spine. 2005;3:86-91.
77. Andaluz N, Zuccarello M, Kuntz C. Long-term follow-up of cervical radiographic sagittal spinal alignment after 1- and 2-level cervical corpectomy for the treatment of spondylosis of the subaxial cervical spine causing radiculomyelopathy or myelopathy: a retrospective study. J Neurosurg Spine. 2012;16:2-7.
78. Uchida K, Nakajima H, Sato R, et al. Cervical spondylotic myelopathy associated with kyphosis or sagittal sigmoid alignment: outcome after anterior or posterior decompression. J Neurosurg Spine. 2009;11:521-8.
79. Klineberg E. Cervical spondylotic myelopathy: a review of the evidence. Orthop Clin North Am. 2010;41:193-202.
80. Deutsch H, Haid RW, Rodts GE, et al. Postlaminectomy cervical deformity. Neurosurg Focus. 2003;15:E5.
81. Kawakami M, Tamaki T, Ando M, et al. Relationships between sagittal alignment of the cervical spine and morphology of the spinal cord and clinical outcomes in patients with cervical spondylotic myelopathy treated with expansive laminoplasty. J Spinal Disord Tech. 2002;15:391-7.
82. Zdeblick T, Bohlman H. Cervical kyphosis and myelopathy. Treatment by anterior corpectomy and strut-grafting. J Bone Joint Surg. 1989;71(2):170-82.

# Section 6

# Cervical Myelopathy in the Setting of Spine Tumors

Chapter 22

# Cervical Myelopathy in the Setting of Metastatic Tumors in the Spine

*Mohamad Bydon, Rafael De la Garza-Ramos, Daniel M Sciubba, Ziya L Gokaslan*

## INTRODUCTION

Cancer is one of the leading causes of mortality worldwide.[44] Currently, it is estimated that approximately one-third of cancer patients will develop spinal metastases.[28] Metastatic lesions in the spine may cause alterations in the spinal integrity, leading to pain, neurological deficits, and/or instability.

Treatment protocols for spinal metastases vary depending on the location of the lesion, tumor histology, and overall patient health status. The purpose of this chapter is to review the epidemiology, presentation, and management of metastatic lesions to the cervical spine, with an emphasis on spinal cord compression causing myelopathy.

## EPIDEMIOLOGY OF SPINAL METASTASES

Although the spine is one of the most common locations for distant metastases, the cervical spine only accounts for approximately 10% of cases, followed by the lumbar spine (20%) and thoracic spine (70%).[1] Nevertheless, with >1.5 million new cases of cancer each year,[28] it is not uncommon to find metastatic lesions in the cervical spine.

Some of the most common primary neoplasms that lead to cervical metastases are breast, prostate, and lung cancer.[29] In a retrospective study of 46 patients with cervical spine metastases, Cho and Chang found that the most common primary tumor was lung cancer, followed by hepatocellular carcinoma and thyroid cancer (Table 22.1).[6] Men are more commonly affected than women, and most cases occur between the fourth and sixth decades of life.[28] Metastatic lesions can reach the cervical spine via direct extension or invasion, hematogenous spread, and cerebrospinal fluid (CSF) seeding.[28]

**Table 22.1:** Most common primary tumors leading to cervical spine metastases in 46 patients. [6]

| *Primary tumor* | *Number of cases* |
|---|---|
| Lung | 12 |
| Hepatocellular | 6 |
| Thyroid | 6 |
| Cholangiocarcinoma | 4 |
| Breast | 4 |
| Unknown | 3 |
| Melanoma | 2 |
| Prostate | 2 |
| Colorectal, advanced gastric, tongue, cervix, chordoma, ovarian, and renal cell carcinoma | 1 each |

## PRESENTATION

Cervical spine metastases can lead to a variety of signs and symptoms, but some patients can present with asymptomatic disease.[17] The most common presenting symptom is localized nonmechanical pain, which affects approximately 90% of patients.[17,26,27,29] Other forms of pain that may affect this group of patients include mechanical and referred pain (due to pathological fracture).

Nonmechanical pain is "often described as not being related to any activities, progressively worsening, and exacerbated in the evening."[28] The pain can also irradiate to the shoulder and trapezial area, and metastatic lesions to the cervical spine should always be included in the differential diagnosis of a patient with neck pain and a history of cancer.

Mechanical pain is exacerbated by motion (loading) and relieved by rest. Metastatic lesions most commonly involve the vertebral bodies of the subaxial cervical spine, causing lysis and/or erosions. In turn, these changes in the cancellous bone lead to a higher risk of vertebral body collapse and angular kyphotic deformity,[17] leading to mechanical pain. Metastases to the atlantoaxial spine do not necessarily result in significant angular kyphosis or flexion/extension instability, but rather in rotational instability from destruction of the transverse ligament and lateral articular masses.[28]

**Table 22.2:** Most common primary tumors leading to metastatic epidural spinal cord compression.[7]

| *Primary tumor* | *Frequency* |
|---|---|
| Lung | 15–20% |
| Breast | 15–20% |
| Prostate | 15–20% |
| Colorectal cancers, sarcomas, unknown | 30% |
| Non-Hodgkin's lymphoma, renal cell carcinoma, multiple myeloma | 5–10% |

Neurologic dysfunction (including myeloradiculopathy) occurs in approximately 10% of patients.[37] Radiculopathy occurs secondary to foraminal invasion and presents as "a burning, dyesthetic type of pain."[28] Myelopathy, however, results in long tract signs such as gait instability, spasticity, high reflexes, loss of hand dexterity, and atrophy of intrinsic hand muscles. Myelopathy secondary to cervical metastases can be due to tumor compression or bone fragments invading the anterior epidural space, and is known as metastatic epidural spinal cord compression (MESCC).

Metastatic epidural spinal cord compression was first described by Spiller in 1925, and affects approximately 5% of all patients with cancer.[7] The most common types of tumors leading to MESCC in adults are summarized in Table 22.2.[7] In children, the most common primary tumors are sarcomas (Ewing), neuroblastomas, Hodgkin's disease, and germ cell tumors.[19,35,41] In approximately 20% of cases, MESCC is the first manifestation of cancer.[36] An estimated 15% of cases of MESCC occur in the cervical spine, 60% in the thoracic spine, and 15% in the lumbosacral spine.[2,8,14]

## PATHOPHYSIOLOGY

Approximately 85% of cases of MESCC occur due to hematogenous spread of neoplastic cells into the vertebral body. Afterward, the tumor grows inside the bone and spreads into the epidural space, causing spinal cord compression. Lytic lesions may cause vertebral body collapse and displacement of tumor/bone fragments into the epidural space.[7]

Metastatic epidural spinal cord compression causes axonal damage, demyelination, and vascular compromise.[7] Animal models have shown "that acute anterior spinal cord compression results in stenosis and occlusion of the epidural venous plexus, which causes breakdown of the blood-spinal cord barrier and results in vasogenic edema."[7] Of note, corticosteroids may partially or completely reverse edema and associated neurological deficits at this stage.[7] However, more advanced stages of compression ultimately lead to spinal cord ischemia and infarction, causing irreversible damage.[18]

**Table 22.3:** Nurick disability score.[30]

| *Grade* | *Signs and symptoms* |
|---|---|
| 0 | Signs or symptoms of root involvement but no evidence of spinal cord disease |
| 1 | Signs of spinal cord disease but no difficulty walking |
| 2 | Slight difficulty in walking that prevented full-time employment |
| 3 | Difficult in walking that prevented full-time employment or the ability to do all housework, but not so severe as to require help to walk |
| 4 | Able to walk only with help or with the aid of a frame |
| 5 | Chair-bound or bedridden |

## INITIAL EVALUATION AND DIAGNOSIS

A high index of clinical suspicion for cervical MESCC is necessary in patients presenting with signs of myelopathy and a history of cancer. As mentioned previously, common symptoms of myelopathy include gait abnormalities and weakness/stiffness of the legs.[3] Signs include hyperactive deep tendon reflexes, upper and lower extremity spasticity, Babinski's sign, Hoffman's sign, and ankle/patellar clonus. Another reflex that may be seen is the pectoralis muscle reflex, elicited by tapping the pectoralis tendon at the level of the deltopectoral groove.[3] This maneuver causes adduction and internal rotation of the shoulder if positive.

Motor examination may reveal triceps and/or hand intrinsic muscle weakness. Typically, patients show atrophy of the thenar muscles and may complain of loss of dexterity, usually with such activities as opening jars, opening doorknobs, or buttoning their shirts. Gait abnormalities include stiff or spastic gait. Two scales that are commonly used to assess myelopathy are the Nurick scale[30] (Table 22.3) and the modified Japanese Orthopedic Association score as proposed by Benzel et al.[4] (Table 22.4).

### Imaging Evaluation

The diagnosis of cervical MESCC also requires visualization of the offending lesion and assessment of spinal

**Table 22.4:** Modified Japanese Orthopedic Association score.[4]

| *Motor dysfunction score of upper extremities* | *Score* |
|---|---|
| Inability to move hands | 0 |
| Inability to eat with a spoon but able to move hands | 1 |
| Inability to button shirt but able to eat with a spoon | 2 |
| Able to button shirt with great difficulty | 3 |
| Able to button shirt with slight difficulty | 4 |
| No dysfunction | 5 |
| *Motor dysfunction score of lower extremities* | *Score* |
| Complete loss of motor and sensory function | 0 |
| Sensory preservation without ability to move legs | 1 |
| Able to move legs but unable to walk | 2 |
| Able to walk on a flat floor with a walking aid | 3 |
| Able to walk up and/or down stairs with handrail | 4 |
| Moderate to significant lack of stability but able to walk up and/or down stairs without handrail | 5 |
| Mid lack of stability but walk unaided with smooth reciprocation | 6 |
| No dysfunction | 7 |
| *Sensation* | *Score* |
| Complete loss of hand sensation | 0 |
| Severe sensory loss or pain | 1 |
| Mild sensory loss | 2 |
| No sensory loss | 3 |
| *Sphincter dysfunction* | *Score* |
| Inability to micturate voluntarily | 0 |
| Marked difficulty with micturition | 1 |
| Mild to moderate difficulty with micturition | 2 |
| Normal micturition | 3 |

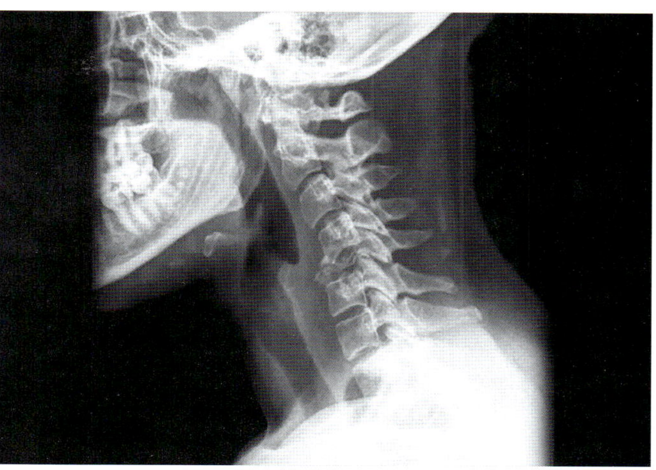

**Fig. 22.1:** A 43-year-old woman with a history of breast cancer presented with a 2-week history of left upper extremity weakness and neck pain. A lateral X-ray of her cervical spine revealed a marked compression deformity at C5, with >75% volume loss and suggestion of retropulsion of fragments posteriorly.

stability. This is achieved via a combination of conventional X-rays, computed tomography (CT), and magnetic resonance imaging (MRI).[17] Conventional X-rays may reveal spinal instability (significant translation or angulation, involvement of >50% of vertebral body, or vertebral body collapse), spinous process erosion, or elevation of soft-tissue shadows (Fig. 22.1).[28]

Computed tomography imaging allows for detailed evaluation of the osseous elements of the cervical spine, including the presence of osteolytic lesions. Magnetic resonance imaging is considered the best imaging modality to assess cervical MESCC, and allows for high-resolution visualization of soft tissues and neural elements. It has an estimated diagnostic sensitivity of 93% and specificity of 97%, with an overall accuracy of 95%.[22] It is recommended that patients undergo a whole-spine MRI, since patients may present with multiple lesions.[7] A prospective study by Husband et al. examined the role of MRI in the diagnosis and treatment of suspected MESCC.[16] Out of 280 patients with clinical suspicion, 201 had MESCC findings on MRI. Moreover, 25% of patients had two or more levels of compression, with 69% of these involving more than one spinal region.[16]

A 6-point grading system was established by Bilsky et al. to assess the degree of MESCC using T2-weighted MRI.[5] A grade of 0 refers to bone-only disease; 1a, epidural impingement without deformation of the thecal sac; 1b, deformation of the thecal sac but with no spinal cord abutment; 1c, abutment of the spinal cord but no compression; 2, spinal cord compression but with visible CSF around the cord; and 3, spinal cord compression with no CSF visible around the cord.[5] T2-weighted images may provide evidence of spinal cord compression (Fig. 22.2) and changes within the spinal cord. T1-weighted images with gadolinium may give further information on tumor margins and extension.

## MANAGEMENT

### Corticosteroids

First-line treatment of cervical MESCC includes the use of corticosteroids, which have been shown to reduce

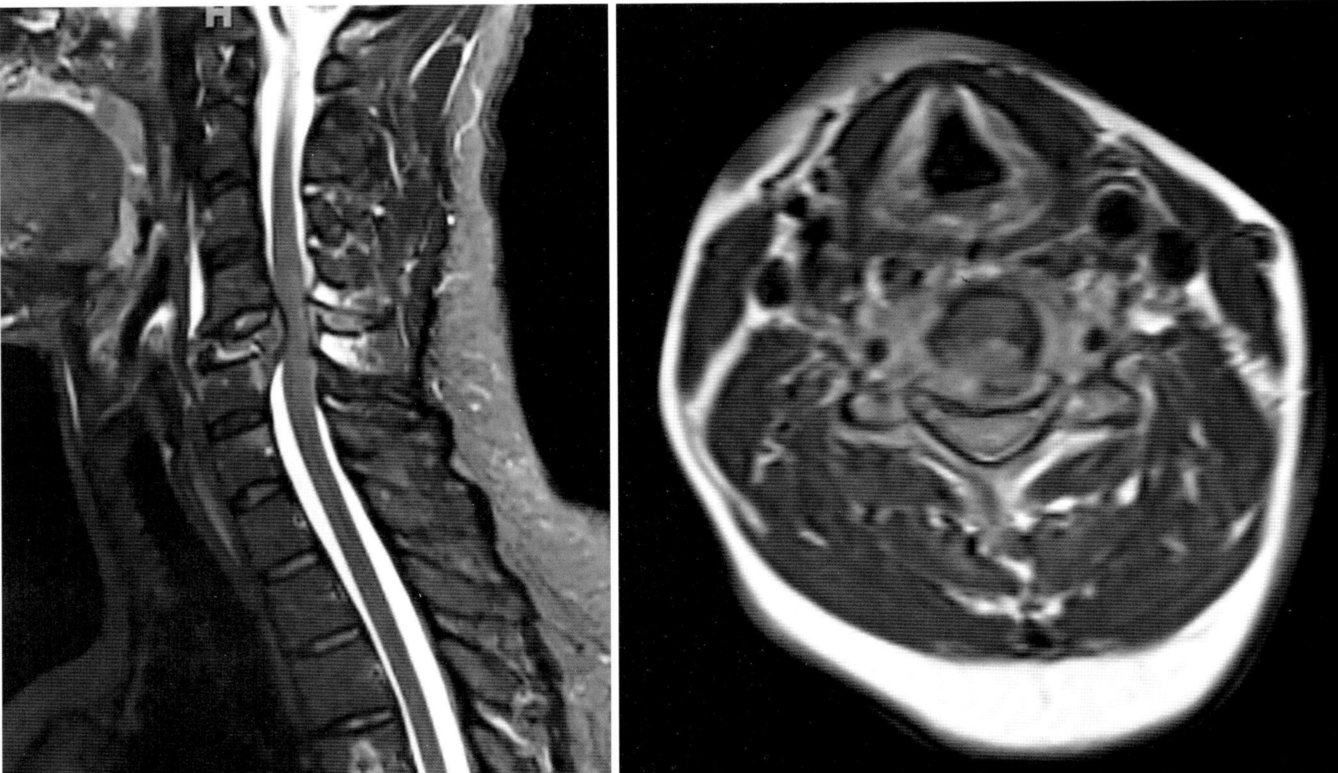

**Fig. 22.2:** T2-weighted magnetic resonance imaging of the same patient in Figure 22.1 showing significant cord compression at the level of C5. According to the Bilsky classification, this would correspond to grade 3 compression.

edema and have a tumoricidal effect on lymphomas and leukemias.[7] Sorensen et al. performed a randomized trial to evaluate the efficacy of dexamethasone versus radiation alone in the treatment of MESCC due to solid tumors.[39] The steroid arm consisted of a 96-mg intravenous bolus of dexamethasone, then 96 mg per day oral dexamethasone for 3 days with a 10-day taper before radiotherapy (RTx). At 3 months, the ambulatory rates were 81% for patients in the steroid group versus 63% in the radiation-only group, and at 6 months the ambulatory rates were 59% and 33%, respectively, in favor of the steroid cohort.

Although Sorensen et al. proved the efficacy of steroids in the treatment of MESCC, the optimum dose has not been established. Animal studies have found that dexamethasone at a dose of 100 mg per kg produces a maximum antiedema effect, and that there is also a positive dose-dependent response at lower doses.[7,9] A randomized trial by Vecht et al. in 1989 compared outcomes of patients receiving an initial bolus of 10 mg IV versus 100 mg IV of dexamethasone, both followed by 16 mg orally.[43] Both treatment groups experienced significant reductions in pain from baseline, but there were no differences in terms of pain reduction, ambulation, or bladder function between cohorts. Although the study was small (only 37 patients), the authors concluded: "Given the absence of a positive effect for the high dose, until other studies have further clarified the issue, we advocate the use of the conventional regimen with an initial bolus of 10 mg IV."[43]

However, animal studies have shown a dose-response effect for steroids. As a result, some authors have proposed that high-dose steroids may be used for severe spinal cord compression (e.g. nonambulant status), and moderate-dose steroids for ambulatory patients with other neurological deficits.[7]

## Radiotherapy

Radiotherapy refers to the administration of external ionizing radiation to relieve MESCC. Broadly speaking, RTx is most effective for "radiosensitive" tumors and in ambulatory patients.[7] Radiosensitive tumors include lymphoma, myeloma, small cell lung carcinoma, breast carcinoma, prostate carcinoma, and thyroid carcinoma.[10] "Radioresistant" tumors include colon cancer, renal cancer, melanoma, sarcoma, and nonsmall cell lung cancer.[10]

Radiotherapy is a widely accepted treatment modality for MESCC, but the optimal dose and regimen are still debated. Rades et al. performed a retrospective review of 1,304 patients with MESCC who underwent RTx.[34] The patients were divided into five groups: single dose of 8 Gy ($n$ = 261, group 1); 5 doses of Gy each in 1 week ($n$ = 279, group 2); 10 doses of 3 Gy each in 2 weeks ($n$ = 274, group 3); 15 doses of 2.5 Gy in 3 weeks ($n$ = 233, group 4); and 20 doses of 2 Gy in 4 weeks ($n$ = 257, group 5). Motor function improved in 26% of patients in group 1, 28% of patients in group 2, 27% of patients in group 3, 31% of patients in group 4, and 28% of patients in group 5, with the difference in rates not being statistically significant. Similarly, post-treatment ambulatory rates were 69%, 68%, 63%, 66%, and 75% ($p$ = 0.578), respectively. Independent factors associated with functional outcomes were age, performance status, primary tumor histology, number of involved vertebrae, interval from cancer diagnosis to MESCC, pretreatment ambulatory status and time to developing a motor deficit. In-field recurrence rates at 2 years of follow-up were 24% for group 1, 26% for group 2, 14% for group 3, 9% for group 4, and 7% for group 5 ($p$ = 0.001). In light of these findings, the authors concluded: "The five RT schedules provided similar functional outcome. The three more protracted schedules seemed to result in fewer in-field recurrences. To minimize treatment time, the following two schedules are recommended: 1 × 8 Gy for patients with poor predicted survival and 10 × 3 Gy for other patients."[34]

Maranzano et al. also evaluated distinct regimens, but in a randomized trial.[24] This study compared 16 Gy over 1 week (two doses of 8 Gy with a 6-day break between doses, group 1) versus 30 Gy over 2 weeks (three doses of 5 Gy and then 5 doses of 3 Gy with a break of 4 days between doses, group 2). Back pain relief was similar between cohorts (56% vs. 59%), as well as preservation of ambulation (68% vs. 71%), and bladder function preservation (90% vs. 89%). In light of these findings, the authors recommended the lower dose treatment.[24]

## Surgery

A number of studies have compared surgery to RTx alone for the treatment of MESCC.[11-13,45] In 2005, a landmark trial by Patchell et al. compared direct decompressive surgery (DDSR) plus postoperative RTx versus RTx alone.[31] Inclusion criteria were patients at least 18 years old with a tissue-proven diagnosis of cancer and evidence of MESCC on MRI. Patients also had to have at least one neurological sign or symptom and "not have been totally paraplegic for >48 hours before study entry."[7] Additionally, MESCC had to be restricted to only one location. The primary end point of Patchell et al., study was the ability to ambulate.

The study aimed to enroll 200 patients, but after an interim analysis recruitment was stopped at 101 because the criterion of a predetermined early stopping rule was met. All patients received 100 mg of dexamethasone, followed by 24 mg every 6 hours until treatment began. Patients were stratified by primary tumor histology, ambulatory status, and spinal stability; afterward they were randomly assigned to one of two treatment groups. Patients in the radiation-only group received 10 doses of 300 cGy within 24 hours of study entry. Patients in the surgical group were operated on within 24 hours of study entry and received RTx within 2 weeks.

Surgical treatment was tailored to each patient, depending on the involved spinal level and the patient's characteristics. Stabilization was done if required via metallic rods, methyl methacrylate, bone grafting, and other fixation devices.

There were 51 patients in the radiation group and 50 patients in the surgery+ radiation group. The most common tumor histology in both groups was lung cancer, followed by prostate and breast cancer. The most common location was between T7 and T12 in 50% of cases. Following treatment, 84% of patients in the surgery + radiation group were able to walk, compared to 57% of patients in the radiation-only group ($p$ = 0.001). Additionally, patients treated with surgery retained the ability to walk for a median of 122 days compared to only 13 days in the radiation group ($p$ = 0.001). The authors of this trial concluded: "[D]irect decompressive surgery plus postoperative RTx is superior to treatment with RTx alone for patients with spinal cord compression caused by metastatic cancer."[31] However, some of the limitations of that study were that there were no subanalyses based on tumor type and that only patients with one area of compression were included. The study included significant crossover between the cohorts. Additionally, radiosensitive tumors such as lymphoma or multiple myeloma were excluded, while patients with instability could be randomized per protocol to either surgery plus radiation or radiation alone.

A recent meta-analysis by Lee et al. analyzed five studies comparing DDSR + RTx versus RTx alone for MESCC.[21] Data were obtained for 238 and 1,137 patients in the DDSR + RTx and RTx-alone groups, respectively.

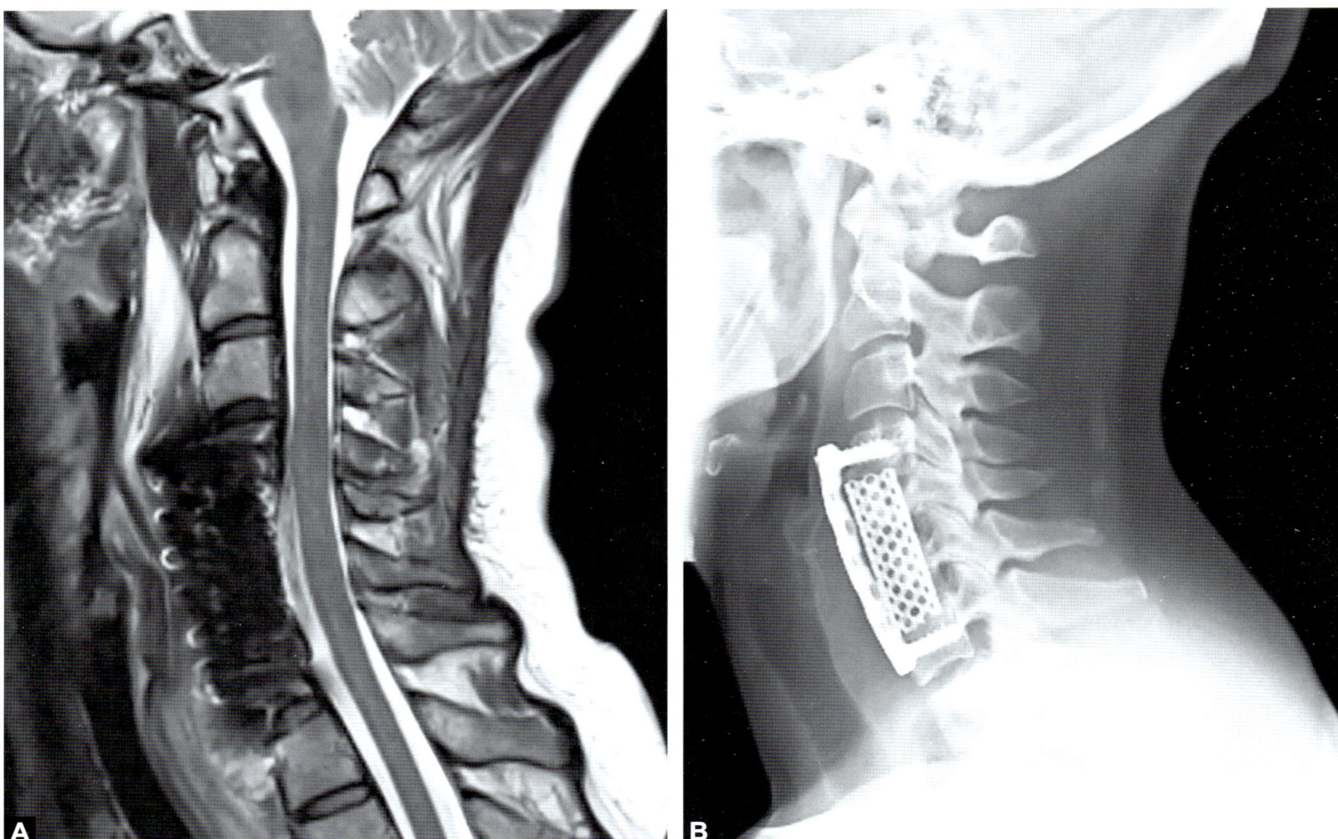


**Figs. 22.3A and B:** Reconstruction of the anterior column of the cervical spine following a C5-C6 corpectomy due to metastatic breast carcinoma. (A) Postoperative T2-weighted magnetic resonance imaging and (B) Postoperative lateral X-ray.

Patients in the DDSR + RTx group were 1.4 times more likely to improve their ambulatory status when compared to patients in the RTx-alone group (relative risk [RR], 1.43; 95% confidence interval [CI], 1.14–1.78). Similarly, the DDSR + RTx group improved significantly their survival rate at 6 months when compared to the RTx-alone group (RR, 1.21; 95% CI, 1.09–1.33). The authors concluded that DDSR + RTx may "produce better clinical improvement of ambulation status and survival than RTx alone in the treatment of MESCC."[21]

Broadly speaking, surgical intervention may be indicated in cases of MESCC, spinal instability, or intractable pain.[28] Surgical treatment options include posterior decompression with or without fusion, or anterior corpectomy with cage and possible plate reconstruction (Figs. 22.3A and B). If a patient has been previously irradiated, the risk of esophageal injury and dysphagia is increased due to radiation-induced scarring, and involving a head and neck surgeon is suggested.[28] Second, highly vascularized metastatic tumors such as renal cell and hepatocellular carcinoma may be evaluated with arteriography prior to surgery, and if required, embolized preoperatively. Finally, multilevel corpectomies or extensive anterior resections may require posterior stabilization as well.[28]

## OUTCOMES

The median survival time for patients with MESCC has been estimated to be between 3 and 6 months.[23,33] Factors associated with longer survival include radiosensitive tumors,[19,20,25,32,33,38] ability to ambulate before and after treatment,[15,20,25,32,38] no visceral or brain metastases,[33,42] and having a single site of spinal cord compression.[40]

The most important prognostic factors associated with post-treatment ambulation are preoperative ambulation, slow onset of motor deficits, and having a radiosensitive tumor (multiple myeloma, germ-cell tumor, lymphoma, small-cell carcinoma, etc.).[8,12,14,15,25,33]

## CONCLUSION

The treatment of cervical MESCC may be challenging. Treatment options include steroids, radiation, and/or surgery via an anterior, posterior, or combined approach. Treatment options should be tailored based on patient functional status, spinal stability, tumor histology, and prognosis.

## REFERENCES


1. Atanasiu JP, Badatcheff F, Pidhorz L. Metastatic lesions of the cervical spine. A retrospective analysis of 20 cases. Spine. 1993;18:1279-84.
2. Bach F, Larsen BH, Rohde K, et al. Metastatic spinal cord compression. Occurrence, symptoms, clinical presentations and prognosis in 398 patients with spinal cord compression. Acta Neurochir (Wien). 1990;107:37-43.
3. Baron EM, Young WF. Cervical spondylotic myelopathy: a brief review of its pathophysiology, clinical course, and diagnosis. Neurosurgery. 2007;60:S35-41.
4. Benzel EC, Lancon J, Kesterson L, et al. Cervical laminectomy and dentate ligament section for cervical spondylotic myelopathy. J Spinal Disord. 1991;4:286-95.
5. Bilsky MH, Laufer I, Fourney DR, et al. Reliability analysis of the epidural spinal cord compression scale. J Neurosurg Spine. 2010;13:324-8.
6. Cho W, Chang UK. Neurological and survival outcomes after surgical management of subaxial cervical spine metastases. Spine. 2012;37:E969-77.
7. Cole JS, Patchell RA. Metastatic epidural spinal cord compression. Lancet Neurol. 2008;7:459-66.
8. Constans JP, de Divitiis E, Donzelli R, et al. Spinal metastases with neurological manifestations. Review of 600 cases. J Neurosurg. 1983;59:111-8.
9. Delattre JY, Arbit E, Thaler HT, et al. A dose-response study of dexamethasone in a model of spinal cord compression caused by epidural tumor. J Neurosurg. 1989;70:920-25.
10. Dodd RL, Gibbs I, Adler JR Jr, et al. Spinal tumors. In: Chin LS, Regine WF (Eds). Principles and Practice of Stereotactic Radiosurgery. New York: Springer; 2008.
11. Findlay GF. Adverse effects of the management of malignant spinal cord compression. J Neurol Neurosurg Psychiatry.1984;47:761-8.
12. Gilbert RW, Kim JH, Posner JB. Epidural spinal cord compression from metastatic tumor: diagnosis and treatment. Ann Neurol. 1978;3:40-51.
13. Greenberg HS, Kim JH, Posner JB. Epidural spinal cord compression from metastatic tumor: results with a new treatment protocol. Ann Neurol. 1980;8:361-6.
14. Helweg-Larsen S. Clinical outcome in metastatic spinal cord compression. A prospective study of 153 patients. Acta Neurol Scand. 1996;94:269-75.
15. Helweg-Larsen S, Sorensen PS, Kreiner S. Prognostic factors in metastatic spinal cord compression: a prospective study using multivariate analysis of variables influencing survival and gait function in 153 patients. Int J Radiat Oncol Biol Phys. 2000;46:1163-9.
16. Husband DJ, Grant KA, Romaniuk CS. MRI in the diagnosis and treatment of suspected malignant spinal cord compression. Br J Radiol. 2001;74:15-23.
17. Jenis LG, Dunn EJ, An HS. Metastatic disease of the cervical spine. A review. Clin Orthop Relat Res. 1999;(359):89-103.
18. Kato A, Ushio Y, Hayakawa T, et al. Circulatory disturbance of the spinal cord with epidural neoplasm in rats. J Neurosurg. 1985;63:260-5.
19. Klein SL, Sanford RA, Muhlbauer MS. Pediatric spinal epidural metastases. J Neurosurg. 1991;74:70-75.
20. Klimo P Jr, Thompson CJ, Kestle JR, et al. A meta-analysis of surgery versus conventional radiotherapy for the treatment of metastatic spinal epidural disease. Neuro Oncol. 2005;7:64-76.
21. Lee CH, Kwon JW, Lee J, et al. Direct decompressive surgery followed by radiotherapy versus radiotherapy alone for metastatic epidural spinal cord compression: a meta-analysis. Spine. 2014;39:E587-92.
22. Li KC, Poon PY. Sensitivity and specificity of MRI in detecting malignant spinal cord compression and in distinguishing malignant from benign compression fractures of vertebrae. Magn Reson Imaging. 1988;6:547-56.
23. Loblaw DA, Laperriere NJ, Mackillop WJ. A population-based study of malignant spinal cord compression in Ontario. Clin Oncol. 2003;15:211-7.
24. Maranzano E, Bellavita R, Rossi R, et al. Short-course versus split-course radiotherapy in metastatic spinal cord compression: results of a phase III, randomized, multicenter trial. J Clin Oncol. 2005;23:3358-65.
25. Maranzano E, Latini P. Effectiveness of radiation therapy without surgery in metastatic spinal cord compression: final results from a prospective trial. Int J Radiat Oncol Biol Phys. 1995;32:959-67.
26. Marchesi DG, Boos N, Aebi M. Surgical treatment of tumors of the cervical spine and first two thoracic vertebrae. J Spinal Disord. 1993;6:489-96.
27. Mazel C, Balabaud L, Bennis S, et al. Cervical and thoracic spine tumor management: surgical indications, techniques, and outcomes. Orthop Clin North Am. 2009;40:75-92, vi-vii.
28. Molina CA, Gokaslan ZL, Sciubba DM. Diagnosis and management of metastatic cervical spine tumors. Orthop Clin North Am. 2012;43:75-87, viii-ix.
29. Moulding HD, Bilsky MH. Metastases to the craniovertebral junction. Neurosurgery. 2010;66:113-8.
30. Nurick S. The pathogenesis of the spinal cord disorder associated with cervical spondylosis. Brain. 1972;95:87-100.
31. Patchell RA, Tibbs PA, Regine WF, et al. Direct decompressive surgical resection in the treatment of spinal cord compression caused by metastatic cancer: a randomised trial. Lancet. 2005;366:643-8.
32. Rades D, Dunst J, Schild SE. The first score predicting overall survival in patients with metastatic spinal cord compression. Cancer. 2008;112:157-61.

33. Rades D, Fehlauer F, Schulte R, et al. Prognostic factors for local control and survival after radiotherapy of metastatic spinal cord compression. J Clin Oncol. 2006;24:3 388-93.
34. Rades D, Stalpers LJ, Veninga T, et al. Evaluation of five radiation schedules and prognostic factors for metastatic spinal cord compression. J Clin Oncol. 2005;23:3366-75.
35. Raffel C, Neave VC, Lavine S, et al. Treatment of spinal cord compression by epidural malignancy in childhood. Neurosurgery. 1991;28:349-52.
36. Schiff D, O'Neill BP, Suman VJ. Spinal epidural metastasis as the initial manifestation of malignancy: clinical features and diagnostic approach. Neurology. 1997;49:452-6.
37. Sciubba DM, Petteys RJ, Dekutoski MB, et al. Diagnosis and management of metastatic spine disease. A review. J Neurosurg Spine. 2010;13:94-108.
38. Sioutos PJ, Arbit E, Meshulam CF, et al. Spinal metastases from solid tumors. Analysis of factors affecting survival. Cancer. 1995;76:1453-9.
39. Sorensen S, Helweg-Larsen S, Mouridsen H, et al. Effect of high-dose dexamethasone in carcinomatous metastatic spinal cord compression treated with radiotherapy: a randomised trial. Eur J Cancer.1994;30A:22-7.
40. Tang SG, Byfield JE, Sharp TR, et al. Prognostic factors in the management of metastatic epidural spinal cord compression. J Neurooncol. 1983;1:21-8.
41. Tasdemiroglu E, Patchell RA, Kryscio R. Neurological complications of childhood malignancies. Acta Neurochir (Wien). 1999;141:1313-21.
42. Tomita K, Kawahara N, Kobayashi T, et al. Surgical strategy for spinal metastases. Spine. 2001;26:298-306.
43. Vecht CJ, Haaxma-Reiche H, van Putten WL, et al. Initial bolus of conventional versus high-dose dexamethasone in metastatic spinal cord compression. Neurology. 1989; 39:1255-7.
44. Yoon PW, Bastian B, Anderson RN, et al. Potentially preventable deaths from the five leading causes of death--United States, 2008-2010. MMWR Morb Mortal Wkly Rep. 2014;63:369-74.
45. Young RF, Post EM, King GA. Treatment of spinal epidural metastases. Randomized prospective comparison of laminectomy and radiotherapy. J Neurosurg. 1980;53:741-8.

Chapter 23

# Cervical Myelopathy in the Setting of Intramedullary Spinal Cord Tumors

*Akwasi Ofori Boah, Donato Pacione, Anthony K Frempong-Boadu*

## INTRODUCTION

Cervical myelopathy can be caused by intramedullary spinal cord tumors. They are relatively rare neoplasms, which account for roughly 2–4% of all central nervous system (CNS) tumors[1,2] and 20–30% of all spinal tumors.[3,4] Myelopathy from these tumors is typically from direct invasion or compression of white matter tracts[5] leading to edema, gliosis, and fiber disruption (Fig. 23.1). Primary intramedullary spinal cord tumors are more common than secondary or metastatic intramedullary spinal cord tumors.

## PRESENTATION

Patients may present with many symptoms; however, pain is the most common initial complaint. More specifically, patients with this diagnosis have neck pain, which has a nocturnal predilection and is often intensified in recumbence or by Valsalva maneuvers. "Medullary pain" may also be a complaint, which is often bilateral, nonradicular, and burning/dysesthetic in quality. Sensory loss with intramedullary spinal cord tumor is typically not painful. Motor symptoms due to myelopathy will typically precede sensory phenomena. Children may present with gait disturbances and ataxia (relative plasticity of CNS), whereas adults can have florid cervical myelopathy, which may be confused with cervical spondylotic myelopathy clinically.

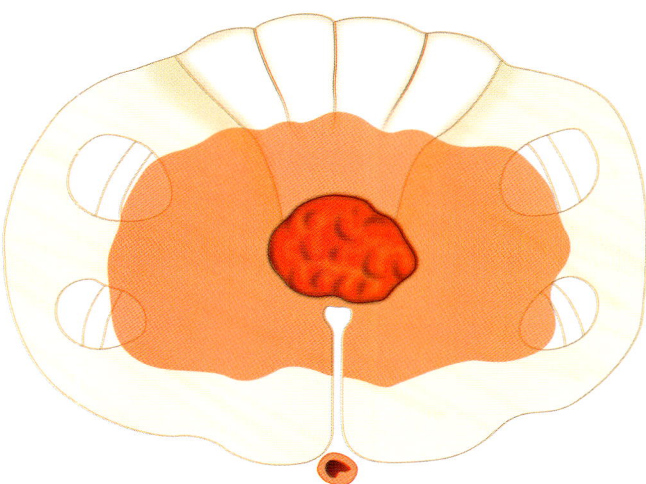

**Fig. 23.1:** Intramedullary spinal cord tumor with surrounding edema and invasion of deep white matter tracts.

## INTRAMEDULLARY TUMORS OF THE CERVICAL SPINAL CORD

There are two main types of cervical intramedullary spinal cord tumors, which are based on their origin:

1. *Primary*: The most common intramedullary tumor type.
2. *Secondary*: The second most common type that includes metastases.

### Primary Glial Spinal Cord Tumors

#### *Ependymoma*

Ependymomas are the most common type of intramedullary spinal cord tumor in adults,[6] accounting for 50–60%[7,8] of all intramedullary tumors (Table 23.1). In pediatric patients, ependymomas and astrocytomas comprise roughly 90% of intramedullary tumors, so our focus will be on the adult population primarily. There is a slight male predominance (56%) with spinal ependymomas.[9] There are two types of spinal ependymomas, cellular and myxopapillary, which are distinguished based on their cellular origin. Cellular ependymomas originate from the ependymal cells of the central canal of the cervical and thoracic spinal cord. They are slightly more aggressive and are often classified as World Health Organization (WHO) grade II or III. Myxopapillary ependymomas originate from cells of the filum terminale and are histologically benign tumors (WHO grade I) and will thus

**Table 23.1:** Incidence of ependymomas versus astrocytomas.

| *Authors* | *Series (n)* | *Age (years)* | *Ependymomas (%)* | *Astrocytomas (%)* |
|---|---|---|---|---|
| Miller | 177 | All > 21 | 53 | 27 |
| Sandalcioglu et al. | 78 | Mean 43 | 41 | 19 |
| Raco et al. | 202 | Mean 42 | 34 | 42 |
| Regelsberger et al. | 78 | Mean 52 | 63 | 18 |
| Shrivastava et al. | 30 | Mean 60 | 83 | 10 |

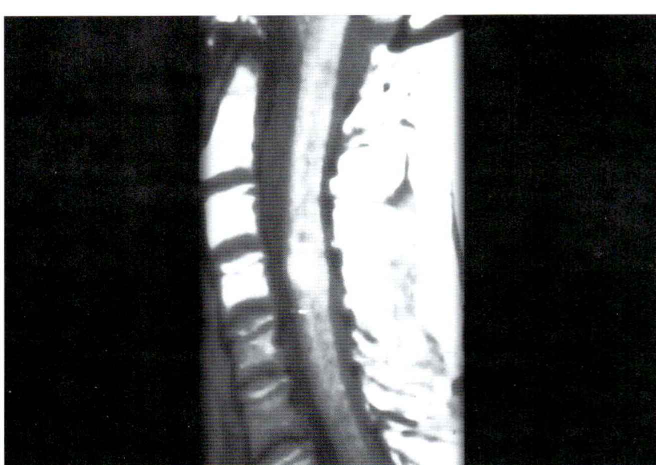

**Fig. 23.2:** C4 level ependymoma on sagittal T1-weighted image post-gadolinium with heterogeneous enhancement.

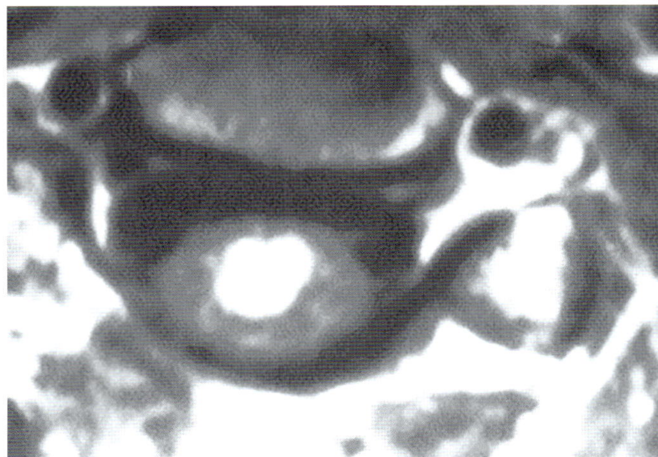

**Fig. 23.3:** C4 level ependymoma on axial T1-weighted image post-gadolinium with associated dilation of central canal.

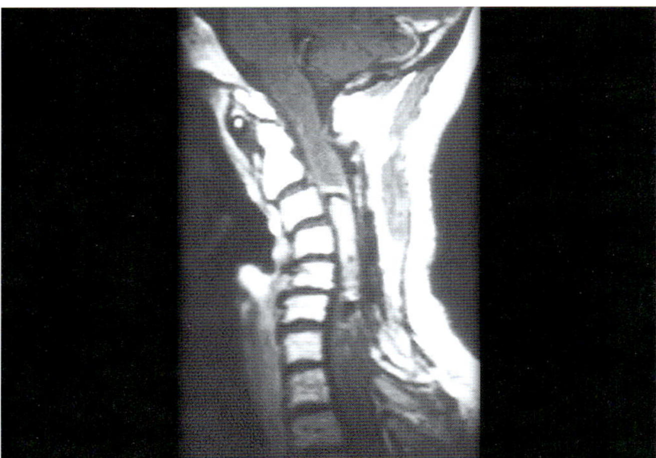

**Fig. 23.4:** C2 through C5 level ependymoma with associated kyphosis of C2-C4 bodies and heterogeneous enhancement. Associated hemosiderin cap sign and syringohydromyelia.

not be discussed further, as they are exclusive to the conus medullaris and filum terminale. On magnetic resonance imaging (MRI) (Figs. 23.2 to 23.4), ependymomas are T2 hyperintense enlargements within the spinal cord and exhibit heterogeneous enhancement on T1 imaging.[2,10] These tumors are also associated frequently with syringohydromyelia (which is a distinguishing feature from astromcytomas[11]) and the hemosiderin cap sign, a cap of T2 hypointensity above and/or below the tumor due to previous hemorrhage (Fig. 23.5). Please note that the cap sign can be associated with other vascular intramedullary tumors such as hemangioblastoma, cavernoma, and paraganglioma. There are only rare case reports of extramedullary spinal ependymomas. Due to the intramedullary nature of these tumors, patients often present with progressive myelopathy and sensory disturbances; however, they may also be asymptomatic.

Because the majority of these tumors are relatively benign in nature, complete surgical resection can be curative. The preoperative McCormick scale (Table 23.2) has been implicated reliably as in important predictor of prognosis and postoperative functionality,[12,13] although some studies do not support this.[14] Resection is generally performed through a posterior approach, either through

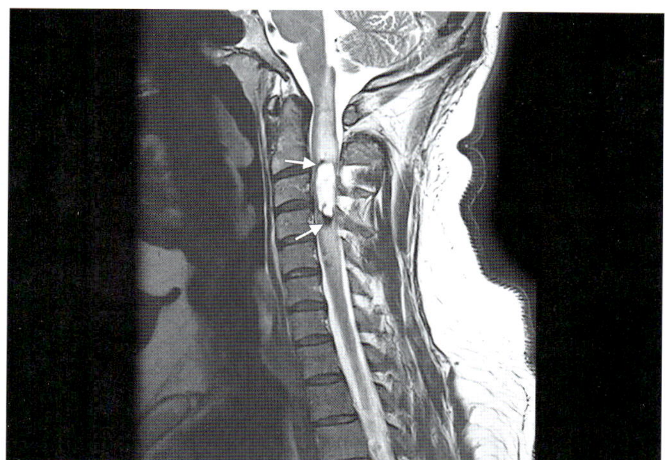

**Fig. 23.5:** C2-C4 level ependymoma with excellent demonstration of hyperintensity on T2-weighted image and hemosiderin cap sign.

laminectomy/laminoplasty or hemilaminotomy or hemilaminectomy (Figs. 23.6 to 23.8). There has also been a developing trend toward minimally invasive approaches for resection of smaller spinal ependymomas. The tumor is usually accessed where it comes to the surface or through a midline myelotomy (Fig. 23.6). Lateralized tumors may be approached through the dorsal root entry zone or posterolateral sulcus. Ependymomas often have a defined plane, which facilitates resection and thus increases the 5-year progression-free survival. However, complete resection may be limited by the degree of spinal cord invasion. As with all spinal cord tumors, intraoperative neurophysiologic monitoring is necessary to assist in determining the limits of the resection. In a recent literature review, gross total resection was achieved in 77% of patients with a 5-year progression-free survival rate of nearly 100%, which has led some institutions to recommend aggressive resection.[2,9,15,16] Subtotal resection has been associated with a 5-year progression-free survival rate of only 45%. The addition of adjuvant radiation therapy was shown to improve the 5-year progression-free survival rate to 65%. As would be expected, subtotal resection is associated with higher-grade tumors and lower rates of progression-free survival. When syndromic, these lesions are classically associated with neurofibromatosis type 2. Sporadic variants have been associated with loss of chromosome 22 as well as loss of 17p.[17]

### *Astrocytoma*

Astrocytomas are the second most common primary intramedullary tumor in adults and the most common in pediatric patients (comprising 90% of intramedullary tumors in patients under 10 years of age and 60% in adolescent patients).[18] There is no gender predominance in these tumors. Tumor grades can range from WHO grade I to grade IV, although WHO grade I intramedullary tumors are much more common. Typically, imaging may demonstrate an infiltrative enhancing tumor often associated with a cystic portion and a syrinx, which can be appreciated as a hypointense focus on T1-weighted image or proton density weighted image (PDWI) (Figs. 23.9 to 23.15). The most common histologic subtype is the fibrillary astrocytoma, which is comprised of a loose fibrillary matrix containing atypical astrocytes that can have minimal cytoplasm with nuclear atypia (Fig. 23.16). World Health Organization grades increase as nuclear atypia, mitotic figures, necrosis, and vascular endothelial proliferation increase. Intramedullary WHO grade IV (spinal cord GBM) tumors histologically resemble their intracranial counterparts in that they can demonstrate nuclear hyperchromasia, pseudopalisading necrosis, and cytologic pleomorphism. In the intramedullary astrocytoma, the most important prognostic factor is tumor grade (includes histology), although location (cervical vs. thoracic), tumor extent (four levels or less vs. greater than four levels), presence of a cyst/syrinx, extent of resection, and higher functional status have also been implicated. These tumors may have a poorly defined plane, which can make their resection more challenging. Prior literature demonstrates that there may be an increased expression of platelet-derived growth factor receptor in spinal cord astrocytomas. When syndromic, these tumors are classically associated with neurofibromatosis type 1.[19] However, sporadic variants, especially with progression to anaplastic astrocytoma, have genetic defects including retinoblastoma gene mutations, chromosome 13q loss, P16 gene

**Table 23.2:** Modified McCormick scale.

| *Grade* | |
|---|---|
| I | Intact neurologically, normal ambulation, minimal dysesthesia |
| II | Mild motor or sensory deficit, functional independence |
| III | Moderate deficit, limitation of function, independent w/external aid |
| IV | Severe motor or sensory deficit, limited function, dependent |
| V | Paraplegia or quadriplegia, even w/flickering movement |

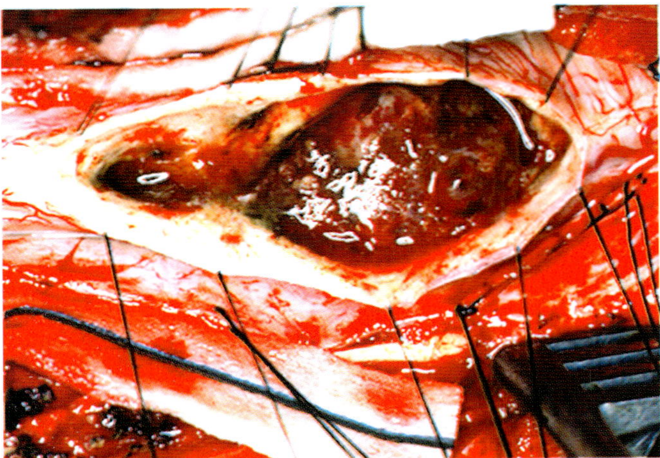

**Fig. 23.6:** Dorsal midline myelotomy with excellent delineation of ependymoma from surrounding parenchyma (note dural and pial tacking sutures).

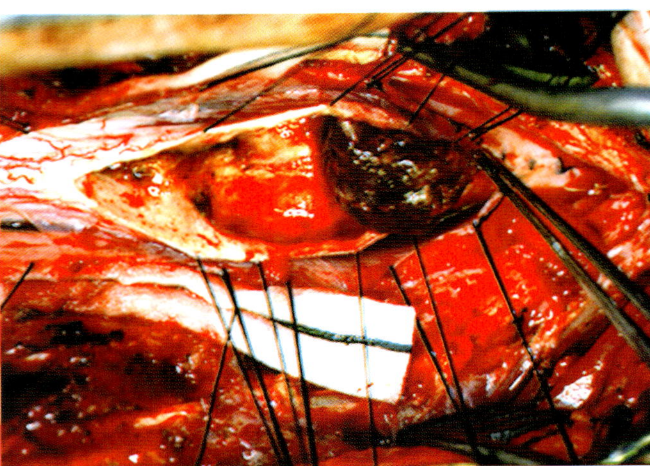

**Fig. 23.7:** Mobilization of ependymoma further demonstrating excellent dissection plane.

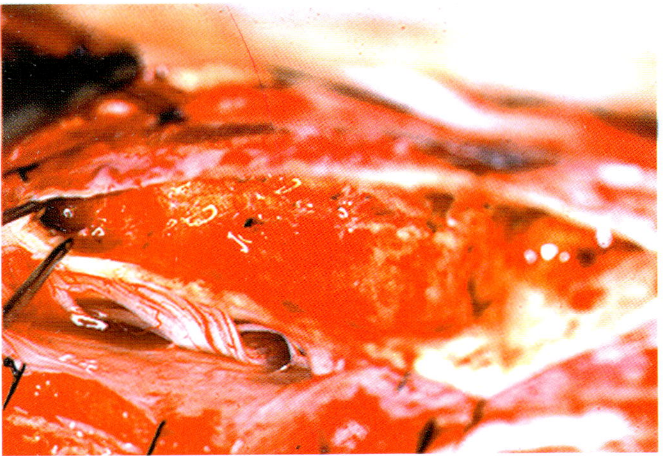

**Fig. 23.8:** Cavitation of dorsal cervical spinal cord after myelotomy and dissection for gross-total resection of ependymoma.

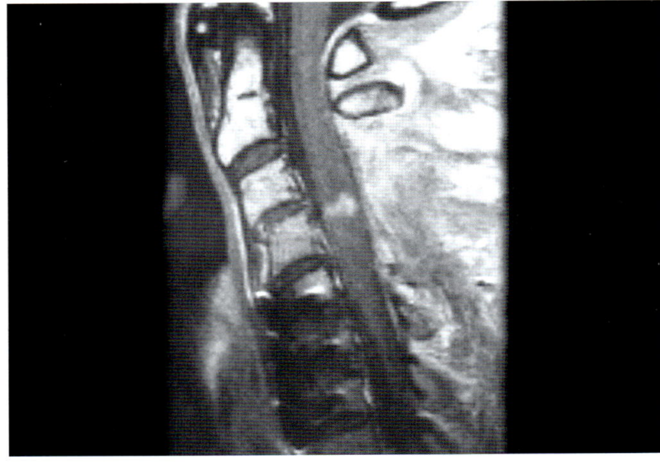

**Fig. 23.9:** C3-C4 level astrocytoma with some enhancement on T1-weighted image post-gadolinium with infiltration and expansion of spinal cord. Note prior C5-C7 anterior cervical discectomy and fusion.

deletions, chromosome 9p loss, and chromosome 19q loss.[17] The transition from anaplastic astrocytoma to glioblastoma has been shown to involve chromosome 10 loss and epidermal growth factor (EGF) receptor gene amplification.[17] Low-grade gliomas are curable with gross total resection. High-grade gliomas (AA and GBM) have been shown to have prognoses of 85% and 59% with aggressive resection (1 and 5 years, respectively) versus 31% and 0% without aggressive resection.[20] Unlike ependymoma and hemangioblastoma, astrocytoma does not have an increased progression-free survival with gross total resection.

### *Hemangioblastoma*

Hemangioblastomas are the third most common intramedullary spinal cord tumor behind ependymoma and astrocytoma, accounting for approximately 3% of intramedullary tumors.[21,22] The majority (75%) are solitary lesions, which occur sporadically, while roughly 33% are associated with von Hippel-Lindau (VHL) disease and multiple CNS lesions or "hemangioblastomatosis." They are more commonly found in males. Patients most commonly present with progressive sensory or proprioceptive deficits.[23,24]

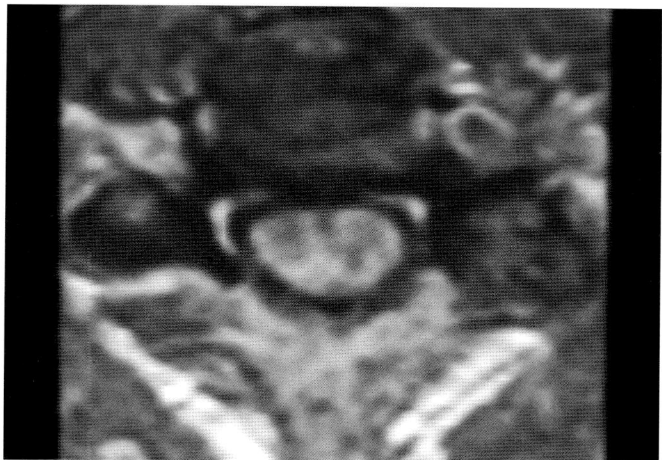

**Fig. 23.10:** T1-weighted image post-gadolinium astrocytoma in axial view demonstrating marked expansion of spinal cord with enhancement.

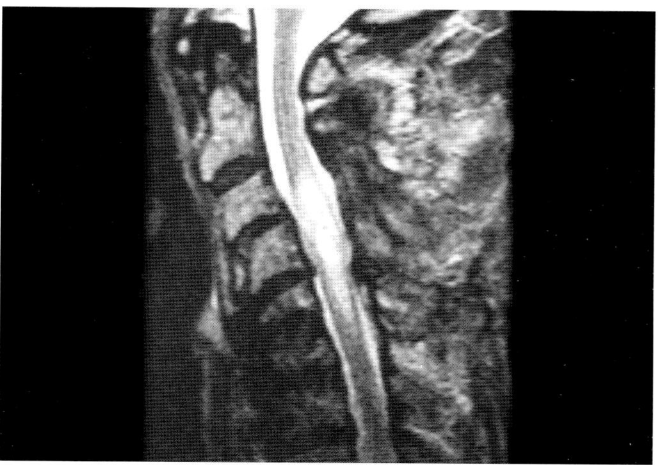

**Fig. 23.11:** T2-weighted image of high-grade C3-C5 level astrocytoma in sagittal view.

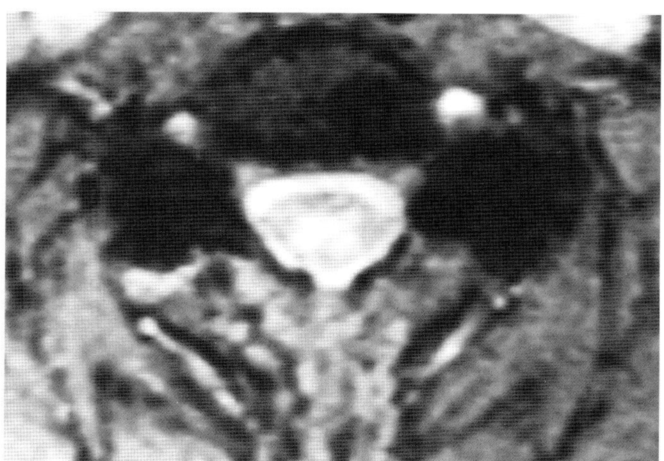

**Fig. 23.12:** Axial T2-weighted image of high grade cervical intramedullary astrocytoma.

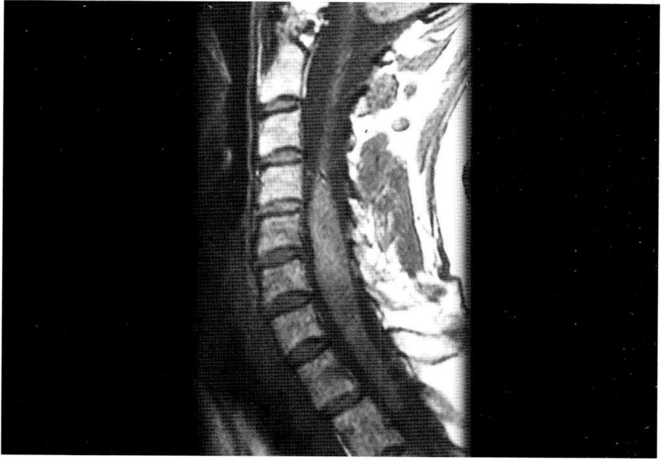

**Fig. 23.13:** C4-C7 level astrocytoma demonstrating marked expansion and infiltration.

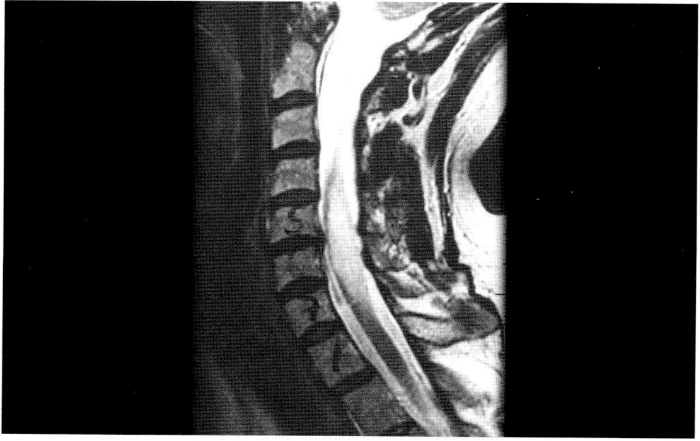

**Fig. 23.14:** T2-weighted image sagittal view demonstrating marked expansion and infiltration by astrocytoma.

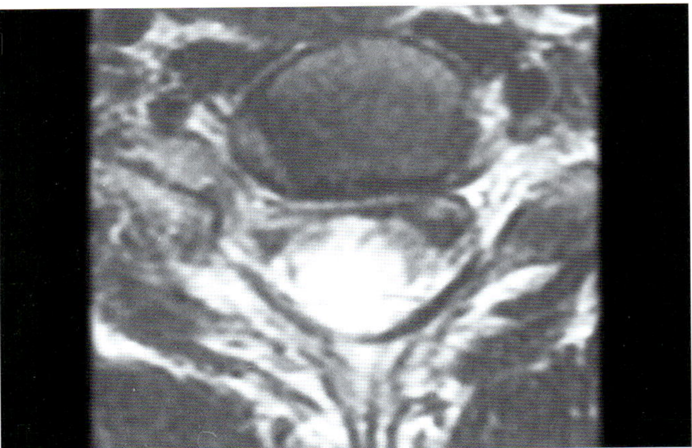

**Fig. 23.15:** Axial T2-weighted image demonstrating high-grade cervical astrocytoma and peripheral invasion/infiltration.

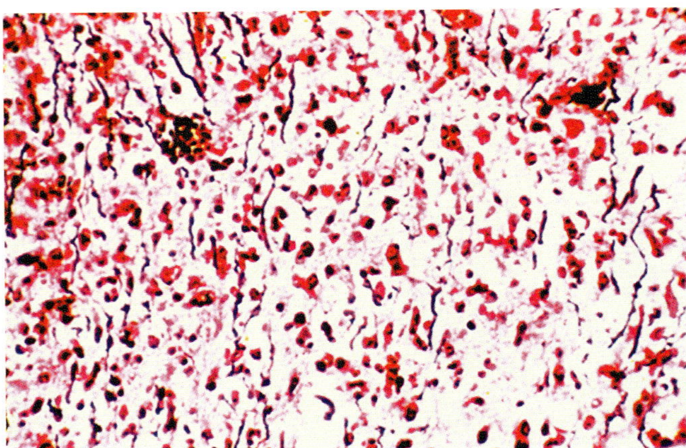

**Fig. 23.16:** Axonal staining demonstrating astrocytoma.

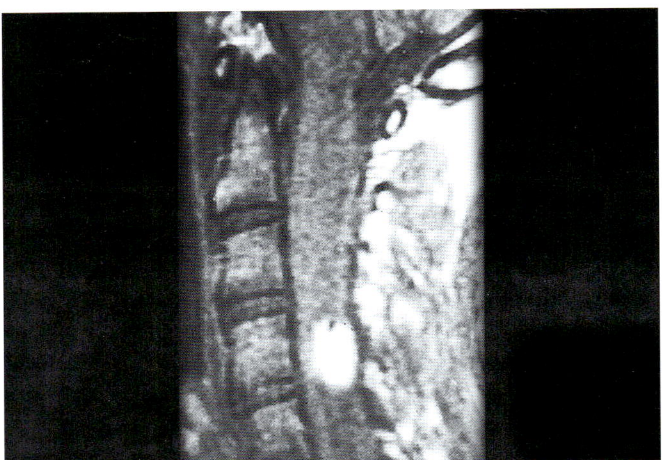

**Fig. 23.17:** Sagittal T1-weighted image post-gadolinium.

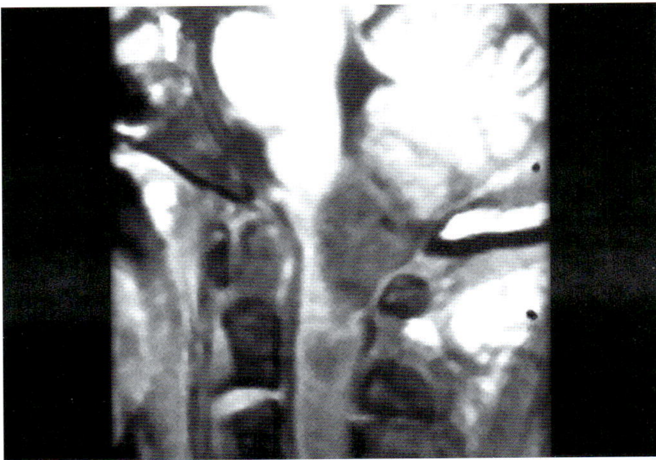

**Fig. 23.18:** Sagittal T1-weighted image cervicomedullary hemangioblastoma located on dorsal brainstem and spinal cord.

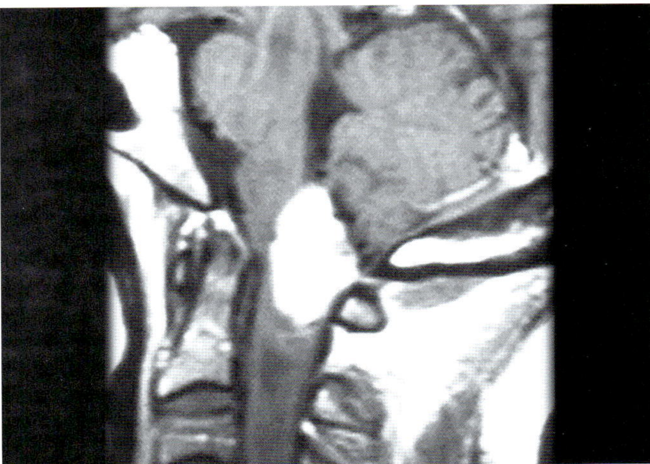

**Fig. 23.19:** Sagittal T1-weighted image post-gadolinium hemangioblastoma located on dorsal brainstem and spinal cord.

Hemangioblastomas are benign lesions made up of stromal cells surrounded by a vascular matrix involving feeding arteries and large draining veins, and usually occur dorsal to the dentate ligament. Magnetic resonance imaging demonstrates a contrast-enhancing nodule that may be associated with a cyst or syrinx (Figs. 23.17 to 23.20). Angiography will demonstrate the hypervascularity of the tumor with large feeding vessels and large draining veins (Fig. 23.21).

Hemangioblastomas are benign lesions. In cases of sporadic tumor development, complete surgical resection is curative. Patients with VHL are prone to recurrence or the development of new lesions throughout their lifetime and should be monitored with serial MRI, despite gross total resection,[22] although the VHL gene has been implicated in both syndromic and sporadic lesions.[17] Surgical

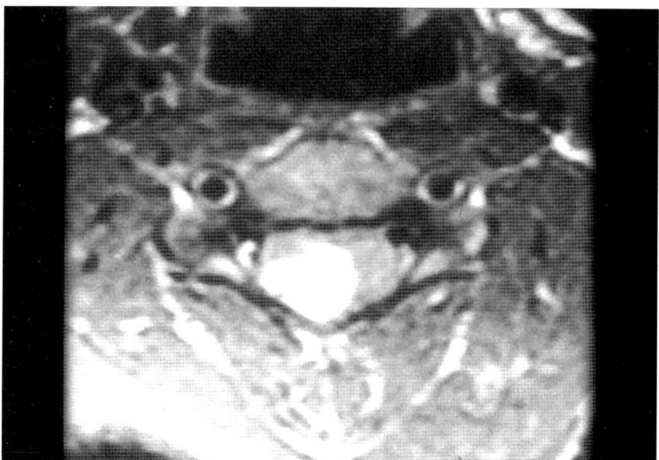

**Fig. 23.20:** Axial T1-weighted image post-gadolinium of cervical hemangioblastoma eccentric to the right side.

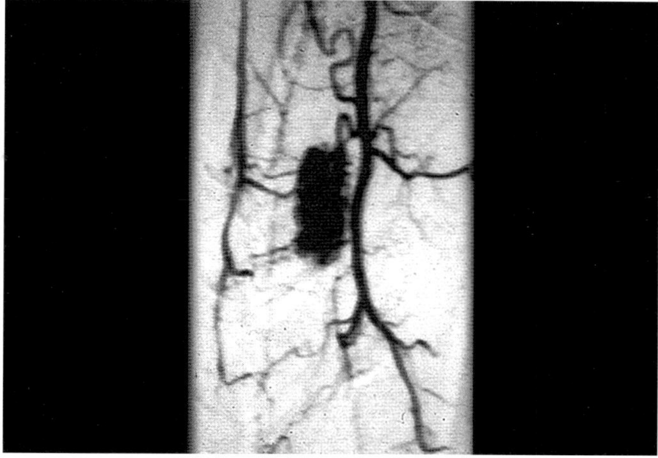

**Fig. 23.21:** Angiography demonstrating large draining vein of cervical hemangioblastoma.

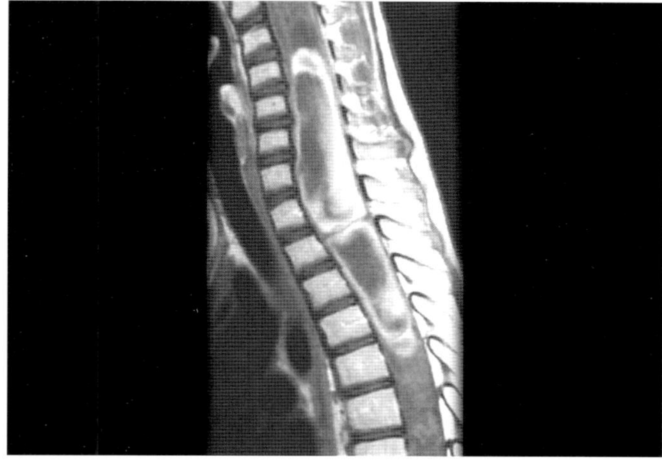

**Fig. 23.22:** Cervicothoracic intramedullary ganglioglioma demonstrating patchy enhancement and septation.

resection is usually carried out through a posterior approach via a laminectomy/laminoplasty or hemilaminotomy or hemilaminectomy due to their typical dorsal location. Care must be taken to identify the borders of the tumor and the associated vascular network. This network of feeding arteries and draining veins should be dissected and coagulated in order to decrease bleeding during dissection of the tumor plane. If the vascular anatomy is favorable, preoperative embolization may be performed in order to reduce intraoperative blood loss and facilitate maintenance of the tumor plane.[25]

Although rare, hemangioblastomas may be located in the ventral aspect of the spinal cord. Approach to these lesions through a standard posterior midline myelotomy or a posterolateral approach may result in neurologic deterioration or subtotal resection. Instead, these lesions may be approached through a more direct anterior approach with a corpectomy and subsequent stabilization. Indocyanine green has been used for augmentation of the extent of resection in intramedullary hemangioblastomas.[26]

Surgical resection is the primary treatment modality of hemangioblastomas, and there is no role for chemotherapy or standard external beam radiation therapy. However, stereotactic radiosurgery may be an effective alternative for VHL patients with multiple lesions, recurrence, or those whose surgical resection may be associated with a high morbidity.[27]

### *Ganglioglioma*

Spinal cord gangliogliomas are rare tumors that account for approximately 1% of all intramedullary tumors.[28,29] They are comprised of a mixture of glial cells, usually astrocytes, and neurons, typically ganglion cells. These tumors are most often found in the pediatric population, with 75% occurring in children <16 years of age.[28] Gangliogliomas can occur anywhere in the spinal cord but have a predilection for the cervicothoracic region.[28] Patients often present with slowly developing symptoms of weakness and sensory disturbances. On MRI, these tumors appear as heterogeneous lesions with T2 hyperintensity and patchy contrast enhancement (Fig. 23.22).[29]

Gangliogliomas are generally considered to be benign, slow-growing tumors (WHO grade I). However, there are case reports of malignant transformation to anaplastic gangliogliomas (WHO grade III).[30,31] Anaplastic gangliogliomas are extremely rare and account for <5% of

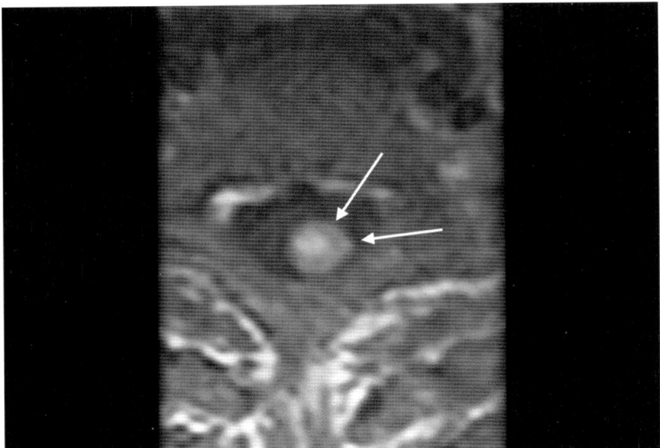

**Fig. 23.23:** Rim sign demonstrated by peripheral rim of enhancement (white arrows) in axial T1-weighted image post-gadolinium.

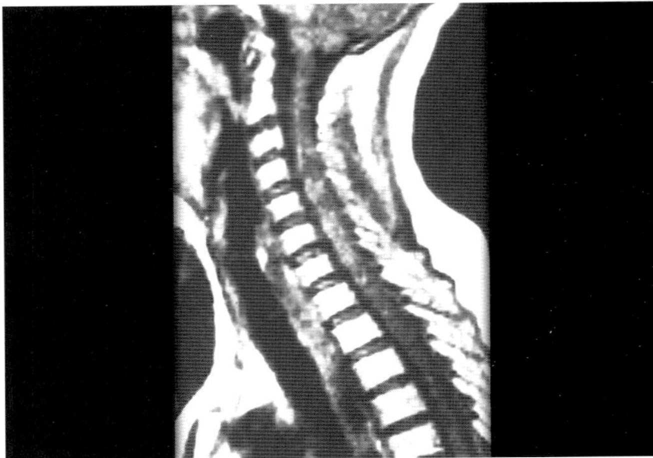

**Fig. 23.24:** C4-T1 level intramedullary metastasis on sagittal T1-weighted image post-gadolinium with inferior flame sign.

gangliogliomas.[30] Surgical resection, with an attempt at gross total resection, is the first-line treatment for these lesions. In a large series, gross total resection was achieved in 82% of patients with a 5-year survival rate of 88% and progression-free survival rate of 67%.[28] Surgical resection of these lesions is through a laminectomy/laminoplasty or hemilaminotomy or hemilaminectomy. As with other intramedullary lesions, resection should be performed with the use of neurophysiologic monitoring. In the case of subtotal resection or recurrence, adjuvant chemotherapy or radiation may be utilized.

### *Others*

A host of other primary intramedullary tumors exist; these are exceedingly rare and include oligodendroglioma (<5% of all primary glial intramedullary spinal cord tumors), melanaocytoma,[32] lipoma, subpendymoma,[33] paraganglioma, schwannoma,[34] meningioma,[35] germinoma,[36] lymphoma,[37] histiocytic sarcoma,[38] and epidermoid.[39] These rare tumors are addressed according to their histology and are generally resectable lesions. The presence of these tumors and clinical behavior with disease progression are reported anecdotally in the literature.

## Secondary Intramedullary Spinal Cord Tumors (Including Metastases)

0.1–0.4% of all cancer patients will experience an intramedullary metastatic lesion, and this figure may include as many as 5% of all spinal metastases, with epidural being the most common.[40] The classic presentation is with rapid neurologic deterioration. Intramedullary spinal metastatic disease is most likely to originate from lung, breast, and to a lesser extent melanoma (5.9%), renal cell carcinoma (5.6%), colorectal carcinoma (5.3%), lymphoma (4.7%), "drop" metastases from primary brain tumor (3.7%), unknown primary origin (3.3%), sarcoma (2.0%), ovarian carcinoma (1.7%), endometrial carcinoma (0.7%), esophageal carcinoma (0.7%), and gastric carcinoma (0.7%).[41] Metastases represent up to 3% of intramedullary tumors[42] and 0.6% of all spinal cord tumors. Drop metastases of primary brain neoplasms to the spinal cord may occur in roughly 1% of cases and are associated with increased mortality and poorer survival.[43] Direct cerebrospinal fluid invasion through the leptomeninges,[40] hematologic spread (arterial and venous routes as Batson's plexus is valveless), or via the ependymal lining have been implicated in the etiology. Intramedullary spinal cord metastases are usually homogenously enhancing, well-circumscribed lesions, which are most easily diagnosed on MRI. Some may be associated with the rim sign (Fig. 23.23) and also with the flame sign—more intense peripheral circumferential enhancement resembling a rim and gradual fading of enhancement on superior and inferior poles, which ends in distinct points resembling a flame (Fig. 23.24).[44] Surgical intervention is best in cases without leptomeningeal dissemination; otherwise, external beam radiation is the treatment of choice due to the very poor prognosis. Prognosis is very poor in this patient group (as high as 6 months with surgery and 5 months without surgery).[42]

## DIAGNOSIS

The diagnosis and evaluation of suspected primary intramedullary and metastatic disease may require multiple modalities, although the best for visualization is MRI.

### Positron Emission Tomography/PET CT

Positron emission tomography with [$^{18}$F]fluorodeoxyglucose (FDG-PET) measures the utilization of glucose and detects regions of high metabolic activity. Positron emission tomography with fluorodeoxyglucose has demonstrated increased metabolic activity within intramedullary foci suspicious for metastases. With sensitivity and specificity >90%, FDG-PET is a useful screening and surveillance tool.[45] Positron emission tomography is limited by its resolution, and further imaging with MRI is necessary after a lesion is identified.

### Computerized Tomography

Computerized tomography (CT) allows for a detailed three-dimensional (3D) view of the bony anatomy of the spinal column; however, it has much poorer resolution of the associated soft tissues compared to MRI. Computerized tomography provides information regarding the degree of bone involvement and destruction by tumor, which is often needed for preoperative planning. Visualization of the spinal cord and neural elements with CT is significantly inferior to that seen on MRI. Computerized tomography scans are often used in conjunction with MRI in the overall assessment of spinal metastases. In the intramedullary spinal cord tumor, the role of contrast-enhanced CT is limited, but it may be employed for patients unable to undergo MRI.

### Magnetic Resonance Imaging

Magnetic resonance imaging (MRI) is the most sensitive imaging modality for early detection of intramedullary spinal cord tumors. Because of its superior 3D soft tissue imaging as well as detailed visualization of soft tissue-osseous interface, MRI is considered the gold standard in evaluation of intramedullary spinal cord tumors and metastases.[46-48] Magnetic resonance imaging also provides high-resolution imaging of the spinal cord and neural elements and is a highly sensitive modality for identifying the area of neurologic compression/invasion. T1 gadolinium-enhanced sequences usually reveal a well-circumscribed, homogenously enhancing lesion within the spinal cord. T2 sequences can be used to assess the degree of surrounding edema and diffusion weighted imaging (DWI) can be used to assess tumoral cellularity. The addition of gadolinium contrast to T1 sequences provides further information as metastatic tumors are often avidly enhancing. Gadolinium contrast is particularly useful in identifying intradural metastases and leptomeningeal involvement. Diffusion tensor tractography[49] also has been shown in the literature to help diagnose these lesions while simultaneously mapping important fiber tracts within the spinal cord funiculi. The use of MRI is an imperative imaging modality for the evaluation of primary intramedullary spinal tumors and metastases. It has been shown to alter therapeutic decision making.

### Angiography

The use of digital subtraction angiography is a valuable adjunct when dealing with intramedullary tumors known to have a high degree of vascularity, such as hemangioblastoma or metastatic lesions from renal cell carcinoma, hepatocellular carcinoma, leiomyosarcoma, thyroid carcinoma, or angiosarcoma. Angiography is used as a diagnostic modality to provide information regarding the vascular supply of the tumor, and also has therapeutic potential through embolization. Preoperative embolization of vascular intramedullary tumors has the potential to reduce intraoperative blood loss, improves tumor resection, and shortens overall operative time.

### Biopsy

Biopsy of intramedullary spinal cord tumors is the most definitive means of diagnosis but is not frequently employed due to its associated morbidity. The histologic tumor type is one of the most important factors influencing the treatment plan. Because biopsies are performed when the histology of the lesion is unknown, the lesion could represent metastatic or primary tumor. This is done through a posterior approach with goals for myelotomy directly over the lesion should it come to the surface dorsally, the posterolateral sulcus, or within the midline.

## TREATMENT OPTIONS

Overall, the prognosis for patients with intramedullary spinal cord tumors is largely dependent on the tumoral histology. At initial presentation, the modified McCormick scale (*see* Table 23.2) is commonly employed to place

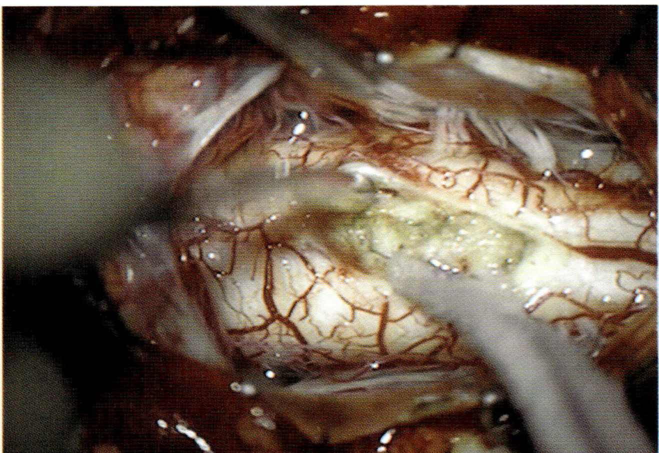

**Fig. 23.25:** Intraoperative photograph during resection of intramedullary metastatic lesion after midline myelotomy.

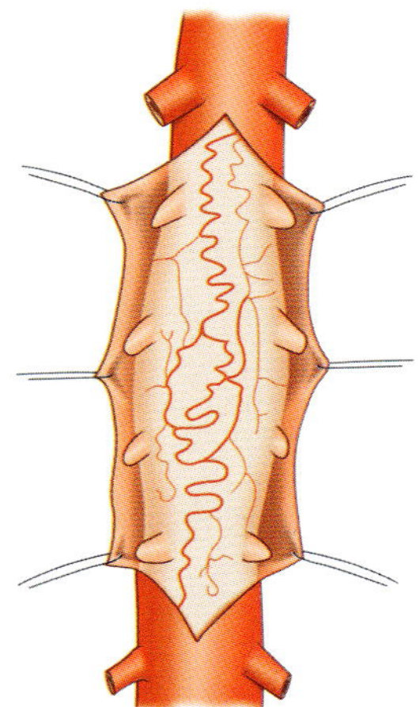

**Fig. 23.26:** Illustration of dorsal view prior to midline myelotomy.

patients in a standardized group according to their individualized levels of function. In many studies, a preoperative McCormick scale and tumor histology are implicated as the most important prognostic factors. Surgical resection, adjuvant radiotherapy (including Cyberknife), adjuvant proton therapy, and chemotherapy are the main treatment modalities.

## Surgical Treatment

Resection of intramedullary spinal cord tumors is typically performed with either laminectomy or laminotomy (can be performed with minimally invasive techniques[27,50,51]) using the operating microscope with premyelotomy ultrasonography[52,53] (shown to increase the extent of resection with a 3D probe). There are isolated reports of anterior approaches[54] and staged posterior approaches;[55] however, this is not the standard. Midline myelotomy (Figs. 23.25 and 23.26) is opted for unless the tumor is lateralized, which facilitates the use of a myelotomy in the posterolateral sulcus or dorsal root entry zone. Resection is typically based on the quality of surgical dissection planes developed around the tumor and can be augmented with intraoperative fluorescence.[56,57] Some reports exist of resection with direct placement of radioactive seeds[58] in the resection cavity as well. Rarely, anterior approaches are employed with a corpectomy. A limiting factor with these approaches is the ability to close the dura.

Intraoperative neurophysiologic monitoring with sensory and motor evoked potentials along with electromyography is the standard of care for resection of these lesions, but has not been unanimously shown in the literature to necessarily increase the extent of resection.[59-61] Placement of an epidural D-Wave catheter has been shown to be as effective as, if not more effective than, evoked potentials.[62] Clear surgical planes are associated with a greater extent of resection, which has been shown to increase the likelihood of gross total resection. Although not necessary for each case involving resection of intramedullary tumors, instrumentation must be considered, particularly when performing a laminectomy of greater than or equal to three levels.[63]

## CONCLUSION

Cervical myelopathy secondary to intramedullary spinal cord tumors is a complex process with several mechanisms that are involved in its pathophysiology. Treatment requires a multidisciplinary approach, including surgery, chemotherapy, and various radiotherapy modalities, with a goal of maintaining quality of life and function. The decision-making process should take into account the histology of the primary tumor, the neurologic manifestations, and the radiographic extent of intramedullary disease, including the systemic tumor burden.

## REFERENCES

1. Beneš III V, Barsa P, Beneš Jr P Jr, et al. Prognostic factors in intramedullary astrocytomas: a literature review. Eur Spine J. 2009;18(10):1397-422.
2. Chamberlain MC, Tredway TL. Adult primary intradural spinal cord tumors: a review. Curr Neurol Neurosci Rep. 2011;11(3):320-8.

3. Manzano G, Green BA, Vanni S, et al. Contemporary management of adult intramedullary spinal tumors-pathology and neurological outcomes related to surgical resection. Spinal Cord. 2008;46(8):540-6.
4. Stein BM, McCormick PC. Intramedullary neoplasms and vascular malformations. Clin Neurosurg. 1992;39:361-87.
5. Nagpal S, Clarke JL. Neoplastic myelopathy. Semin Neurol. 2012;32(2):137-45.
6. Brotchi J, Fischer G. Spinal cord ependymomas. Neurosurg Focus. 1998;4:e2.
7. Boström A, von Lehe M, Hartmann W, et al. Surgery for spinal cord ependymomas: outcome and prognostic factors. Neurosurgery. 2011;68(2):302-8; discussion 309.
8. Lee J, Parsa AT, Ames CP, et al. Clinical management of intramedullary spinal ependymomas in adults. Neurosurg Clin North Am. 2006;17(1):21-7.
9. Oh MC, Ivan ME, Sun MZ, et al. Adjuvant radiotherapy delays recurrence following subtotal resection of spinal cord ependymomas. Neuro Oncol. 2013;15(2):208-15.
10. Abul-Kasim K, Thurnher MM, McKeever P, et al. Intradural spinal tumors: current classification and MRI features. Neuroradiology. 2008;50(4):301-14.
11. Kim DH, Kim JH, Choi SH, et al. Differentiation between intramedullary spinal ependymoma and astrocytoma: a comparative MRI analysis Clin Radiol. 2014; 69(1):29-35.
12. Alkhani A, Blooshi M, Hassounah M. Outcome of surgery for intramedullary spinal ependymoma. Ann Saudi Med. 2008;28(2):109-13.
13. Bansal S, Ailawadhi P, Suri A, et al. Ten years' experience in the management of spinal intramedullary tumors in a single institution. J Clin Neurosci. 2013;20 (2):292-8.
14. Gepp Rde A, Couto JM, Silva MD, et al. Intramedullary tumors in children: analysis of 24 operated cases. Arq Neuropsiquiatr. 2010;68(3):396-9.
15. Figueiredo N, Brooks N, Resnick DK. Evidence-based review and guidelines for the management of myxopapillary and intramedullary ependymoma. J Neurosurg Sci. 2013;57(4):327-41.
16. Shrivastava RK, Epstein FJ, Perin NI, et al. Intramedullary spinal cord tumors in patients older than 50 years of age: management and outcome analysis. J Neurosurg Spine. 2005;2(3):249-55.
17. Parsa AT, Chi JH, Acosta FL Jr, et al. Intramedullary spinal cord tumors: molecular insights and surgical innovation. Clin Neurosurg. 2005;52:76-84.
18. Tihan T, Chi JH, McCormick PC, et al. Pathologic and epidemiologic findings of intramedullary spinal cord tumors. Neurosurg Clin North Am. 2006;17(1):7-11.
19. Taleb FS, Guha A, Arnold PM, et al. Surgical management of cervical spine manifestations of neurofibromatosis Type 1: long-term clinical and radiological follow-up in 22 cases. J Neurosurg Spine. 2011;14(3):356-66.
20. McGirt MJ, Goldstein IM, Chaichana KL, et al. Extent of surgical resection of malignant astrocytomas of the spinal cord: outcome analysis of 35 patients. Neurosurgery. 2008;63(1):55-60; discussion 60-1.
21. Chamberlain MC, Tredway TL. Adult primary intradural spinal cord tumors: a review. Curr Neurol Neurosci Rep. 2011;11(3):320-8.
22. Lonser RR, Weil RJ, Wanebo JE, et al. Surgical management of spinal cord hemangioblastomas in patients with von Hippel-Lindau disease. J Neurosurg. 2003; 98(1):106-16.
23. Ebner FH, Schittenhelm J, Roser F, et al. Management of holocord pilocytic astrocytomas in children and adolescents: an update. Pediatr Neurosurg. 2012;48(3): 133-40.
24. Guo L, Zhong C, Jiang J, et al. A rare intramedullary spinal cord metastasis from prostate carcinoma. Neurol India. 2013;61(4):444-6.
25. Guss ZD, Moningi S, Jallo GI, et al. Management of pediatric spinal cord astrocytomas: outcomes with adjuvant radiation. Int J Radiat Oncol Biol Phys. 2013;85(5):1307-11.
26. Hao S, Li D, Ma G, et al. Application of intraoperative indocyanine green videoangiography for resection of spinal cord hemangioblastoma: advantages and limitations J Clin Neurosci. 2013;20(9):1269-75.
27. Haji FA, Cenic A, Crevier L, et al. Minimally invasive approach for the resection of spinal neoplasm. Spine (Phila Pa 1976). 2011;36(15):E1018-26.
28. Jallo GI, Freed D, Epstein FJ, et al. Spinal cord gangliogliomas: a review of 56 patients. J Neurooncol. 2004;68:71-7.
29. Mechtler LL, Nandigam K. Spinal cord tumors: new views and future directions. Neurol Clin. 2013;31(1):241-68.
30. Schneider C, Vosbeck J, Grotzer MA, et al. Anaplastic ganglioglioma: a very rare intramedullary spinal cord tumor. Pediatr Neurosurg. 2012;48(1):42-7.
31. Zakaria Z, Fenton E, Jansen M, et al. The occult nature of intramedullary spinal cord metastases from renal cell carcinoma. BMJ Case Rep. 2012;2012. pii: bcr2012007476.
32. Muthappan M, Muthu T, Hussain Z, et al. Cervical intramedullary melanocytoma: a case report and review of literature. J Clin Neurosci. 2012;19(10):1450-3.
33. Jain A, Amin AG, Jain P, et al. Subependymoma: clinical features and surgical outcomes. Neurol Res. 2012;34(7):677-84.
34. Lee SE, Chung CK, Kim HJ. Intramedullary schwannomas: long-term outcomes of ten operated cases. J Neurooncol. 2013 May;113(1):75-81.
35. Hafiz MG, Rahman MR, Yeamin MB. Intradural intramedullary spinal cord meningioma in a seven years old female child. Mymensingh Med J. 2013;22(1): 180-5.
36. Madhukar M, Maller VG, Choudhary AK, et al. Primary intramedullary spinal cord germinoma. J Neurosurg Pediatr. 2013;11(5):605-9.
37. Lin YY, Lin CJ, Ho DM, et al. Primary intramedullary spinal cord lymphoma. Spine J. 2012;12(6):527-8.
38. Toshkezi G, Edalat F, O'Hara C, et al. Primary intramedullary histiocytic sarcoma. World Neurosurg. 2010;74(4-5):523-7.
39. Agarwal A, Bhake A, Kakani A. Cervical intramedullary epidermoid cyst with liquid contents. Asian Spine J. 2011; 5(1):59-63.
40. Hrabalek L. Intramedullary spinal cord metastases: review of the literature. Biomed Pap Med Fac Univ Palacky Olomouc Czech Repub. 2010;154(2):117-22.

41. Sung WS, Sung MJ, Chan JH, et al. Intramedullary spinal cord metastases: a 20-year institutional experience with a comprehensive literature review. World Neurosurg. 2013; 79(3-4):576-84.
42. El-Fiki M. Intramedullary spinal deposits: overview and perspective. World Neurosurg. 2013;79(3-4):445-6.
43. Gepp Rde A, Couto JM, Silva MD, et al. Mortality is higher in patients with leptomeningeal metastasis in spinal cord tumors. Arq Neuropsiquiatr. 2013;71(1):40-45.
44. Rykken JB, Diehn FE, Hunt CH, et al. Rim and flame signs: postgadolinium MRI findings specific for non-CNS intramedullary spinal cord metastases. AJNR Am J Neuroradiol. 2013;34(4):908-15.
45. Tomura N, Ito Y, Matsuoka H, et al. PET findings of intramedullary tumors of the spinal cord using [18F] FDG and [11C] methionine. AJNR Am J Neuroradiol. 2013; 34(6):1278-83.
46. McCormick WF. Intramedullary spinal cord schwannoma. A unique case. Arch Pathol. 1964;77:378-82.
47. McGirt MJ, Chaichana KL, Atiba A, et al. Resection of intramedullary spinal cord tumors in children: assessment of long-term motor and sensory deficits. J Neurosurg Pediatr. 2008;1(1):63-7.
48. McGirt MJ, Chaichana KL, Atiba A, et al. Neurological outcome after resection of intramedullary spinal cord tumors in children. Childs Nerv Syst. 2008;24(1):93-7.
49. Radek M, Wiśniewski K, Grochal M, et al. [Spinal cord diffusion tensor tractography as a diagnostic tool in difficult cases of spinal cord intramedullary tumours]. Neurol Neurochir Pol. 2013;47(1):74-9.
50. Xie T, Qian J, Wu X, et al. Unilateral, multilevel, interlaminar fenestration in the removal of a multisegment cervical intramedullary ependymoma. Spine J. 2013;13(7):747-53.
51. Yeo DK, Im SB, Park KW, et al. Profiles of spinal cord tumors removed through a unilateral hemilaminectomy. J Korean Neurosurg Soc. 2011;50(3):195-200.
52. Regelsberger J, Fritzsche E, Langer N, et al. Intraoperative sonography of intra- and extramedullary tumors. Ultrasound Med Biol. 2005;31:593-8.
53. Shamov T, Eftimov T, Kaprelyan A, et al. Ultrasound-based neuronavigation and spinal cord tumour surgery-marriage of convenience or notified incompatibility? Turk Neurosurg. 2013;23(3):329-35.
54. Pluta RM, Iuliano B, DeVroom HL, et al. Comparison of anterior and posterior surgical approaches in the treatment of ventral spinal hemangioblastomas in patients with von Hippel-Lindau disease. J Neurosurg. 2003;98(1):117-24.
55. Yokota H, Yokoyama K, Noguchi H, et al. Two-stage operation for high cervical intramedullary ependymoma in young adult. Br J Neurosurg. 2012;26(4):540-1.
56. Eicker SO, Floeth FW, Kamp M, et al. The impact of fluorescence guidance on spinal intradural tumour surgery. Eur Spine J. 2013;22(6):1394-401.
57. Inoue T, Endo T, Nagamatsu K, et al. 5-aminolevulinic acid fluorescence-guided resection of intramedullary ependymoma: report of 9 cases. Neurosurgery. 2013;72(2 Suppl Operative):159-68; discussion 168.
58. Colnat-Coulbois S, Klein O, Braun M, et al. Management of intramedullary cystic pilocytic astrocytoma with rhenium-186 intracavitary irradiation: case report. Neurosurgery. 2010;66(5):E1023-4; discussion E1024.
59. Kobayashi S, Matsuyama Y, Shinomiya K, et al. A new alarm point of transcranial electrical stimulation of motor evoked potentials for intraoperative spinal cord monitoring: a prospective multicenter study from the Spinal Cord Monitoring Working Group of the Japanese Society for Spine Surgery and Related Research J Neurosurg Spine. 2014; 20(1):102-7.
60. Rajshekhar V, Velayutham P, Joseph M, et al. Factors predicting the feasibility of monitoring lower-limb muscle motor evoked potentials in patients undergoing excision of spinal cord tumors. J Neurosurg Spine. 2011;14(6):748-53.
61. Sala F, Palandri G, Basso E, et al. Motor evoked potential monitoring improves outcome after surgery for intramedullary spinal cord tumors: a historical control study. Neurosurgery. 2006;58(6):1129-43; discussion 1129-43.
62. Costa P, Peretta P, Faccani G. Relevance of intraoperative D wave in spine and spinal cord surgeries. Eur Spine J. 2013; 22(4):840-8.
63. Sciubba DM, Chaichana KL, Woodworth GF, et al. Factors associated with cervical instability requiring fusion after cervical laminectomy for intradural tumor resection. J Neurosurg Spine. 2008;8(5):413-9.

## SUGGESTED READING

1. Aghakhani N, David P, Parker F, et al. Intramedullary spinal ependymomas: analysis of a consecutive series of 82 adult cases with particular attention to patients with no preoperative neurological deficit. Neurosurgery. 2008; 62(6):1279-85; discussion 1285-6.
2. Aghayev K, Vrionis F, Chamberlain MC. Adult intradural primary spinal cord tumors. J Natl Compr Canc Netw. 2011;9(4):434-47.
3. Ahmed R, Menezes AH, Awe OO, et al. Long-term disease and neurological outcomes in patients with pediatric intramedullary spinal cord tumors. J Neurosurg Pediatr. 2014;13(6):600-12.
4. Ambrossi GL, McGirt MJ, Mehta VA, et al. Factors associated with progression-free survival and long-term neurological outcome after resection of intramedullary spinal cord tumors: analysis of 101 consecutive cases. J Neurosurg Spine. 2009;11:591-9.
5. Angevine PD, Kellner C, Haque RM, et al. Surgical management of ventral intradural spinal lesions. J Neurosurg Spine. 2011;15(1):28-37.
6. Angevine PD, McCormick PC. Spinal deformity and pediatric intramedullary spinal cord tumors. J Neurosurg. 2007;107(6 Suppl):460-2; discussion 462.
7. Antoniadis G, Engelhardt M, Börm W, et al. [Spinal intramedullary tumors. When is surgical treatment indicated?] Nervenarzt. 2005;76(2):186-92.
8. Ardeshiri A, Chen B, Hütter BO, et al. Intramedullary spinal cord astrocytomas: the influence of localization and tumor

extension on resectability and functional outcome. Acta Neurochir (Wien). 2013;155(7):1203-7.
9. Arishima H, Takeuchi H, Tsunetoshi K, et al. Intraoperative and pathological findings of intramedullary amputation neuroma associated with spinal ependymoma. Brain Tumor Pathol. 2013;30(3):196-200.
10. Arrifin A, Kaliaperumal C, Keohane C, et al. 'Serpent in the spine': a case of giant spinal ependymoma of cervicothoracic spine. BMJ Case Rep. 2012;2012:5890.
11. Babu R, Owens TR, Karikari IO, et al. Spinal cavernous and capillary hemangiomas in adults. Spine (Phila Pa 1976). 2013;38(7):E423-30.
12. Belaid I, Jlassi H, Debbiche G, et al. [Lung adenocarcinoma with intramedullary spinal cord metastasis: a case report and review of the literature]. Rev Pneumol Clin. 2013;69(3):149-51.
13. Brotchi J, Bruneau M, Lefranc F, et al. Surgery of intraspinal cord tumors. Clin Neurosurg. 2006;53:209-16.
14. Brotchi J. Intramedullary astrocytomas surgery in adult patients: the rationale for cautious surgery. World Neurosurg. 2013;80(5):e139-40.
15. Brotchi J. Intrinsic spinal cord tumor resection. Neurosurgery. 2002;50:1059-63.
16. Cavanaugh DA, Utter PA, Jawahar A, et al. Intramedullary space occupying lesion of the cervical cord: when magnetic resonance imaging is not possible. Spine J. 2013;13(2):206-7.
17. Cemil B, Gokce EC, Kirar F, et al. Intramedullary spinal cord involvement from metastatic gastric carcinoma: a case report. Turk Neurosurg. 2012;22(4):496-8.
18. Chang UK, Choe WJ, Chung SK, et al. Surgical outcome and prognostic factors of spinal intramedullary ependymomas in adults. J Neurooncol. 2002;57:133-9.
19. Connolly ES Jr, Winfree CJ, McCormick PC, et al. Intramedullary spinal cord metastasis: report of three cases and review of the literature. Surg Neurol. 1996; 46(4):329-37; discussion 337-8.
20. Constantini S, Miller DC, Allen JC, et al. Radical excision of intramedullary spinal cord tumors: surgical morbidity and long-term follow-up evaluation in 164 children and young adults. J Neurosurg. 2000;93:183-93.
21. Cooper PR. Outcome after operative treatment of intramedullary spinal cord tumors in adults: intermediate and long-term results in 51 patients. Neurosurgery. 1989;25:855-9.
22. Coumans JV, Walcott BP, Nahed BV, et al. Multimodal therapy of an intramedullary cervical primitive neuroectodermal tumor in an adult. J Clin Oncol. 2012;30(2):e15-8.
23. Ding D, Fullard M, Jarrell HS, et al. Intramedullary spinal cord metastases from salivary ductal carcinoma of the parotid gland mimicking transverse myelitis in a patient with radiologically isolated syndrome. J Neurol Sci. 2014; 336(1-2):265-8.
24. Ebner FH, Roser F, Falk M, et al. Management of intramedullary spinal cord lesions: interdependence of the longitudinal extension of the lesion and the functional outcome. Eur Spine J. 2010;19(4):665-9.
25. Ellis JA, Canoll P, McCormick PC 2nd, et al. Platelet-derived growth factor receptor (PDGFR) expression in primary spinal cord gliomas. J Neurooncol. 2012;106(2):235-42.
26. Endo T, Aizawa-Kohama M, Nagamatsu K, et al. Use of microscope-integrated near-infrared indocyanine green videoangiography in the surgical treatment of intramedullary cavernous malformations: report of 8 cases. J Neurosurg Spine. 2013;18(5):443-9.
27. Eroes CA, Zausinger S, Kreth FW, et al. Intramedullary low grade astrocytoma and ependymoma. Surgical results and predicting factors for clinical outcome. Acta Neurochir (Wien). 2010;152(4):611-8.
28. Fakhreddine MH, Mahajan A, Penas-Prado M, et al. Treatment, prognostic factors, and outcomes in spinal cord astrocytomas. Neuro Oncol. 2013;15(4):406-12.
29. Ferrante L, Mastronardi L, Celli P, et al. Intramedullary spinal cord ependymomas—a study of 45 cases with long-term follow-up. Acta Neurochir (Wien). 1992; 119:74-9.
30. Fiorentino A, Caivano R, Chiumento C, et al. Radiotherapy and bevacizumab for intramedullary and leptomeningeal metastatic glioblastoma: a case report and review of the literature. Int J Neurosci. 2012;122(11):691-4.
31. Garber ST, Bollo RJ, Riva-Cambrin JK. Pediatric spinal pilomyxoid astrocytoma. J Neurosurg Pediatr. 2013;12(5):511-6.
32. Garces-Ambrossi GL, McGirt MJ, Mehta VA, et al. Factors associated with progression-free survival and long-term neurological outcome after resection of intramedullary spinal cord tumors: analysis of 101 consecutive cases. Journal of neurosurgery. Spine. 2009;11(5):591-9.
33. Goh KY, Velasquez L, Epstein FJ. Pediatric intramedullary spinal cord tumors: is surgery alone enough? Pediatr Neurosurg. 1997;27(1):34-9.
34. Gonzalez R, Spears J, Bharatha A, et al. Spinal capillary hemangioma with an intramedullary component. Clin Neuropathol. 2014;33(1):38-41.
35. Grah JJ, Katalinic D, Stern-Padovan R, et al. Leptomeningeal and intramedullary metastases of glioblastoma multiforme in a patient reoperated during adjuvant radiochemotherapy. World J Surg Oncol. 2013;11:55.
36. Harrop JS, Ganju A, Groff M, et al. Primary intramedullary tumors of the spinal cord. Spine. 2009;34:S69-S77.
37. Houten JK, Cooper PR. Spinal cord astrocytomas: presentation, management and outcome. J Neurooncol. 2000;47: 219-24.
38. Ito T, Sawakami K, Ishikawa S, et al. Progression of paralysis is the most useful factor for differentiating malignant from benign intramedullary tumors. Spinal Cord. 2013;51(4): 319-21.
39. Jeon MJ, Kim TY, Han JM, et al. Intramedullary spinal cord metastasis from papillary thyroid carcinoma. Thyroid. 2011; 21(11):1269-71.
40. Joaquim AF, Santos MJ, Tedeschi H. Surgical management of intramedullary spinal ependymomas. Arq Neuropsiquiatr. 2009;67(2A):284-9.
41. Kang K, Lee JH, Kim HG. Contralateral referred pain in a patient with intramedullary spinal cord metastasis from extraskeletal small cell osteosarcoma. J Spinal Cord Med. 2013;36(6):695-9.
42. Karikari IO, Nimjee SM, Hodges TR, et al. Impact of tumor histology on resectability and neurological outcome in

primary intramedullary spinal cord tumors: a single-center experience with 102 patients. Neurosurgery. 2011;68(1):188-97; discussion 197.
43. Kawanabe Y, Sawada M, Yukawa H, et al. Radiation-induced spinal cord anaplastic astrocytoma subsequent to radiotherapy for testicular seminoma. Neurol Med Chir (Tokyo). 2012;52(9):675-8.
44. Klekamp J, Samii M. Intramedullary tumors. In: Klekamp J, Samii M (Eds). Surgery of Spinal Tumors. Berlin: Springer-Verlag; 2007. pp. 20-131.
45. Klekamp J. Treatment of intramedullary tumors: analysis of surgical morbidity and long-term results. J Neurosurg Spine. 2013;19(1):12-26.
46. Kothbauer KF. Neurosurgical management of intramedullary spinal cord tumors in children. Pediatr Neurosurg. 2007; 43(3):222-35.
47. Kucia EJ, Bambakidis NC, Chang SW, et al. Surgical technique and outcomes in the treatment of spinal cord ependymomas, part 1: intramedullary ependymomas. Neurosurgery. 2011;68(1 Suppl Operative):57-63; discussion 63.
48. Lee SH, Chung CK, Kim CH, et al. Long-term outcomes of surgical resection with or without adjuvant radiation therapy for treatment of spinal ependymoma: a retrospective multicenter study by the Korea Spinal Oncology Research Group. Neuro Oncol. 2013;15(7):921-9.
49. Lefranc F, Brotchi J. Surgical strategy in spinal cord hemangioblastomas. Oper Tech Neurosurg. 2003;6:24-31.
50. Lin GZ, Wang ZY, Liu B. [Application of intraoperative neurophysiological monitoring in spinal cord surgery]. Beijing Da Xue Xue Bao. 2012;44(5):776-9.
51. Madhugiri VS, Pandey P, Indira Devi B, et al. Intramedullary metastasis in a case of vermian medulloblastoma. Br J Neurosurg. 2012;26(2):278-80.
52. Maira G, Amante P, Denaro L, et al. Surgical treatment of cervical intramedullary spinal cord tumors. Neurol Res. 2001;23(8):835-42.
53. Mandigo CE, Ogden AT, Angevine PD, et al. Operative management of spinal hemangioblastoma. Neurosurgery. 2009;65(6):1166-77.
54. Matsui Y, Mineharu Y, Satow T, et al. Coexistence of multiple cavernous angiomas in the spinal cord and skin: a unique case of Cobb Syndrome J Neurosurg Spine. 2014;20(2):142-7.
55. Matsuyama Y, Sakai Y, Katayama Y, et al. Surgical results of intramedullary spinal cord tumor with spinal cord monitoring to guide extent of resection. J Neurosurg Spine. 2009; 10(5):404-13.
56. McCormick PC, Stein BM. Intramedullary tumors in adults. Neurosurg Clin North Am. 1990;1(3):609-30.
57. McCormick PC, Torres R, Post KD, et al. Intramedullary ependymoma of the spinal cord. J Neurosurg. 1990;72(4): 523-32.
58. Mehta AI, Mohrhaus CA, Husain AM, et al. Dorsal column mapping for intramedullary spinal cord tumor resection decreases dorsal column dysfunction. J Spinal Disord Tech. 2012;25(4):205-9.
59. Mehta VA, Kretzer RM, Orr B, et al. Primary intramedullary spinal germ cell tumors. World Neurosurg. 2011;76(5):478.e1-6.
60. Melcher C, Wegener B, Niederhagen M, et al. An intramedullary capillary hemangioma of the spine with an underlying plasmacytoma. Spine J. 2013;13(7):e1-4.
61. Miller D. Surgical pathology of intramedullary spinal cord neoplasms. J Neurooncol. 2000;47:189-94.
62. Minehan KJ, Brown PD, Scheithauer BW, et al. Prognosis and treatment of spinal cord astrocytoma. Int J Radiat Oncol Biol Phys. 2009;73(3):727-33.
63. Mirone G, Cinalli G, Spennato P, et al. Hydrocephalus and spinal cord tumors: a review. Childs Nerv Syst. 2011;27(10):1741-9.
64. Moon HJ, Shin BK, Kim JH, et al. Adult cervical intramedullary teratoma: first reported immature case. J Neurosurg Spine. 2010;13(2):283-7.
65. Murakami T, Koyanagi I, Kaneko T, et al. Progression of paralysis is the most useful factor for differentiating malignant from benign intramedullary tumors J Neurosurg Spine. 2013;18(2):184-8.
66. Nakamura M, Tsuji O, Iwanami A, et al. Central neuropathic pain after surgical resection in patients with spinal intramedullary tumor. J Orthop Sci. 2012;17(4): 352-7.
67. Park J, Chung SW, Kim KT, et al. Intramedullary spinal cord metastasis in renal cell carcinoma: a case report of the surgical experience. J Korean Med Sci. 2013; 28(8):1253-6.
68. Parsa AT, Fiore AJ, McCormick PC, et al. Genetic basis of intramedullary spinal cord tumors and therapeutic implications. J Neurooncol. 2000;47(3):239-51.
69. Raco A, Esposito V, Lenzi J, et al. Long-term follow-up of intramedullary spinal cord tumors: a series of 202 cases. Neurosurgery. 2005;56:972-81.
70. Rao A, Griffiths R, Arnaoutakis K. Paralyzed by a rare cause: an unusual case of metastatic diffuse large B cell lymphoma of the intramedullary spinal cord. Ann Hematol. 2014;93(2):337-8.
71. Rostami R, Safarpour D, Tavassoli FA, et al. Intramedullary metastasis in breast cancer—a comprehensive literature review. J Neurol Sci. 2013;332(1-2):16-20.
72. Ryu SI, Kim DH, Chang SD. Stereotactic radiosurgery for hemangiomas and ependymomas of the spinal cord. Neurosurg Focus. 2003;15(5):E10.
73. Safavi-Abbasi S, Senoglu M, Theodore N, et al. Microsurgical management of spinal schwannomas: evaluation of 128 cases. J Neurosurg Spine. 2008;9(1):40-7.
74. Sandalcioglu I, Gasser T, Asgari S, et al. Functional outcome after surgical treatment of intramedullary spinal cord tumors: experience with 78 patients. Spinal Cord. 2005;43:34-41.
75. Sari O, Kaya B, Kara Gedik G, et al. Intramedullary metastasis detected with 18F FDG-PET/CT. Rev Esp Med Nucl Imagen Mol. 2012;31(5):299-300.
76. Schneider C, Hidalgo ET, Schmitt-Mechelke T, et al. Quality of life after surgical treatment of primary intramedullary spinal cord tumors in children. J Neurosurg Pediatr. 2014;13(2):170-7.
77. Schwartz TH, McCormick PC. Intramedullary ependymomas: clinical presentation, surgical treatment strategies and prognosis. J Neurooncol. 2000;47(3):211-8.

78. See-Sebastian EH, Marks ER. Spinal cord intramedullary cavernoma: A case report. W V Med J. 2013;109(3):28-30.
79. Serban D, Exergian F. Intramedullary hemangioblastoma - local experience of tertiary clinic Chirurgia (Bucur). 2013;108(3):325-30.
80. Setzer M, Murtagh RD, Murtagh FR, et al. Diffusion tensor imaging tractography in patients with intramedullary tumors: comparison with intraoperative findings and value for prediction of tumor resectability. J Neurosurg Spine. 2010;13 (3):371-80.
81. Shirzadi A, Drazin D, Gates M, et al. Surgical management of primary spinal hemangiopericytomas: an institutional case series and review of the literature. Eur Spine J. 2013;22 Suppl 3:S450-9.
82. Shofty B, Roth J, Ben-Sira L, et al. Massive hematomyelia following intramedullary spinal cord tumor surgery. Acta Neurochir (Wien). 2012;154(4):751-2.
83. Soltani-Arabshahi R, Vanderhooft S, Hansen CD. Intractable localized pruritus as the sole manifestation of intramedullary tumor in a child: case report and review of the literature. JAMA Dermatol. 2013;149(4):446-9.
84. Su HY, Wu YT, Liu MY, et al. Concomitance of cervical intramedullary traumatic neuroma and cervical cord herniation in a tetraplegic woman. J Back Musculoskelet Rehabil. 2013;26(3):251-4.
85. Sundaresan N, Rothman A, Manhart K, et al. Surgery for solitary metastases of the spine: rationale and results of treatment. Spine (Phila Pa 1976). 2002;27 (16):1802-6.
86. Tan LA, Kasliwal MK, Nag S, et al. A rare intramedullary spinal cord metastasis from uterine leiomyosarcoma. J Clin Neurosci. 2013;20(9):1309-12.
87. Thakar S, Rao A, Mohan D, et al. Metachronous occurrence of an intramedullary abscess following radical excision of a cervical intramedullary pilocytic astrocytoma. Neurol India. 2013;61(3):322-4.
88. Tobias ME, McGirt MJ, Chaichana KL, et al. Surgical management of long intramedullary spinal cord tumors. Childs Nerv Syst. 2008;24(2):219-23.
89. Tovar Martín MI, López Ramírez E, Saura Rojas E, et al. Spinal cord astrocytoma: multidisciplinary experience. Clin Transl Oncol. 2011;13(3):185-8.
90. Tseng HM, Kuo LT, Lien HC, et al. Prolonged survival of a patient with cervical intramedullary glioblastoma multiforme treated with total resection, radiation therapy, and temozolomide. Anticancer Drugs. 2010;21(10):963-7.
91. Tsuji O, Nakamura M, Fujiyoshi K, et al. Cervical intramedullary ependymoma masquerading as cervical spondylotic myelopathy on MRI analysis. J Orthop Sci. 2013;18(2):355-8.
92. Veeravagu A, Lieberson RE, Mener A, et al. CyberKnife stereotactic radiosurgery for the treatment of intramedullary spinal cord metastases. J Clin Neurosci. 2012;19(9):1273-7.
93. Waters JD, Peran EM, Ciacci J. Malignancies of the spinal cord. Adv Exp Med Biol. 2012;760:101-13.
94. White JB, Miller GM, Layton KF, et al. Nonenhancing tumors of the spinal cord. Neurosurg Spine. 2007;7(4):403-7.
95. Winograd E, Pencovich N, Yalon M, et al. Malignant transformation in pediatric spinal intramedullary tumors: case-based update. Childs Nerv Syst. 2012;28 (10):1679-86.
96. Wu L, Deng X, Yang C, et al. Intramedullary spinal capillary hemangiomas: clinical features and surgical outcomes: clinical article. J Neurosurg Spine. 2013; 19(4): 477-84.
97. Wu L, Yao N, Chen D, et al. Preoperative diagnosis of intramedullary spinal schwannomas. Neurol Med Chir (Tokyo). 2011;51(9):630-4.
98. Yao KC, McGirt MJ, Chaichana KL, et al. Risk factors for progressive spinal deformity following resection of intramedullary spinal cord tumors in children: an analysis of 161 consecutive cases. J Neurosurg. 2007;107(6 Suppl):463-8.
99. Zhang Y, Huang Y, Wang X, et al. Intramedullary spinal cord metastasis detected with whole body diffusion-weighted imaging. Neurol India. 2013;61(5):555-6.

Chapter 24

# Role of Total Disk Replacement for the Treatment of Cervical Myelopathy

*Emmanuel N Menga, Shaleen Vira, John A Bendo*

## INTRODUCTION

Multiple treatment modalities have been described when treating cervical myelopathy, including surgical and nonsurgical management. Surgical options include anterior discectomy with or without fusion, cervical disk replacement/arthroplasty (CDA), laminectomy with or without fusion, laminoplasty, corpectomy with fusion, and combined procedures. The utilization of nonfusion cervical spine techniques has increased worldwide.[1,2]

Total disk replacement, also referred to as CDA, cervical disk replacement, cervical artificial disk replacement, or anterior cervical discectomy and replacement, aims to restore height and to preserve range of motion (ROM) of the intervertebral disk after decompression. This feature potentially has a multifaceted benefit to the spinal column.

There is a growing appreciation of the concept that limiting motion at one segment of the spine via fusion has a negative effect on adjacent segments. The use of a prosthesis for spinal disk arthroplasty was first documented and reported in 1966 by the Swedish surgeon Ulf Fernstrom, who used a stainless-steel ball-bearing implant in the cervical and lumbar spine after discectomy.[3] During the same period, Reitz and Joubert in 1964 also reported the use of stainless steel balls in the cervical spine for the treatment of severe neck pain and headaches.[4] However, due to the unacceptable failure rates, cervical arthroplasty diminished in favor of arthrodesis as described by Smith and Robinson.

The success of lumbar disk arthroplasty in the 1980s led to the re-emergence of the concept of cervical disk replacement. Cummins, in 1989, developed the metal-on-metal stainless steel device known as the Cummins-Bristol disk; this is currently known as the Prestige disk.[5] The device was also associated with poor clinical outcomes, leading to the design of a second-generation implant to reduce constraint and allow for increased freedom of translation and rotation. The success of this device led to the development of other designs, including the Pointillart disk, the Bryan disk, the Porous Coated Motion (PCM) disk, the ProDisc-C, and the Secure-C. There are currently six Food and Drug Administration (FDA)-approved CDA designs, including the Prestige ST, ProDisc-C, Bryan disk, Secure-C, PCM, and Mobi-C.[6] These devices allow for variable motion of the cervical spine at the level of disk replacement and at the adjacent levels, and are believed to favorably impact the overall biomechanics of the cervical spine. Preserved motion using rigorous radiographical analysis was reported using 30-year follow-up data in CDA compared to anterior discectomy and fusion (ACDF).[7]

## INDICATIONS FOR CERVICAL DISK REPLACEMENT

Cervical disk arthroplasty is currently FDA-approved and indicated for skeletally mature patients for disk replacement at the C3-C7 levels following single-level discectomy for radiculopathy and/or myelopathy secondary to disk herniation or spondylosis.[6] It is contraindicated in patients with multilevel spondylosis, instability, and retrovertebral pathology.[2] Figures 24.1A to E demonstrate the pre- and postoperative radiographs of a 37-year-old man with C5-C6 degenerative disk disease with myelopathic findings on physical exam who underwent CDA.

## BIOMECHANICS

It is well accepted that limiting motion at one or more segments increases stress in adjacent segments. Chapter 3 outlines the importance of regional and focal cervical alignment and the pathologic factors that lead to and exacerbate cervical myelopathy.

Multiple studies have demonstrated increase in motion and intradiscal pressure at the segments adjacent to

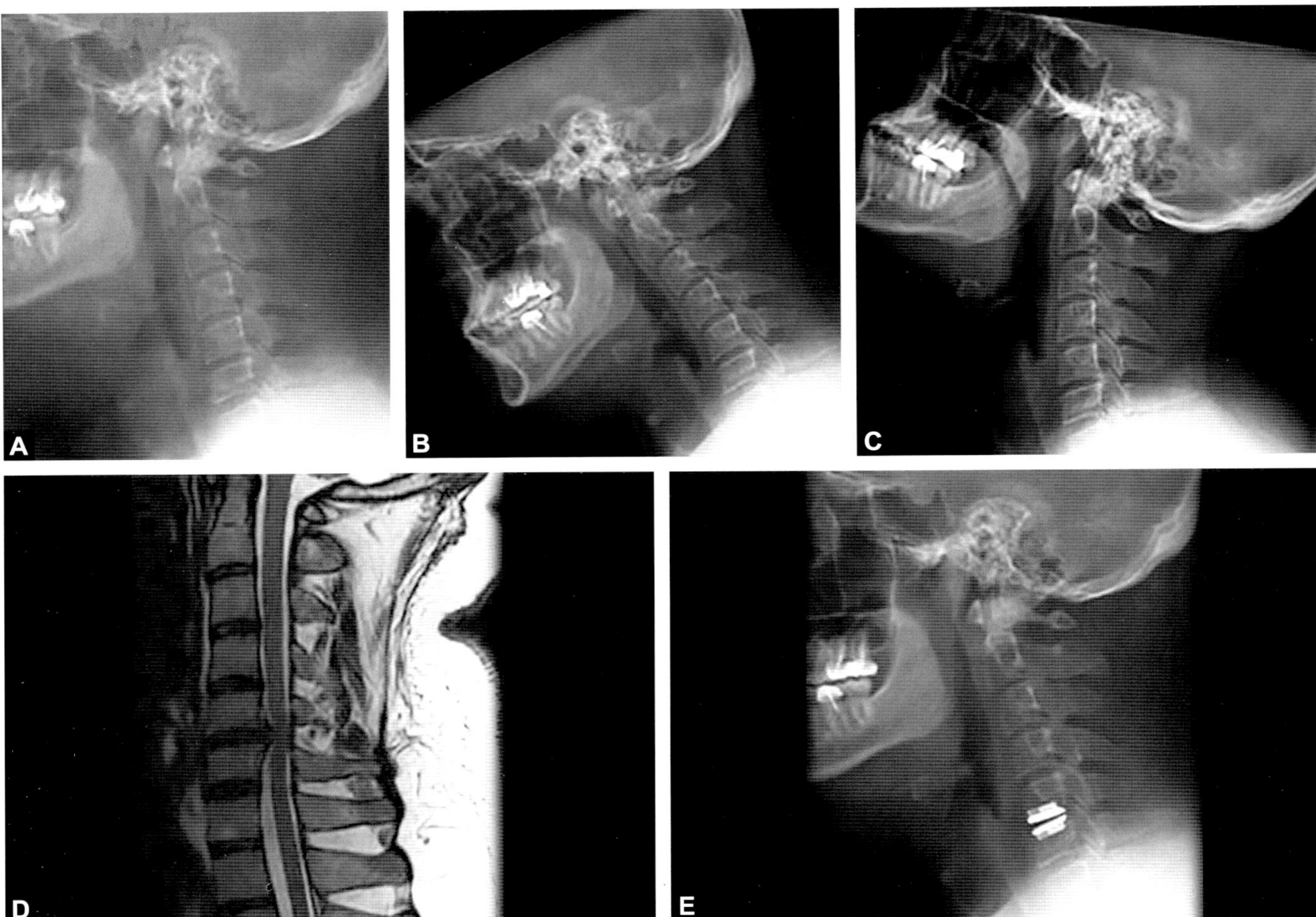


**Figs. 24.1A to E:** A 37-year-old man with C5-6 degenerative disk disease with myelopathic findings on physical exam. He underwent cervical disk arthroplasty. (A) Preoperative neutral X-ray; (B) preoperative flexion X-ray; (C) preoperative extension X-ray; (D) preoperative magnetic resonance imaging; and (E) postoperative neutral X-ray.

the fused level after ACDF.[8-10] Eck et al. performed a biomechanical study on fused cadaveric cervical spine segments and found increased intradiscal pressure with flexion only. There is a statistically significant increase in pressure during flexion with the greatest increase in intradiscal pressure observed at the cephalad-adjacent level.[11] In their study, the increase in intradiscal pressure with flexion at the cephalad-adjacent level also coincided with increase in motion at the adjacent cephalad level. There were no statistically significant changes in intradiscal pressure at the adjacent levels during extension despite the statistically significant increase in motion at the caudal segment adjacent to the fused level.

However, some studies evaluating spinal motion after disk replacement have demonstrated spinal motion comparable to the intact native spine. Puttlitz et al. evaluated changes in spinal kinetics after CDA, comparing intact cervical spine versus cervical spine with disk replacement. They reported no change in physiologic motion at the affected and adjacent levels. They concluded that disk arthroplasty with a ball-and-socket disk had comparable kinetic properties to the intact spine.[12] Zhu et al. compared the clinical outcomes between ACDF, dynamic cervical implant, and cervical total disk replacement (CTDR) for cervical spondylotic myelopathy. They demonstrated that ROM was reduced following ACDF, whereas there was no significant change between pre- and postoperative ROM after CTDR. These findings suggest that CTDR can successfully preserve motion.[13]

Burkus et al. performed a prospective randomized control between ACDF and the Prestige CTDR for single-level cervical disk disease. Sagittal angular motion was effectively maintained above the implant for the CTDR group, whereas this was slightly decreased for the ACDF group. In contrast, angular motion below the implant was not found to be superior in the CTDR group. At 84-month follow-up, the rates of reoperations and need for supplemental fixation procedures were much lower for the CTDR than the ACDF group. However, the specific rate of adjacent segment procedures was not found to be statistically different between the two groups.[14] Indeed, whether CTDR truly prevents symptomatic adjacent segment degeneration requiring intervention is still unclear.

The increase in motion and intradiscal pressure at the segments adjacent to the fused level after ACDF have been postulated as potential risk factors for adjacent level disease associated with ACDF. It is theorized that CDA eliminates these stresses and hence reduces the risk of adjacent level disease.

## ADJACENT SEGMENT DISEASE

### Pathophysiology

The pathophysiology of adjacent segment degeneration is complex, but can be simplified as an accelerated development of arthritic changes as the body attempts to adapt to greater motion requirements in the adjacent segments. Risk factors for adjacent segment disease include smoking and female sex.[15]

There is a wide variability in the reported incidence of adjacent segment degeneration.[16] One important factor that has complicated appropriate comparison between these studies is the variable definition of adjacent segment degeneration. Adjacent segment degeneration can refer to isolated radiographic changes versus new onset clinical symptoms referable to adjacent levels after spinal fusion. Using radiographic parameters, Katsuura, et al. reported adjacent segment disease in half of their patient cohort at 9.8 years following ACDF.[17] Other studies have described adjacent segment disease as the development of new radiculopathy or myelopathy referable to a motion segment adjacent to the site of a previous arthrodesis in the cervical spine.[2,16] A generally acceptable estimate of adjacent segment cervical disease is that it occurs in approximately 3% of patients per year, with an expected incidence of 25% within the first 10 years following fusion.[2] This risk of adjacent segment disease has been reported to be higher for those undergoing single-level cervical fusion than those going for multilevel fusion.[18]

Whether CDA protects against the need for revision surgery for adjacent segment disease is controversial. In a meta-analysis, Yu et al. found a 2.8% revision rate in the CDA population versus a 7.5% reoperation rate in the ACDF group.[1] Robertson et al. compared the Bryan cervical disk replacement with single-level ACDF and found a radiographic odds ratio and clinical odds ratio for adjacent segment disease of 2.44 and 35.8, respectively. They conclude that CTDR can protect against adjacent segment disease.

In contrast, some authors advocate that the changes deemed to be adjacent segment degeneration are simply part of the natural aging process and that arthrodesis does not definitively increase adjacent segment degeneration.[18] Recently, using a database of 1,358 patients (albeit only 378 with myelopathic signs), Lee et al. found no differences in adjacent segment pathology among the following groups: posterior decompression, anterior arthrodesis, and arthroplasty. Posterior fusion, however, resulted in a higher risk of reoperation for adjacent segment pathology. They explain that one possible reason for this finding is that posterior fusion typically requires dissection of ligaments, facet capsule, and muscle, which results in progressive kyphosis over time, eventually requiring revision surgery.[15] Indeed, controversy exists as to whether motion-preserving technologies such as CDA truly reduce adjacent segment disease requiring intervention.

## OUTCOMES FOR CERVICAL DISK REPLACEMENT IN MYELOPATHY

There has been great interest in understanding the clinical outcomes of this promising technology.[1] Cervical disk replacement for radiculopathy has demonstrated equivalent outcomes to cervical arthrodesis. While most studies report on the outcomes after CDA for radiculopathy, very few studies have reported patient outcomes stratified to the specific diagnosis of myelopathy.[19-21] Cummings et al. reported stable or improved symptoms after disk replacement in 16 patients with myelopathy in their group of 20 patients with neck pain, radiculopathy, and myelopathy.[22] Goffin et al. reported excellent outcome at 6-month follow-up in 3 of 7 (44%) of patients with myelopathy and 3 of the 3 (100%) patients at 1-year follow-up.[23] Their study was limited by the short follow-up and <50% follow-up rate in all patients with myelopathy at 6 months and 1 year following surgery.

Case series have also been reported on the use of disk replacement in myelopathic patients. Sekhon reported on the use of CDA in 11 patients with myelopathy, with 8 of the 11 patients also having some symptoms of radiculopathy. He reported a 91% good to excellent outcome with a statistically significant decrease in the Nurick scores (Nurick grade from 2 ± 1 to 1.09 ± 0.3 ($p < 0.001$ for all four preceding comparisons) at mean 18 months follow-up.[24] Sekhon also reported outcomes in 11 patients with isolated cervical myelopathy undergoing CDA. Despite the short-term follow-up, he reported good to excellent outcomes with radiographic evidence of cord decompression and improvement in clinical myelopathy at a mean follow-up of 6.29 months (range 1–17 months).[25]

Using the visual analog pain scale (VAS) of neck and arm pain, the Japanese Orthopaedic Association scores and Nurick scores for cervical myelopathy as outcome measures, Fay et al. reported on the outcomes of CDA for treatment of cervical spondylotic myelopathy compared to patients with radiculopathy at mean 36.4 months (range 24–56 months) follow-up. They reported significant improvement in myelopathic symptoms after CDA in patients with cervical spondylotic myelopathy caused by degenerative disk disease. The Nurick score for the patients in the myelopathy group improved from a mean 2.5 ± 0.9 preoperatively to 1.0 ± 1.0 ($p < 0.001$) after cervical arthroplasty. The outcome was comparable to patients with isolated cervical radiculopathy.[26]

Finally, Riew et al. reported comparable outcomes between disk replacement in 106 patients and arthrodesis in 93 patients with myelopathy. They reported significant improvement in the Neck disability index, Short form-36, and specific arm and neck pain VAS scores at all times point in patients undergoing single-level CDA.[27] This study represents the largest cohort of patients with isolated myelopathy using two types of cervical disk replacement prosthesis with an arthrodesis-controlled group. In summary, CDA has successfully been used to alleviate the symptoms of myelopathy from cervical spondylosis.

## COMPLICATIONS

The complications associated with CDA appear to be comparable to complications associated with ACDF. Complications from CDA include dysphagia,[28] dysphonia, neurologic events,[29] dural tears,[30] heterotopic ossification,[31] implant migration,[29] wear debris,[32] and medical complications. As long-term data become available, accurate assessment of the relative incidences of these complications can be better understood.

## ON THE HORIZON

### Cost Considerations

With health care costs on the rise, any new technology must be rigorously evaluated for its benefits with respect to its costs and outcome. The average cost of an arthroplasty implant is $4,000 versus the interbody device and plate for ACDF reported at $2,500.[33] This cost difference may be offset by cost reductions from a lower rate of reoperations for adjacent segment degeneration and earlier return to work. This concept has not been quantitatively demonstrated and is certainly a fertile area for future research.

### Two-Level CDA

Currently, the FDA only approves CDA for one-level use. Recent research has shown encouraging results for two-level CDA.[30,34] Future regulations may adapt to new data on this rapidly evolving technology. Indeed, long-term clinical data are only beginning to become available, and efforts are required to understand the long-term implications of CDA.

## CONCLUSION

Successful treatment of orthopedic conditions depends upon a versatile armamentarium of surgical techniques and procedures that can be adapted to each patient's unique needs. Cervical disk arthroplasty appears to be limited to retrodiscal cord/nerve root compression and spondylotic changes, which allow for adequate anterior interbody decompression while maintaining the integrity of the bony endplate. Cervical disk replacement is a valid option for treating cervical myelopathy with attempts to preserve cervical ROM. While long-term outcome studies are pending, most studies report comparable outcomes between CDA and arthrodesis for the treatment of myelopathy. The goals for the treatment remain critical, with the ultimate goal to decompress and stabilize the spinal cord. As with any new technology, appropriate patient selection is critical to successful utilization of this technique.

## KEY POINTS

- Spine fusion and its resulting limitation of spinal motion have been found to be associated with adjacent segment degeneration. Consequently, novel motion-preserving techniques such as CDA have been developed.

- Cervical disk replacement has been found to have at least equivalent results in terms of pain and disability outcome scores as fusion techniques for the treatment of cervical spondylotic myelopathy
- Whether motion preservation results in a lower incidence of adjacent segment degeneration is unclear. Future research efforts consisting of studies with large data sets and longer-term follow-up are required to truly assess whether motion-preserving technologies prevent iatrogenic degeneration of adjacent segments.
- Recent studies demonstrate encouraging 4-year clinical outcomes of performing two-level cervical disk replacements. These positive findings must be tempered with the higher costs of performing the procedure.

## REFERENCES


1. Yu L, Song Y, Yang X, et al. Systematic review and meta-analysis of randomized controlled trials: comparison of total disk replacement with anterior cervical decompression and fusion. Orthopedics. 2011;34:e651-8.
2. Cho SK, Riew KD. Adjacent segment disease following cervical spine surgery. J Am Acad Orthop Surg. 2013;21:3-11.
3. Fernstrom U. Arthroplasty with intercorporal endoprosthesis in herniated disc and in painful disc. Acta Chir Scand. 1966;357:154-9.
4. Reitz H, Joubert M. Intractable headache and cervicobrachialgia treated by complete replacement of cervical intervertebral discs with a metal prosthesis. South African Med J. 1964;38:881-4.
5. Chen F, Yang J, Ni B, et al. Clinical and radiological follow-up of single-level Prestige LP cervical disc replacement. Arch Orthop Trauma Surg. 2013;133:473-80.
6. http://www.fda.gov. Accessed: 12/6/14 n.d.
7. Yang H, Lu X, Yuan W, et al. Artificial disk replacement in the treatment of degenerative cervical disk disorder: a 30-year follow-up study. Spine (Phila Pa 1976). 2014;39:1564-71.
8. Weinhoffer S, Guyer RD, Herbert M, et al. Intradiscal pressure measurements above an instrumented fusion. A cadaveric study. Spine (Phila Pa 1976). 1995; 20:526-31.
9. Shono Y, Kaneda K, Abumi K, et al. Stability of posterior spinal instrumentation and its effects on adjacent motion segments in the lumbosacral spine. Spine (Phila Pa 1976). 1998;15:1550-8.
10. Burkus JK, Haid RW, Traynelis VC, et al. Long-term clinical and radiographic outcomes of cervical disc replacement with the Prestige disc: results from a prospective randomized controlled clinical trial. J Neurosurg Spine. 2010;13: 308-18.
11. Eck JC, Humphreys SC, Lim TH, et al. Biomechanical study on the effect of cervical spine fusion on adjacent-level intradiscal pressure and segmental motion. Spine (Phila Pa 1976). 2002;27:2431-4.
12. Puttlitz CM, Rousseau MA, Xu Z, et al. Intervertebral disc replacement maintains cervical spine kinetics. Spine (Phila Pa 1976). 2004;29:2809-14.
13. Zhu R, Yang H, Wang Z, et al. Comparisons of three anterior cervical surgeries in treating cervical spondylotic myelopathy. BMC Musculoskelet Disord. 2014; 15:233.
14. Burkus JK, Traynelis VC, Haid RW, et al. Clinical and radiographic analysis of an artificial cervical disc: 7-year follow-up from the Prestige prospective randomized controlled clinical trial. J Neurosurg Spine. 2014:1-13.
15. Lee JC, Lee SH, Peters C, et al. Risk-factor analysis of adjacent-segment pathology requiring surgery following anterior, posterior, fusion, and nonfusion cervical spine operations: survivorship analysis of 1358 patients. J Bone Joint Surg Am. 2014;96:1761-7.
16. Lawrence BD, Hilibrand AS, Brodt ED, et al. Predicting the risk of adjacent segment pathology in the cervical spine: a systematic review. Spine (Phila Pa 1976). 2012;37:S52-64.
17. Katsuura A, Hukuda S, Saruhashi Y, et al. Kyphotic malalignment after anterior cervical fusion is one of the factors promoting the degenerative process in adjacent intervertebral levels. Eur Spine J. 2001;10:320-4.
18. Hilibrand AS, Carlson GD, Palumbo MA, et al. Radiculopathy and myelopathy at segments adjacent to the site of a previous anterior cervical arthrodesis. J Bone Joint Surg Am. 1999;81:519-28.
19. Mummaneni PV, Burkus JK, Haid RW, et al. Clinical and radiographic analysis of cervical disc arthroplasty compared with allograft fusion: a randomized controlled clinical trial. J Neurosurg Spine. 2007;6:198-209.
20. Murrey D, Janssen M, Delamarter R, et al. Results of the prospective, randomized, controlled multicenter Food and Drug Administration investigational device exemption study of the ProDisc-C total disc replacement versus anterior discectomy and fusion for the treatment of 1-level symptomatic cervi. Spine J. 2009;9:275-86.
21. Sasso RC, Anderson PA, Riew KD, et al. Results of cervical arthroplasty compared with anterior discectomy and fusion: four-year clinical outcomes in a prospective, randomized controlled trial. J Bone Joint Surg Am. 2011;93:1684-92.
22. Cummins BH, Robertson JT, Gill SS. Surgical experience with an implanted artificial cervical joint. J Neurosurg. 1998;88:943-8.
23. Goffin J, Casey A, Kehr P, et al. Preliminary clinical experience with the Bryan cervical disc prosthesis. Neurosurgery. 2002;51:840-5; discussion 845-7.
24. Sekhon LHS. Cervical arthroplasty in the management of spondylotic myelopathy: 18-month results. Neurosurg Focus. 2004;17:E8.
25. Sekhon LHS. Cervical arthroplasty in the management of spondylotic myelopathy. J Spinal Disord Tech. 2003;16: 307-13.

26. Fay LY, Huang WC, Wu JC, et al. Arthroplasty for cervical spondylotic myelopathy: similar results to patients with only radiculopathy at 3 years' follow-up. J Neurosurg Spine. 2014;21:400-10.
27. Riew KD, Buchowski JM, Sasso R, et al. Cervical disc arthroplasty compared with arthrodesis for the treatment of myelopathy. J Bone Joint Surg Am. 2008;90: 2354-64.
28. McAfee PC, Cappuccino A, Cunningham BW, et al. Lower incidence of dysphagia with cervical arthroplasty compared with ACDF in a prospective randomized clinical trial. J Spinal Disord Tech. 2010;23:1-8.
29. Goffin J, van Loon J, Van Calenbergh F, et al. A clinical analysis of 4- and 6-year follow-up results after cervical disc replacement surgery using the Bryan Cervical Disc Prosthesis. J Neurosurg Spine. 2010;12:261-9.
30. Pimenta L, McAfee PC, Cappuccino A, et al. Superiority of multilevel cervical arthroplasty outcomes versus single-level outcomes: 229 consecutive PCM prostheses. Spine (Phila Pa 1976). 2007;32:1337-44.
31. Leung C, Casey AT, Goffin J, et al. Clinical significance of heterotopic ossification in cervical disc replacement: a prospective multicenter clinical trial. Neurosurgery. 2005; 57:759-63.
32. Cavanaugh DA, Nunley PD, Kerr EJ, et al. Delayed hyper-reactivity to metal ions after cervical disc arthroplasty: a case report and literature review. Spine (Phila Pa 1976). 2009;34:E262-5.
33. Singh K, Vaccaro AR, Albert TJ. Assessing the potential impact of total disc arthroplasty on surgeon practice patterns in North America. Spine J. 2004;4: 195S-201S.
34. Davis RJ, Nunley PD, Kim KD, et al. Two-level total disc replacement with Mobi-C cervical artificial disc versus anterior discectomy and fusion: a prospective, randomized, controlled multicenter clinical trial with 4-year follow-up results. J Neurosurg Spine. 2015;22(1):15-25.

# Index

*Note*: Page numbers followed by *f* and *t* refer to figures and tables, respectively.


## A

Abumi's technique 125, 126*f*
Achilles tendonitis 99
Achondroplasia 111, 133
American Rheumatological Association 95
American Spinal Injury Association Classification 36*f*
Amyotrophic lateral sclerosis 38, 88
Anderson's technique 184
Angiography 140
Ankylosing spondylitis 100, 118
Anterior cervical
  corpectomy and fusion 91
  decompression and fusion 90
  discectomy and fusion 105, 149, 152
  hybrid decompression and fusion 152
Anticonvulsants 68
Apparent sensory loss 123
Arm, disabilities of 74
Arrhythmia 45
Arterial blood sample 130
Articulation disorder 122
Asymptomatic degenerative compressive cervical stenosis 63
Ataxia 122
Athetoid cervical myelopathy 161*f*
Atlantial socket 16*f*
Atlantoaxial dislocation 117, 117*f*, 118, 121*f*, 123*f*, 125*f*
  etiology of 118*t*
  surgical classification of 124*f*
Atlantoaxial fixation 124
Atlantoaxial joint 18, 117
  biconcave structure of 16*f*
  subluxation 93, 94, 98
Atlantodental interval measurement 118*f*
Atlanto-occipital joint 17
Atrophy 47
Autosomal dominant disorder 111

## B

Babinski sign 36, 95, 214
Bacteria 118
Bamboo spine 101
Basilar artery 195
Basilar invagination 133
Berg balance scale 74
Biceps brachii 51*f*
Bilsky classification 216*f*
Biplanar system, setup of 20*f*
Bispectral index monitor 53
Bladder function 123
Bony dislocation 123
Brachialgia 33
Brachioradialis 35
Brain, tumors of 38
Breast 213, 214
  cancer 215*f*
Brown-Séquard syndrome 33

## C

Cancer 151, 189, 213
Carotid sheath 150
Carpal tunnel syndrome 90
Central cord syndrome 33, 104
Central nervous system tumors 38
Cerebral artery, anterior 195
Cerebral ischemia 130
Cerebrospinal fluid 137, 213
  leak 105, 129, 150
Cerebrovascular accident 38
Cervical alignment 25
Cervical amyotrophy 87
Cervical axial rotation 18*t*
Cervical biomechanics 15
Cervical canal stenosis 157
Cervical cord, compression of 105*f*
Cervical deformities 199, 201
Cervical disk
  arthroplasty 149, 151, 152
  replacement 241
Cervical flexion-extension 18*t*
Cervical fusion 158
Cervical immobilization 68
Cervical kyphosis 192*f*, 202
Cervical laminectomy 157, 158, 161, 162
  procedure 163
  with fusion 157, 162
  without fusion 157
Cervical laminoplasty 167, 173
Cervical lateral bending 19*t*
Cervical lordosis 31*f*, 202
Cervical myelopathy 37*t*, 43, 45, 47, 69, 74*t*, 77, 112, 123, 191*f*, 192*f*, 199, 201, 211, 213
  clinical diagnosis of 33
  deterioration of 79*f*
  diagnosis of 43
  surgical treatment of 73
Cervical pedicle screw 161
  fixation 157, 184
Cervical region 26
Cervical sagittal vertical axis 31*f*
Cervical spine 15*f*, 99-101, 122, 143, 157
  congenital abnormalities of 143
  disease 94
  magnetic resonance imaging of 89*f*
  metastases 213*t*
  pathology 177
  rheumatologic disorders of 93
Cervical spondylosis 33, 87, 167, 168
Cervical spondylotic amyotrophy 87, 90
Cervical spondylotic myelopathy 33, 40, 57, 59, 60, 60*f*, 64, 67, 68*t*, 74, 76*f*, 77, 149, 162, 190*f*, 201
  surgical management of 149
Cervical sympathetic chain 150
Cervical traction 138
Cervical vertebra 177, 185
Cervicomedullary angle 96, 119
  measurement 119*f*
Cervicomedullary compression 140*f*
Cervicomedullary junction, compression of 137*f*
Cervix 213
Chamberlain's line 96, 136
Chemical arachnoiditis 68
Chin-brow angle 101
Chin-brow vertical
  angle 26, 26*f*
  axis 31*f*
Cholangiocarcinoma 213
Chordoma 213
Chronic inflammatory autoimmune disorder 93
Circle of Willis 194, 195, 195*f*
Clark's stations 96
Clonus 37
Colorectal cancers 214
Combination disease-modifying antirheumatic drug therapy 97

Combined syndrome 33
Communicating artery, anterior 195
Compound muscle action potential 45, 89
Computed tomography 38, 104, 106, 112, 168
  scans 18, 97, 118, 136
Computer assisted software 21
Congenital anomalies 177
Congenital scoliosis 143
Congenital theory 109
Congestive heart failure 68
Constipation 68
Cord lamina angle 193*f*
Cord syndrome 33
Coronal computed tomography 135*f*
Corpectomy 149-150
Corticosteroids 215
Coupled motions 19
Cranial settling 94, 99
Craniocervical region 25
Craniovertebral junction 109, 117, 138
  compressive disease 123*t*
Cruciate ligament, visualization of 139*f*
Crutchfield's skull traction 63
Cubital-Tunnel syndrome 90
Cyclo-oxygenase-2 inhibitors 67
Cytoskeletal protein permitting 111

## D

Daily living scale, activities of 69
Decompression 78
Deep tendon reflexes 35
Deep vein thrombosis 129
Deformity 151
Degenerative disease 177
Delayed deep infection 129
Diabetes mellitus 38
Diffuse idiopathic skeletal hyperostosis 99
Dingman mouth retractor 138
Diplopia 122
Direct decompressive surgery plus 217
Dizziness 68
Dome laminectomy 172
Double-door laminoplasty 168, 171
Double-layer sign 104*f*
Down syndrome 110, 118
Dry mouth 68
Dubousset's conus of economy 202
Dural puncture 68
Dyspepsia 68
Dysphagia 99

## E

Ectopic kidney 143
Electromyography 43, 52, 89
Ellipsoid joint 17*f*
En bloc laminoplasty 168, 171
Endochondral bone formation 111
Epidemiology 189, 193
Epidural corticosteroid injection 68
Epidural venous plexus engorgement 90
Esophageal injury 150
Esophagus 150
European Myelopathy Scale 74
Eustachian tubes 138
Extension functional radiographs 21*f*
Extension, X-ray of 119*f*

## F

Facet joints 95
  degeneration of 151
Fixation techniques 179
Focal cervical spinal stenosis 62*f*
Foramen magnum
  dorsal border of 96
  ventral border of 96
Foraminal diameter 193
Foraminotomy 172
Fractures, acute 101
French-door laminoplasty 172
Functional magnetic resonance imaging 19
Fusion failure 129

## G

Gait abnormalities 214
Gardner-Wells cranial traction 123
Gastropathy 68
Germ cell tumors 214, 218
Goldenhar syndrome 118
Gravity, center of 25, 31*f*
Green-stick fracture 172
Grip strength 74
Grisel syndrome 118
Guillain-Barré syndrome 38, 46

## H

Harms technique 182
Hattori's method 167*f*
Hematosepsis 129, 130
Hemostatic tamponade 130
Hirayama's disease 90
Hodgkin's disease 214
Hoffman's sign 95, 214
Hoffmann reflex 36
Horseshoe kidney 143
Hybrid discectomy 149
Hyperkyphotic deformity 100
Hyperreflexia 35
Hypertension 68
Hyposmia 129

## I

Iatrogenic vertebral artery injury 193
Immobile segments 151
Incision infection 129
Infections 177
Inflammatory arthritidies 177
Inflammatory arthritis 100
Internal carotid artery 195
Intervertebral foramina 191
Intraoperative neurophysiologic monitoring 43, 47, 48
Inverted radial reflex 36, 37
Irreducible dislocation 127, 128*f*
Ischemic stroke 129

## J

Japanese Orthopaedic Association 69, 74, 123
Japanese Orthopaedic Association cervical myelopathy evaluation questionnaire 74
Japanese Orthopaedic Association Score 58, 59*f*, 173, 240
Jaw jerk 37
  reflex 36
Juvenile muscular atrophy 90

## K

Klippel-Feil anomaly 111
Klippel-Feil fusions 111
Klippel-Feil syndrome 110, 143
Kyphosis 122, 169, 201, 202
Kyphotic alignment 160*f*
Kyphotic deformity 171

## L

Laminectomy 77, 105, 170
Laminoplasty 75, 77, 90, 100, 105, 167, 172, 173, 191*f*
  technique 171, 173
Larsen syndrome 111
Lateral mass screw 157, 195
  fixation 183
Lateral syndrome 33
Leg hyper-reflexia 47
Lhermitte's sign 35, 95
Ligamentous anatomy 178
Ligamentum flavum 99, 172
  ossification of 77
Longitudinal ligament, ossification of 61*f*, 77, 103, 104, 105, 167
Longus capitis muscles 128*f*
Longus colli muscles, bilateral 128*f*
Lordosis, loss of 169*f*
Lower cervical spine 22*t*
  resulting pathology of 121

Lower cranial nerve 123
dysfunction 122
Lower extremities, motor dysfunction score of 58, 215
Lumbar lordosis 202
loss of 30*f*
Lumbar subarachnoid drainage 140
Lung 213, 214
Lymphoma 218

## M

Magerl's technique 114, 184
Magerl's transarticular screw technique 98
Magnetic resonance imaging 38, 60, 69, 75, 77, 87, 90, 96, 104, 105, 117*f*, 119, 134*f*, 136, 140*f*, 160*f*, 168, 190*f*, 203, 215
Manual muscle test 88, 190
Mayfield head holder 124
McGregor's line 96, 97, 136
McGregor's slope 26
McRae's line 96, 136
Median nerve sensory conduction study 47*f*
Median nerve somatosensory-evoked potential 44*f*, 50*f*
Melanoma 213
Mental component summary 153
Metastatic breast carcinoma 218*f*
Metastatic epidural spinal cord compression 214, 214*t*
Metastatic tumors, setting of 213
Minimal sensory loss 123
Modified Japanese Orthopaedic Association Scale 36, 37*t*, 74
Modified Japanese Orthopaedic Association Score 58, 58*t*, 76*f*, 215*t*
Modified Magerl technique 124
Monomelic amyotrophy 90
Morquio syndrome 110, 118
Motor system syndrome 33
Motor-evoked potentials 43, 45, 51, 62, 191
Mucopolysaccharidosis 110
Multilevel laminectomy 157
Multiple myeloma 214, 218
Multiple sclerosis 38
Muscle relaxants 67, 68
Myelopathy 34*t*, 37, 100
disability index 74
hand 130

## N

Neck
disability index 74, 153, 202
movement restriction 122
pain 122
Nerve
conduction studies 43, 45
root, tethering of 189
Neurological dysfunction, predictors of 62
Neurosurgical cervical spine scale 106
Non-Hodgkin's lymphoma 214
Nonopioid analgesics 68
Nonsteroidal anti-inflammatory drugs (NSAIDs) 67, 68
Normal cervical
alignment 28
lordosis 169*f*
values 28*t*
sagittal vertical axis 29*t*
Normal pressure hydrocephalus 38
Nurick classification 35, 35*t*
Nurick grade 74, 204
Nurick scale 59, 59*t*, 214*t*
Nystagmus 122

## O

Obstructive sleep apnea 100
Occipitocervical fixation 179
Odontoid, fracture of 118
Old odontoid fracture 118
Open-door laminoplasty 167, 171-173
Opioid 67
analgesics 68
Ossiculum terminale 110
Osteoporosis 151
Ovarian 213

## P

Pain, management of 68*t*
Paralysis 123
Parsonage-Turner syndrome 90
Pavlov's index 61, 64
Pedicle screw 195
Pelvic incidence 27
Pelvic retroversion 30*f*
Persistent dysphagia 150
Posterior atlantodental interval 94
Posterior cerebral artery, first segment of 195
Posterior communicating artery 195
Posterior foraminotomy 90
Posterior interosseous nerve palsy 90
Posterior longitudinal ligament 61, 71, 103, 167
cervical ossification of 74, 79*f*
continuous ossification of 104*f*
ossification of 105
segmental ossification of 104*f*
Posterior vertebral body line 168*f*
Postlaminectomy kyphosis 162, 163
Postoperative iatrogenic foraminal stenosis 191*f*
Primary axial rotation 20t
Progressive degenerative disease 149
Prostate 213, 214
Pseudarthrosis 162
Pseudoachondroplasia 111
Pseudostabilization 95
Psoriatic arthritis 100
Pulmonary embolism 129
Pyramidal signs 122

## R

Radiotherapy 216
Ranawat index 96
Ranawat method 96
Recurrent laryngeal nerve 150
palsy 150
Redlund-Johnell value 96
Reflexes, loss of 47
Renal cell carcinoma 213, 214
Renal failure 68, 151
Renal malrotation 143
Reperfusion injury 190
Respiratory distress 122, 129
Rheumatoid arthritis 74, 80*f*, 93, 118, 134*f*, 135*f*, 151
Rheumatoid spine 93
Romberg test 34
Rotation
axes of 205
center of 21, 21*f*, 205
instantaneous
axis of 205
centers of 21
Roy-Camille technique 184

## S

Sagittal plane translation 29
Sarcomas 214
Scapulohumeral reflex 36, 37
Sedation 68
Segmental spinal motion, reproduction of 20f
Semmes-Weinstein monofilament 38
Sensation 58
Sensory dysfunction upper extremities 37
Several classification systems 95
Severe canal stenosis 105
Skeletal traction test 123
Small cell carcinoma 218
Smith-Robinson approach 149, 151
Snake eyes 88
lesion 89*f*
Somatosensory-evoked potentials 43, 49, 62

Spastic gait 47
Sphincter disturbances 122
Sphincter dysfunction 37, 215
  score 58
Spinal alignment, significance of 25
Spinal column 38
Spinal cord
  compression 60*f*, 87
  evoked potentials 77
  injury 43, 171
Spinal headache 68
Spinal kyphosis, influence of 77
Spinal metastases, epidemiology of 213
Spine tumors, setting of 211
Spinolaminar line 168*f*
Spondyloepiphyseal dysplasia 118
Spondylolisthesis 206
Spondylosis 61*f*, 201
Sprengel's deformity 143
Stiff neck 68
Subaxial cervical spine 19, 178, 183, 185
Subaxial kyphosis 129
Subaxial subluxation 95, 99
Surgery 217
Swallow dysfunction 129
Swan-neck deformity 122
Synovial joints 94
Syringomyelia 38

## T

Takayasu's technique 186
Thalamus, ventral posterolateral nucleus of 49
Thoracic inlet angle 27
Thoracic kyphosis 202
Thyroid 213
Tibial nerve somatosensory-evoked potential 44*f*, 50*f*
Tinnitus 122
Tongue 213
Torg-Pavlov ratio 168*f*
Transarticular screw fixation 185
Transoral atlantoaxial joint 127
Transoral odontoidectomy 127, 128*f*, 140*f*
Transverse lesion syndrome 33
Trauma 177
Triceps brachii 51*f*
Tuberculosis 118
Tumors 177

## U

Ulcers 68
Ulnar nerve motor conduction study 46*f*
Unilateral renal agenesis 143
Upper extremities, motor dysfunction score of 215
Upper limb assessment 74
Urinary frequency 47
Urinary retention 68

## V

Vascular anatomy 178
Vascular complication 193
Vascular syndrome 33
Vertebral artery 119, 129, 150, 195
  injury 151, 193
Vertigo 122
Visual analog pain scale 240
Vulnerable anatomic structures 150

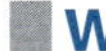

## W

Weakness 47
Weight gain 68
Wildervanck syndrome 144
Wound hematoma 150

## Y

Yellow ligament, ossification of 157

## Z

Zygapophyseal joints 17, 17*f*, 20, 100